Cutaneous Disorders

of the

Lower Extremity

CUTANEOUS DISORDERS
of the
LOWER EXTREMITY

GARY L. DOCKERY, D.P.M.

Medical Director
Washington Center for Specialty Surgery
Seattle, Washington

Private Practice, Seattle Foot and Ankle Clinic
Seattle, Washington

with the editorial assistance of

MARY ELIZABETH CRAWFORD, D.P.M.

Director of Education and Surgical Residency Training
Waldo Residency Program Washington Center for Specialty Surgery
Seattle, Washington

Private Practice, Ankle and Foot Clinic of Everett
Everett, Washington

W.B. SAUNDERS COMPANY
A Division of Harcourt Brace & Company
Philadelphia   London   Toronto   Montreal   Sydney   Tokyo

W.B. SAUNDERS COMPANY
A Division of Harcourt Brace & Company

The Curtis Center
Independence Square West
Philadelphia, Pennsylvania 19106

Library of Congress Cataloging-in-Publication Data

Dockery, Gary L.
    Cutaneous disorders of the lower extremity / Gary L. Dockery; with the editorial assistance of Mary Elizabeth Crawford.—1st ed.

    p.   cm.

    ISBN 0-7216-5034-1

    1. Skin—Diseases.   2. Extremities, Lower—Diseases.
I. Crawford, Mary Elizabeth.   II. Title
    [DNLM: 1. Leg Dermatoses.   WR 140 D637c 1997]

RL72.D63 1997 616.5—dc20

DNLM/DLC   95-43899

CUTANEOUS DISORDERS OF THE LOWER EXTREMITY   ISBN 0-7216-5034-1

Printed in the United States of America

Last digit is the print number: 9   8   7   6   5   4   3   2   1

PREFACE

Dermatology is one of those subjects that many practitioners find interesting but very intimidating. I have taught and lectured for many years on skin conditions involving the lower extremities, and I am constantly amazed at the number of times physicians have approached me after one of these seminars and stated that they learned more from my talk than they did in medical school. Many people have told me that I should publish my collection of color slides on dermatological conditions of the feet and legs, and I have always responded with "maybe someday."

This book is written for all of those practicing physicians, residents, and students who have requested it. I have attempted to combine current and comprehensive therapeutic information with classic clinical illustrations and variations of many conditions seen in clinical practice. Some obvious topics are missing from this text, such as complete sections on connective tissue disorders and the rather bizarre dermatological conditions, because I have not seen many of these conditions or because these particular topics are covered in greater detail in other texts.

The photographs taken for this project were all made with the Lester Dine 35-mm close-up camera with built-in flash (Lester A. Dine, Inc., Palm Beach Gardens, FL) using 200 ASA color slide film or the Nikon FE-2 camera with a Nikon Micro-Nikkor 55-mm lens and Nikon SB-E flash (Nikon, Torrance, CA) using 100 ASA color slide film. This equipment for close-up technique provides maximum detail and full color reproduction of most lesions. Nothing is less helpful than a black-and-white photograph or a drawing of a skin condition.

Cutaneous Disorders of the Lower Extremity is designed to be studied from the beginning to the end. This process involves reviewing and learning the primary and secondary lesions and studying the differential diagnosis of the lesions presented. This text is not intended to be a "picture book" only. Learning how to be a good observer of the skin and understanding basic principles will make the reader a better diagnostician and practitioner.

ACKNOWLEDGMENTS

My special thanks and deep appreciation to my assistant editor and contributing author, Dr. Mary Elizabeth Crawford, for the many hours spent finding articles for references, organizing materials, reading and rewriting segments of chapters, and poring over thousands of color slides to select the best examples presented herein.

CONTENTS

ANATOMY OF THE SKIN

INTRODUCTION

The skin is the largest human organ, and its structure varies greatly over different areas of the body. Human skin weighs about 10 pounds in the average man and about 7 pounds in the average woman. The area of the skin equals up to 15,000 square inches (approximately 9 by 12 feet). The skin is thicker on the dorsal, plantar, and extensor surfaces than on the ventral and flexor surfaces. However, it is also thin with occasional hairs on the dorsal foot as compared with the thick and hairless skin on the plantar foot.

Considerable regional variation occurs in skin structure, with wide variations noted in different parts of the body. Skin is either glabrous (smooth and without hair) or hairy. Glabrous skin covers the surfaces of the plantar foot and portions of the foot and ankle, whereas most other areas of the lower extremities are covered with hair-producing skin. The surface of the skin is irregular with marked areas of complex creases, ridges, and changes in thickness.

The skin has a large range of diverse functions. It covers the body; provides thermoregulation, waterproofing, and protection against injury; and aids in fluid conservation. It acts as a protective barrier against bacterial assault, provides detection of sensory stimuli, and is important in the absorption of ultraviolet radiation and the production of vitamin D. The skin is divided into three layers (Fig. 1–1): the epidermis, the dermis, and the subcutaneous tissue. The skin also arises from three embryonic levels: the ectoderm, mesoderm, and neuroectoderm. The epidermis and its appendages arise from ectoderm; the dermis, with the underlying subcutaneous fat and vascular structures, is derived from mesoderm. The nerves and melanocytes are of neuroectodermal origin.

Epidermis

The epidermis (also called the epithelial layer) is composed of at least four cell types: melanocytes (synthesize pigment), keratinocytes (produce keratin), Merkel's cells (probable storage granules), and Langerhans' cells (an element in immune reaction of the skin). The epidermal layer of the skin is also composed of four layers or strata, with the exception of on the palms and soles where there is a fifth stratum (Fig. 1–2). These are the outer or horny layer (stratum corneum), the lucid layer (stratum lucidum), the granular layer (stratum granulosum), the prickle cell layer (stratum spinosum), and the basal cell layer (stratum basale or germinativum).

STRATUM GERMINATIVUM. The columnar cell layers all start at the single-row basilar layer. The epidermal transit time from cell production to completion or sloughing is somewhere between 27 and 30 days. The germinative cells rest upon the basement membrane and dermis and contain an ovoid nucleus that is deeply basophilic. These cells are primarily directed toward replication or keratinization. Mitotic activity is greatest at night and can be accelerated as a response to removal of the stratum corneum, injury, and tissue repair. Basal cells divide to form keratinocytes (prickle cells), which in turn make up the spinosum layer.

STRATUM SPINOSUM. Cells of the spinosum layer become progressively flattened and orient parallel to the surface of the skin as they proceed outward. These polygonal cells form a mosaic pattern when laid down. They were originally thought to be connected to each other by intercellular bridges or spines, which appear histologically as lines. No true bridges occur, but this appearance is perceived with regular microscopy. Spinosal cells contain one or more nuclei and protein granules, called *keratohyaline* granules. These cytoplasmic granules eventually become a major component of the outer stratum corneum.

STRATUM GRANULOSUM. The granular cell layer is characterized by the acquisition of a large number of deep basophilic keratohyaline granules. Granulosum cells are flat, diamond-shaped cells with a bulging nucleus. The cells continue to flatten, and further maturation leads to loss of nuclei until the flattened plates of the keratin layer are fully formed. The three living layers (stratum basale, stratum spinosum, and stratum granulosum) are collectively termed the *stratum malpighii.*

STRATUM LUCIDUM. The lucid layer is present only on the palms and soles. It is composed of a translucent line of flat cells. This transitional layer of the epidermis acts as a barrier for prevention of water loss and protection against the absorption of noxious substances.

STRATUM CORNEUM. The stratum corneum is thickest on the palmar and plantar areas and thinnest on the eyelids. This is a nonliving layer that forms a protective shell against external injury and hinders penetration of microorganisms and solvents into the deeper layers. This stratified layer of compressed, flattened, and dead keratinized cells is constantly shedding. Keratin cells have the ability to absorb large amounts of water, which is readily noted during bathing when the soles become swollen and white (macerated).

BASEMENT MEMBRANE. The basement membrane, or basal lamina, separates the dermis and epidermis layers. This dermoepidermal junction consists of an area of extracellular materials underlying the basal cells and extending into the upper layers of the dermis. This bilaminar structure is composed of the lamina densa (an electron-dense region) and the lamina lucida (an adjacent and less dense region). The dermoepidermal membrane is divided into three separate zones. The first zone contains the tonofilament-hemidesmosome complex of the basal cells and extends through the lamina lucida to the lamina densa. The second zone completely contains the lamina densa itself, and the third zone extends from the lamina densa to the upper dermis.

Dermis

The dermal layer, also called the corium, is the primary supporting layer of the epidermis and consists of papil-

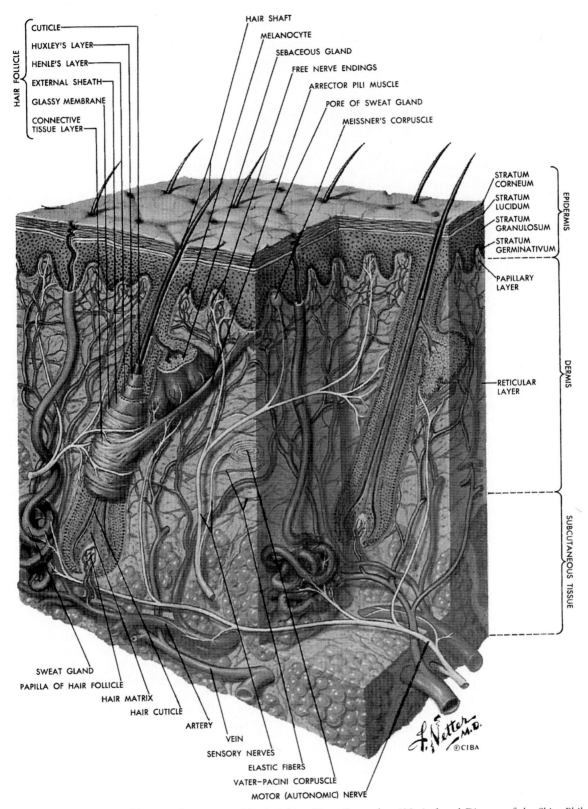

Figure 1–1 · Cross section of layers and structures of human skin. (From Domonkos AN: Andrews' Diseases of the Skin. Philadelphia, WB Saunders, 1971.)

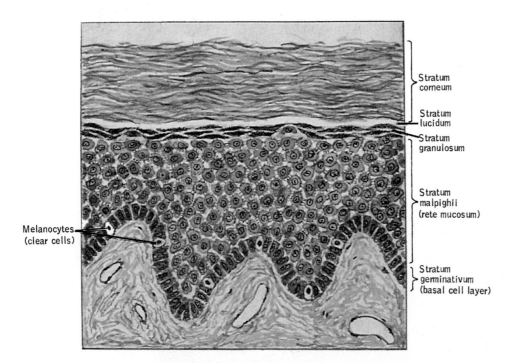

Stratum corneum

Stratum lucidum

Stratum granulosum

Stratum malpighii (rete mucosum)

Stratum germinativum (basal cell layer)

Melanocytes (clear cells)

Figure 1–2 Diagram of epidermis. (From Domonkos AN: Andrews' Diseases of the Skin. Philadelphia, WB Saunders, 1971.)

lary and reticular layers. The papillary layer is bordered above by the epidermis and below by the reticular zone. The dermis contains a fibrous component of elastin and collagen together with the ground substance or interfibrillar matrix. Lying within the dermis are the epidermal appendages and neurovasculature (e.g., blood vessels, hair follicles, nerves). Also contained in the dermis are three cellular elements of mesodermal cells: a reticulohistiocytic group, a myeloid group, and a lymphoid group. The reticulocytic group consists of histiocytes, fibroblasts, and mast cells. The myeloid group consists of polymorphonuclear leukocytes and eosinophilic leukocytes. The lymphoid group contains lymphocytic and neolymphocytic cells.

Subcutaneous Layer

The subcutaneous layer is sometimes included with the dermal layer, and it serves as the receptacle for the production and storage of the fat cells. It supports the blood vessels and nerves passing from the deep layers through to the dermis. The fat is divided into lobules by fibrous septa, and its cells contain large volumes of lipid that compress the nucleus into the cytoplasmic membrane. The subcutaneous fat layer is important in the nutritional storage of the body as well as in thermoinsulation.

Adnexa

The adnexa consists of appendages, glands, vessels, hair, and nails.

Eccrine Sweat Glands

These secretory glands are found throughout the skin but are not present in the mucous membranes or on the nail beds. They are maximally distributed on the palms and soles and are prominent factors in hyperhidrosis and bromhidrosis.

The main function of the eccrine sweat glands is to produce water for evaporation to regulate body temperature. They respond primarily to psychogenic stimulation on the forehead, palms, and soles. The eccrine glands on the hairy surfaces respond mostly to thermal stimulation. Thermal sweating is dependent on an intact hypothalamus, and psychogenic sweating is thought to be under the control of the limbic system.

The eccrine glands may be divided into four distinct parts: the coiled secretory portion, the straight dermal duct, the coiled dermal duct, and the coiled intraepidermal duct. The dermal sweat duct system has a biological function in modifying the secretion with resorption of water. The coiled secretory gland is found deep in the reticular dermis or the subcutaneous-dermal junction. The gland opens into a duct system, which passes through the dermal layer, enters the epidermis between the papillae, and continues as a corkscrew-like channel to the outer layer of the epidermis, where it terminates in a trumpet-shaped pore. Sweat from the eccrine system, which may also contain sodium, chloride, potassium, lactate, and urea, is a clear hypotonic solution that ranges from 4 to 6.8 on the pH scale.

Vascular System

A large continuous arteriovenous network perforates the subcutaneous layer and extends into the dermis

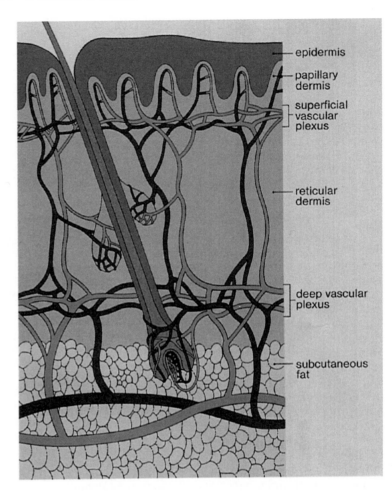

epidermis

papillary dermis

superficial vascular plexus

reticular dermis

deep vascular plexus

subcutaneous fat

Figure 1-3 Diagram showing the relationship of the superficial and deep vascular plexuses. (From McKee PH: The structure and function of normal skin. In du Vivier A [ed]: Atlas of Clinical Dermatology, p 12. Philadelphia, WB Saunders, 1986.)

(Fig. 1–3). These blood vessels form three networks within the skin. They are of all sizes and are present in each level and plane of the skin and appendages. The deepest and largest layer is located within the subcutaneous tissues and sends blood vessels to the middle network within the dermis. These vessels then branch and send additional smaller vessels upward to the most superficial layer located at the papillary-reticular junction of the dermis. This is frequently termed the *superficial vascular plexus*. Small offshoot loops of capillaries enter into each papillary convolution. A similar three-network venous system is present that starts as collecting vessels from the papillary dermis. Within the papillary plexus are direct communications between the arteries and veins called arteriovenous shunts. Additionally, the lymphatic vessels form a rich network in the papillary layer to the subcutaneous layer where the lymph vessels have valves. This complex vascular system appears to be primarily responsible for the regulation of heat, blood pressure of the body, and nutrition of the skin.

Within the tips of the fingers and toes and under the nails is a special vascular body termed the *glomus*. This body contains a specialized cutaneous arteriovenous anastomosis called the Sucquet-Hoyer canal. This canal is a shunt system that connects an arteriole with a venule directly without intervening capillaries. These anastomoses enable the capillary plexus of the superficial dermis to be bypassed, which increases the venous return from the extremities. This effect results in a great increase in the blood flow through the skin. When this system is injured or grows abnormally, it results in a red, swollen, and very painful condition termed a *glomus tumor*. This lesion is usually located under the fingernail but may occur under toenails, commonly of the great toe, or on any other part of the body. It has to be removed surgically (see Chapter 9).

Cutaneous Nerve Supply

Both sensory (the afferent system) and motor (the efferent system) nerves supply the skin. The efferent system is responsible for control of the blood supply of the skin and for control of the skin appendages derived from the sympathetic division of the autonomic nervous system. The afferent system is responsible for appreciation of sensation (touch, temperature, itch, pain) to the skin. There are three different types of afferent receptors: free nerve endings, hair nerve endings, and encapsulated nerve endings. The low-conduction free nerve endings are responsible for the perception of temperature, itch, and pain. Hair nerve endings are composed of myelinated fibers of both free nerve endings and encapsulated nerve endings, associated with tactile disks that function as touch receptors. Encapsulated nerve endings include specialized tactile corpuscles of Meissner (Wagner-Meissner) and Pacini (Vater-Pacini). The Meissner corpuscles are found in the dermal papillae of the hands and feet and enable appreciation of both light and soft sensations of touch. The pacinian corpuscles, found on the palms, soles, and digits, are responsible for the appreciation of deep firm touch or pressure sensation. These cells are located within the subcutaneous fat layers, and they are also thought to be responsible for the perception of vibratory sensation.

Hair

Hair is developed from ectoderm derived from hair follicles of the epidermis. It grows on most of the human body with the exception of the palms, soles, and ventral aspects of the fingers and toes. There is usually no hair growth on the glans penis, inner aspect of the prepuce, and inner parts of the female external genitalia. Hormones influence the various types of hair growth. This cyclic hair growth pattern has several phases: growing (anagen phase), involution (catagen phase), and resting (telogen phase).

Hair color depends on melanosomes, with dark hair containing large amounts of melanosomes, blond hair containing a decreased number of partially pigmented melanosomes, and white hair containing none at all. In red hair the melanosome is structurally and chemically different from the melanosome of black hair.

Hair is not of much importance in thermoregulation for the human body. It does, however, serve some function in touch reception.

There are two main types of adult human hair: vellus (fine) hair and terminal (coarse) hair. Vellus hairs are short, fine hairs of the body that are usually not pigmented. The terminal hairs are coarse, thick, and pigmented hairs that are found most extensively on the scalp, eyebrows, and extremities.

Nails

The toenail is a very specialized keratinized appendage with a primary function of protection for the distal phalanx (Fig. 1–4). It is capable of only a limited number of pathological responses, many of which are reviewed in Chapter 6. Unlike skin or hair, the nail does not shed or desquamate and is not cyclical. Nails are very hard because of a relative lack of water content as compared with the stratum corneum. Water flux across the nail is 10 times that across skin; however, the nail plate is unable to hold water because of its very low (less than 5% by weight) lipid content. The relatively high sulfur content in nails, predominantly in the form of cystine, appears to contribute to their hardness. Because the nail is hard and does not desquamate, many of the conditions involving the nails become more difficult to treat either with medication or by surgical means.

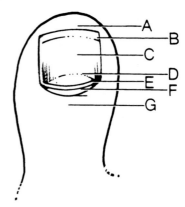

Figure 1–4 Illustration of toenail: A, free nail edge; B, point of separation of nail from bed; C, nail plate; D, lunula; E, cuticle; F, eponychium; G, skin overlying posterior nail fold. (From Dockery GL: Nails. In McGlamry ED, Banks AS, Downey MS [eds]: Comprehensive Textbook of Foot Surgery, 2nd ed, p 277. Baltimore, Williams & Wilkins, 1987.)

The nail consists of a nail plate, the free nail border, the matrix (root), and the supporting tissues surrounding it. Nail growth appears to be continuous with very little change in the overall rate. Normal toenails extend distally 0.03 to 0.05 mm per day. The thickness of the toenail is between 0.05 and 1.0 mm. Nail growth can be inhibited during serious illnesses (especially with a high fever) or with advancing age, increased with certain types of stress or nail biting, and altered by systemic disease and dermatitis.

The toenail is set on the dorsal surface of the distal end of the toes in grooves that are referred to as the lateral and proximal nail grooves. These grooves are covered by corresponding folds, known as the lateral and proximal nail folds (Fig. 1–5).

The nail bed is an epidermis-like stratified squamous epithelium base upon which the nail plate rests. The nail plate itself appears translucent in areas where it is not attached to the underlying nail bed. The areas of the nail that are attached to the underlying adherent and vascular nail bed appear pink, as the result of the transmission of color from this area.

The white semicircular lunula at the proximal end of the nail plate is the topographical marker of the nail matrix. The lunula represents the junction points between the nail matrix and the nail bed. The matrix, which synthesizes the nail plate substance, extends proximally under the nail fold 5 to 10 mm in depth. The region underlying the free edge of the nail plate distal to the nail bed and proximal to the epidermis of the tip of the digit is the *hyponychium*. Overlapping the matrix of the nail is the proximal nail fold, the stratum corneum of which is prolonged distally as a thin cuticular fold, the *eponychium*. Below the nail lies the germinative zone that, together with the subjacent corium, forms the nail bed. The nail plate lies on a highly vascularized nail bed that is continuous proximally with the nail matrix.

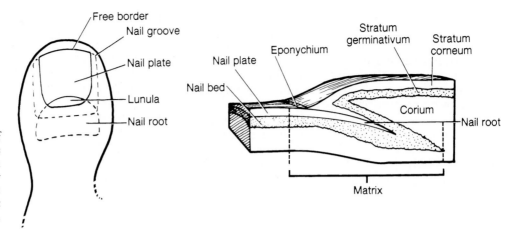

Figure 1–5 Anatomy of the nail with longitudinal cross section of the toenail. (From Dockery GL: Nails. In McGlamry ED, Banks AS, Downey MS [eds]: Comprehensive Textbook of Foot Surgery, 2nd ed, p 277. Baltimore, Williams & Wilkins, 1987.)

Histological Factors

EPIDERMIS. The pathological processes involving the epidermis center on two categories: acquired and congenital. The acquired processes can be further divided into two types: limited and diffuse. An example of a limited acquired epidermal condition would be the callus or hyperkeratosis tissue buildup. An example of the diffuse acquired epidermal condition would be palmar-plantar hyperkeratosis or pityriasis rubra pilaris.

The pathological processes primarily involving the epidermis due to congenital conditions may be localized, as in keratoderma palmare et plantare, or generalized, as in ichthyosis. The epidermis may undergo hypertrophy as a whole or in one of its component cellular layers: keratinocytes or melanocytes. Pathological changes in the epidermis therefore depend on what happens on a cellular layer involving the keratinocytes and melanocytes.

Keratinocyte. Changes in the keratinocytic properties may be due to alterations in function, alterations from an injury, or alterations in normal growth. Alterations in function are represented by three pathological processes: hyperkeratosis, parakeratosis, and dyskeratosis. *Hyperkeratosis* is an increased thickness or hypertrophy of the stratum corneum. This condition is localized or diffuse and may be primary or secondary. Primary hyperkeratoses are seen in hereditary conditions. Secondary hyperkeratoses are due to thickening of the epidermis because of stimulation or intermittent pressure or are neurocutaneous syndromes. Corns, calluses, and plantar keratomas typically fit into this classification. *Parakeratosis* is an accelerated level of keratinocyte activity usually secondary to inflammation of the skin. The resulting cells are not mature when they reach the external layer and therefore retain their nuclei. If there is parakeratosis, the stratum granulosum is not developed. *Dyskeratosis* is applied to indicate imperfect keratinocyte activity. Some of the malpighian cells undergo premature and abnormal keratinization. Benign dyskeratosis is seen in Darier's disease and many other common dermatoses. Malignant dyskeratosis is seen in Bowen's disease and squamous cell carcinoma.

Alterations from injury usually involve the malpighian layer as the principal site of change and are characteristic of the blistering diseases. Alterations in growth are represented by overgrowth of the keratinocytes, such as in benign seborrheic keratoses and verrucae formation. Malignant overgrowth of the keratinocyte is seen in basal and squamous cell epitheliomas.

Melanocyte. Alterations in function secondary to melanocyte hyperfunction are seen in tanning, freckles, and postinflammatory hyperpigmentation. Loss of pigmentation in the melanocytes causes leukoderma and vitiligo.

DERMIS. There are many different pathological changes that occur in the dermal layer, and, in general, these changes may be divided into three classifications: connective tissue changes, cellular changes, and matrix changes.

Connective Tissue Changes. These changes may be secondary to alterations in elastic fibers, which may be degenerative, scarce, or absent, causing scarring. Marked changes in the elastic fibers may be seen in atrophy. Calcareous or fatty deposits may also occur within the connective tissues. Collagen fibers may also undergo chemical degenerative changes.

Cellular Changes. These changes are due to acute or chronic inflammation, granulomas, or neoplasms. Inflammatory changes are characterized by a perivascular infiltration of various cell types. The infiltrate is composed of polymorphonuclear leukocytes in the acute phase and lymphocytes, monocytes, and histiocytes in the chronic phase. Plasma cells may also be increased in deeper chronic inflammatory reactions. The relative number of these cells is influenced by the cause of the inflammation and the individuality of the patient.

Granulomatous changes are due to a special tissue response to cellular infiltration in which large cells with abundant cytoplasm develop. Granulomas consist of plasma cells, epithelioid cells, and multinucleated giant cells. Granulomas composed mostly of plasma cells are called plasmomas. Other types of granulomas include nonspecific types due to mechanical or chemical irritation, foreign body types, and infectious types. Infectious granulomas are distinctive histologically, and they usually contain substances that help in their identification.

Neoplasms of the dermis are characterized by cellular infiltrations that correspond to the cells of origin, and they may be benign or malignant. Dermal fibromas are benign alterations, and fibrosarcomas are malignant alterations in the connective tissue cells. Carcinomas resemble the basal cell or prickle cell layers, or both, of the epidermis. Melanomas show the greatest activity at the dermoepidermal junction, and the tumor cells show large, irregularly densely stained nuclei and nucleoli.

Matrix Changes. Cellular matrix changes are related to chemical alterations in hyaluronic acid and chondroitin sulfate. The cutaneous mucinoses are a group of heterogeneous disorders that feature the dermal deposition of mucin. In the dermis, mucin is mostly acid mucopolysaccharide, hyaluronic acid, and chondroitin sulfate. Under normal circumstances, hyaluronic acid is produced by the fibroblasts. Excessive production of hyaluronic acid and chondroitin sulfate characterizes the primary and secondary forms of mucinoses.

SUBCUTANEOUS LAYER. Pathological changes within the subcutaneous layer are classified into noninflammatory and inflammatory disorders. The noninflammatory conditions include low-protein edema (renal and cardiac), high-protein edema (lymphedema), and cold injury (immersion foot or frostbite). The inflammatory conditions consist of traumatic (physical, mechanical, and chemical injury), infectious (tuberculosis and leprosy), and unknown etiologies (erythema nodosum and nodular vasculitis).

COMMON PATHOLOGICAL TERMS

Acanthosis–Hyperplasia of the epidermis (prickle cell layer or malpighian layer). Diffuse acanthosis of the prickle cell layer of the epidermis occurs in eczema and psoriasis.

Acantholysis–Loss of cohesiveness between the cells due to dissolution of the intercellular bonds in the prickle cell layer of the epidermis. The cells become separated and lie singly in vesicles within the epidermis (intraepidermal). One type of acantholysis is seen in herpes simplex and another in epidermolysis bullosa.

Anaplasia–Loss of differentiation of cells and of their orientation to one another and their axial framework. This is the atypical proliferation of cells that usually occurs in neoplasms or malignancies. The anaplastic cells have large nuclei that produce unusual mitotic figures, such as in Bowen's disease.

Dyskeratosis–Imperfect keratinization in which some of the malpighian cells undergo a premature and abnormal keratinization. Benign dyskeratosis is seen in Darier's disease, and malignant dyskeratosis is found in epidermoid carcinoma in situ (Bowen's disease).

Liquefaction Degeneration–A type of degeneration resulting in vacuolization (converting into a liquid) of basal cells. This occurs in dermatomyositis and lichen sclerosus et atrophicus.

Microabscess–A minute intraepidermal abscess with differing cell types. Those containing polymorphonuclear leukocytes are seen in psoriasis and are termed *Munro's microabscesses;* those with mononuclear cells seen in mycosis fungoides are called *Pautrier's abscesses;* and those multilocular microabscesses containing neutrophils are seen in Reiter's disease and impetigo herpetiformis and are referred to as *Kogoj's pustules* or *microabscesses.*

Parakeratosis–Persistence of the nuclei of the keratinocytes into the stratum corneum of the skin. Because of the immaturity of the cells, the nuclei are retained in the outer layers.

Spongiosis–A spongy appearance of the rete caused by intercellular edema between the keratinocytes. This condition is seen in inflammatory disorders such as eczema. Spongiosis often secondarily produces parakeratosis.

BIBLIOGRAPHY

Brenner MA, Kalish SR: Glomus tumors with special reference to children's feet. J Am Podiatr Assoc 68:715–720, 1978.

Burgeson RE: Basement membranes. In Fitzpatrick TB, Eisen AZ, Wolff K, Freedberg IM, Austen KF (eds): Dermatology in General Medicine, pp 288–303. New York, McGraw-Hill, 1987.

Dockery GL: Nails. In McGlamry ED, Banks AS, Downey MS (eds): Comprehensive Textbook of Foot Surgery, pp 277–303. Baltimore, Williams & Wilkins, 1987.

Habif TP: Clinical Dermatology: A Color Guide to Diagnosis and Therapy, pp 1–10. St. Louis, CV Mosby, 1990.

McCarthy DJ: Cutaneous anatomy. In McCarthy DJ, Montgomery R (eds): Podiatric Dermatology, pp 1–15. Baltimore, Williams & Wilkins, 1986.

McKee PH: The structure and function of normal skin. In du Vivier A: Atlas of Clinical Dermatology, pp 1–12. Philadelphia, WB Saunders, 1986.

Potter GK, Ward KS: Tumors. In McGlamry ED, Banks AS, Downey MS (eds): Comprehensive Textbook of Foot Surgery, pp 1136–1190. Baltimore, Williams & Wilkins, 1987.

Sauer GC: Manual of Skin Diseases, pp 1–7. Philadelphia, JB Lippincott, 1973.

2

History and Physical Examination in Dermatological Patients

INTRODUCTION

A large number of diseases involve only the skin, but many lesions of the skin are also clues to serious underlying medical problems. With such large numbers of lesions, the physician is often overwhelmed and unable to differentiate those lesions that are the clues to internal disease from the localized conditions. One needs to learn to "read" the skin as efficiently as one interprets a roentgenogram or reads a laboratory report.

The physician is concerned when a patient has a painful lower extremity condition and will develop a differential diagnosis and search for an explanation by history, physical examination, and special tests. That same physician often, however, may disregard irregular, discolored lesions on the leg or purpuric papules on the feet. A physician should know enough about skin lesions to be able to discern which lesions can be overlooked and which ones need to be treated.

It is just as important for the physician to develop good visual skills to diagnose dermatological entities as it is to develop and refine other diagnostic and surgical skills. The detection of clues to diagnose disease by examination of the skin is a skill that must be acquired through experience, study, and refinement of technique. One must train oneself to become a good observer.

The problem in dermatological diagnosis is largely related to the examiner's inability to recognize specific lesions. Too often, the medical student does not have a chance to get thoroughly acquainted with the various skin lesions. Although a student may be introduced to them, he or she catches only a fleeting glance and never gains enough familiarity with the various lesions to allow recognition of even the most common of them. In time, by not recognizing the lesions, the physician develops the habit of disregarding the skin and its presentations. I have often visited a colleague's office and heard the statement, "I don't see those types of problems in my practice." But while I was there, several interesting dermatological cases were identified. My colleague was probably right—he just did not "see" those problems when the patient came into the office.

In the remaining portions of this text dermatological conditions of the lower extremities are presented from several different points of view. The evaluation based on a complete history and physical examination is reviewed. Then localization of lesions is discussed, which compares those diseases limited strictly to the skin, diseases due to acquired conditions, and those that are heritable. A review of diagnosis using a technique designed to place lesions into specific categories of primary, secondary, and elementary lesions is presented. A large number of clinical cases are presented throughout the text in group classifications such as infections, vascular disorders, eczematous dermatitis, and papulosquamous diseases. There is considerable overlap of information throughout this text to show the interrelationship of dermatological conditions and to provide the reader with a better understanding of how to approach the patient with a cutaneous disorder.

Medical History

The medical history of a patient with a cutaneous disorder should be obtained in the same manner and with the same care as it would be gathered from a patient with any other physical condition presenting to the office for treatment. As mentioned earlier, some practitioners will all too often assess skin lesions as trivial or unimportant and believe that there is simply no need to obtain a history or perform a thorough physical examination on a patient. The history, however, may provide the details necessary to make the final diagnosis. In comparison, some lesions are so distinct and typical in their characteristics and appearance that it seems unlikely that the physician need spend excessive time with the initial history and physical examination. For this reason, the diagnosis may be made early on by presentation and a brief preliminary history may be adequate. If the dermatological condition is not readily distinguishable, a more complete history is warranted.

At the beginning of obtaining the history from the patient it is important to ask several specific questions. When was the problem first noticed? What did it look like and how did it feel? Has this problem ever been noticed in the past? Is the patient taking any medication now or before the appearance of the lesion? A question that must be asked for all skin lesions on the lower extremities is whether the patient has ever or is currently applying any topical medications to the area in question. Topical medications and lotions can significantly change the texture and general appearance of skin lesions and make visual identification very difficult.

Further questions regarding any symptoms, such as itching (pruritus) or pain, may also be helpful in the differential diagnosis. A basic problem with symptoms involves the mistaken attitude of some physicians that if a condition does not itch it cannot be an allergic reaction or if it hurts it must be related to a nerve condition. This simplified approach more often than not leads most practitioners down the wrong diagnostic or treatment pathway.

Specific information obtained from the patient should include the type of skin problem and whether it is localized or diffused. It is important to find out if the problem is located on any other area besides the lower extremity. It may be difficult for some practitioners to ask the patient to disrobe to evaluate the abdomen or back when the patient presents with a problem on the legs or feet. This may be done during the questioning portion of the history or during the physical examination. Often I have asked a patient if there are any similar lesions on other parts of the body and he or she responds with a negative reply. But, during the examination it was quite evident that there were lesions located on the back or in the scalp hairline. At that point the patient would say, "Oh, I've had this other problem for years."

During the history it is helpful to ascertain whether there is a family history of similar problems, whether the patient has any past or present allergies, what the patient does for a living, whether there is any chance of exposure to chemicals or caustic agents, what composes the patient's general diet and oral supplements, and whether there is a history of any previous treatments. Is the problem acute or chronic? Specifically, how long has it been present? The objectives of obtaining the history in a patient with skin conditions are to trace the development of the disease as accurately as possible, to find any elements in the history that may be related to the present condition, and to compare and evaluate the relationship of the patient's condition with his or her personal and occupational environment. Additional information regarding the current psychic and emotional status may also be helpful. The patient may have a theory as to the underlying cause of the current skin condition, and this information may be very helpful in establishing a cause for the disorder.

Family History

A history of arthritis, diabetes, cardiovascular disease, psoriasis, or other familial incidence of allergies may be important. Along with conditions and illnesses, it is usually necessary to ask specific questions, such as are there any family members who get hives or rashes or have eczema or asthma? Additional questions should be asked about congenital anomalies, hereditary traits, acne, rosacea, and vascular ulcers. Finding out if current family members are well or have a similar skin condition may be useful. Some conditions, such as scabies or impetigo, usually affect several family members, only one of whom may present to the medical office for evaluation.

Ethnic Background

Ethnicity is rarely a crucial determining factor in making a diagnosis of skin conditions, but certain conditions show a greater prevalence in some groups. Blacks have a greater tendency to lichenification and follicular disorders; Asians are more prone to atopic dermatitis or lichen simplex chronicus of the ankles. Because there are very few specific conditions seen only in certain ethnic groups it is difficult to use this information to any advantage. Understanding ethnic background is probably more of a matter of general interest and not a determining factor in developing the diagnosis of skin conditions.

Age

In the consideration of classification of dermatological conditions, age of the patient is as nonspecific as is the determination of ethnic background. There are some conditions that appear more prevalent in certain age groups, and sometimes it will be helpful in the overall formation of a differential diagnosis. Young children are more prone to impetigo and ringworm of the scalp. Older children have a predilection for atopy, and adolescents tend to be predisposed to acne. However, all of these conditions may be seen in other age groups. Keratoses and dermal atrophy appear much more commonly in elderly patients; nevertheless, they may sometimes appear in younger adults. Age should not be a great determining factor in arriving at the diagnosis of skin conditions of the feet or legs but may be helpful in the overall presentation of the disease.

Time of Year

Many conditions, including *Rhus* dermatitis (poison ivy and poison oak), miliaria, papular urticaria, photosensitivity reactions, and insect bites, are much more common during the summer. In winter, conditions such as ichthyosis, fissured heels, and generalized pruritus are exacerbated. In comparison, some conditions improve at certain times of the year. Acne, psoriasis, atopic dermatitis, and pediatric winter itch may resolve during the summer. Stinging insects (honeybees, hornets, wasps, yellow jackets) are most active in the spring and summer, and it is unusual for reports of stings in the late fall or winter. Rocky Mountain spotted fever is reported in 95% of patients as having an onset between April 1 and September 30, the time when ticks are the most active. This information, by itself, is not very important, but it may help when trying to isolate certain conditions or develop the differential diagnosis.

Geographical Area

Some dermatological conditions are endemic to certain regions and totally absent in others. *Rhus* dermatitis (poison ivy and poison oak), for example, is common in the southern United States but is not seen in England because these plants do not grow there. Other conditions, such as creeping eruptions or cutaneous larva migrans, are commonly found in the southeastern United States or may be seen in patients after visits to warm sandy beaches.

Occupational and Environmental Factors

Understanding the patient's occupation may help, for example, if plastic or rubber boots are worn all day at work; if work is done in a wet environment; if there is exposure to harsh chemicals or materials; or if work is done outdoors. Contact dermatitis from plants obviously is seen more frequently in those patients who are exposed to the incriminating substance on a regular basis. Working in wet places or wearing protective footgear predisposes patients to immersion conditions, infections, and contact dermatitis.

General Medical Conditions

The patient must be asked about any other health-related conditions. Patients frequently do not mention medications or health problems when they are seeing a physician about skin conditions because they do not see any correlation between the two problems. Because they do not want to waste the physician's time, or their own, they may not offer any additional insight into any present illnesses. For this reason, it is important to ascertain if there is any past or present problem with hypertension, heart disease, diabetes, kidney disease, liver disease, alcoholism, or any other medical condition. Specific questions should include when the patient last had a complete physical examination, who the physician was who performed it, and what treatments were provided. Patients also should be asked what medication they may be currently taking. Many patients will say that they are not taking any medications but on further questioning they will say, for example, that they are taking birth control pills, water pills, aspirin, ibuprofen, estrogen, thyroid pills, or megavitamins. They do not consider these substances as medications but simply something they take daily for some unrelated condition.

Psychosocial History

The psychological factors of skin diseases are covered in detail in Chapter 17. Factitial dermatitis and self-induced skin conditions are sometimes discovered during a review of mental health status. Disturbances in the psychic background may vary greatly in seriousness and presentation. The simplest form of self-induced dermatitis is lichen simplex chronicus or lichenification of skin due to excessive rubbing or scratching. Other problems may include the creation of skin conditions for the purpose of getting attention, the creation of dermal excoriation lesions with fingernails, the application of caustic agents to cause skin injury, and the severe forms of self-mutilation. Parasitophobia and delusions of parasitosis are also expressions of psychic disorders. Social issues should also include the patient's use of prescription medications, narcotics, and illicit drugs. The history of alcohol consumption and smoking are important for a complete evaluation of the patient.

Pruritus

Pruritus is a symptom complex and not a dermatological condition. It is important to ascertain the exact nature of the itching as part of the gathering of historical information. The intense discomfort produced by itching is probably the primary reason that patients come into the office for treatment. Pruritus may be noted only in certain phases of the dermatoses and may be the predominant feature and may precede all other symptoms. Mechanical injury to the skin may follow pruritus and result in excoriations or lichenification. Pruritus is a very common symptom with many skin diseases, and the primary treatment is relief of the itching. However, it is important to try to discover the cause of the problem because it might be a cardinal symptom of general medical significance; for example, it may be the earliest sign of Hodgkin's disease, primary biliary cirrhosis, or occult carcinoma. The itch-scratch cycle is not well defined, but a simple model shows the process from a primary stimulus that causes the pruritus through the transition to scratching or rubbing, which in turn causes an irritation (inflammation) to the skin, continuing the cycle (Fig. 2–1).

CLINICAL EXAMINATION

The clinical examination follows the preliminary history. The clinical physical evaluation includes visual examination, palpation of the lesions, determination of the distribution of lesions, and a description of the characterization of the appearance of the condition. The physician should always wear an examination glove when inspecting the oral mucosa, open or draining wounds, or obviously infected lesions. For all other inspections the ungloved fingers provide greater tactile information and aid in accurate palpation sensation.

Visual inspection of the skin involves a complete evaluation of the mucocutaneous system. It is essential that the physician begin with examination of the present problem and then evaluate the rest of the patient. It is important to evaluate the entire mucocutaneous system. The patient should be carefully examined with a meticulous visual check of the entire skin, scalp, and mouth areas. Some patients may be reluctant to have their back or abdomen evaluated when they have presented with a skin problem on the foot or ankle area. They should be assured that it is important to evaluate other areas to confirm the presence of any additional skin problems and to check for other signs that might help confirm the diagnosis. It is not usually necessary to examine the groin or breast area. Do not forget to

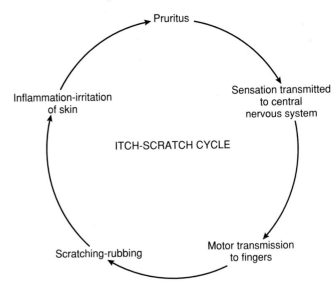

Figure 2–1 Mechanism of pruritus through the perpetual itch-scratch cycle.

examine the hands carefully because many lower extremity conditions are also expressed on the palms. With this complete visual inspection the physician may develop a sense of the distribution of the dermatological condition as well as a determination of the configuration or arrangement of patterns of the condition. Often this information alone is all that is necessary to make an accurate diagnosis, but one must always consider the fact that atypical distributions occur with all disorders.

For a complete evaluation, the patient must be carefully examined under full illumination. Natural daylight provides the best source of light for examining skin conditions. Ordinary incandescent light from at least a 60-watt bulb is also satisfactory for skin evaluation. Fluorescent lighting alone may distort color presentations but if bright enough will be adequate for most situations. All of these lighting sources may be used together for the best exposure to illuminating the skin. Side-lighting with a movable lamp or penlight is useful to determine if a lesion is elevated or irregular. When the overhead lighting is dimmed the side-lighting may reveal the extent or contour of the lesion much more clearly. This lighting source is also useful for examining the mouth, usually an area that is overlooked. Such lighting may also aid in examining between the toes and in illuminating the toenails. Another light source that is very helpful in the examination of skin is the Wood's lamp, which may also be helpful in diagnosing erythrasma or accentuating pigmentary changes in the skin.

During the clinical examination of the skin and the evaluation of dermal conditions it may be helpful to use a magnification lens. Several types of hand lenses are available from the local stationery store or university book store. They range from simple 1:2 magnification lenses to variable lenses that can be adjusted to different magnification powers. There are also lenses that have a small light source attached that allows illumination during inspection under magnification. The type of lens used to inspect stamp collections is very useful and is easily carried in the physician's lab coat or kept in the examination equipment drawer in each treatment room. Magnification may aid in clarifying the presence of scales, telangiectasia, or small satellite lesions.

Once the patient has been prepared for the examination, the lighting has been adjusted, and the physician has performed the visual portion of the examination, it is time to actually start the physical examination. This involves palpation of the dermatological process. During this part of the examination the physician may be able to assess the texture of the lesions and determine the consistency of the problem, evaluate the underlying subcutaneous layers for palpable conditions, and determine whether the lesions are tender. During the "hands-on" portion of the physical examination the physician may be able to determine the firmness or softness of lesions, whether they move or are adherent, and the depth of the condition. During palpation of mucous membrane lesions, moist or open areas, or around obvious infected lesions, the examiner should wear protective gloves. For examination of most other lesions the physician learns more and can assess the involved area better if the palpation of the skin is done without gloves.

Once the extent of the dermatological process has been determined, it is time to characterize the appearance of the lesion. This is one of the most important parts of the overall examination process. Proper characterization of lesions eventually leads to the most correct classification scheme and ultimately the differential diagnosis. Once the characterization (or morphology) is identified, the clinical correlation of the lesion can then be made.

CLINICAL CHARACTERIZATION OF LESIONS

Types of Skin Lesions

To clearly evaluate the skin and its conditions the physician must recognize the basic lesions. To arrive at a differential diagnosis, one must know what these lesions represent, how they are arranged or distributed, and how they behave. Knowing generalized and basic terminology helps in this classification scheme. (An excellent source is *Dermatology* by Samuel L. Moschella and Harry J. Hurley, published by W. B. Saunders Company, 1992; see plates I and II on pages 206 and 207.)

Primary lesions are those that occur as a result of direct expression of the disease process. Examples of primary lesions include macules, papules, plaques, nodules, wheals, vesicles, bullae, pustules, cysts, and tumors. *Secondary lesions* (or sequential lesions) are those lesions that follow the disease process. The evolution of individual lesions results in the formation of sequential lesions such as scales, crusts, excoriations, fissures, ulcers, erosions, scars, and atrophy. Other lesions that are unique skin reactions are sometimes classified as *elementary lesions.* These include comedones, burrow, lichenification, purpura, and telangiectasia. The elementary lesions are frequently listed with either the primary or secondary lesions for ease of classification. The evolution of a primary lesion into a secondary lesion is illustrated on the flow chart. Often, the identification of the *type* of primary or secondary lesion is all that is needed to establish a correct diagnosis. In many instances, however, the skin condition is changing and it may be necessary to observe the entire evolution before an accurate diagnosis can be made.

Descriptions of Lesions

Primary, secondary, and elementary lesions may be listed based on the clinical appearance of flat, elevated, or depressed lesions when compared with the level plane of the surrounding skin (Table 2–1).

Primary Lesions

MACULES. A macule is an alteration in the color of the skin that is not visibly raised or depressed; therefore, the macule is a flat, circumscribed lesion that differs in color from the surrounding skin. Some lesions may appear as macules but are shown to be slightly elevated by oblique lighting. Macules may have any size, shape, or color. They may be the result of changes in blood vessels (vascular abnormalities), changes in pigment (hypopigmentation or hyperpigmentation), or changes due to other causes (infection, internally or externally produced products).

Erythema and purpura are frequently classified as macular. The application of pressure over a red macule with a small glass slide (termed *diascopy*) is a simple method of differentiating erythema due to vascular dilatation from purpura due to red blood cells extravasated into the skin (Fig. 2–2). If the redness stays visible through the glass slide during pressure, the lesion is purpuric. Macules may be pigmented and present in a variety of colors, such as red, blue, or brown. Red lesions may be due to fixed drug reactions, capillary hemangiomas, or conditions such as juvenile rheumatoid arthritis or rheumatic fever. Blue lesions are secondary to nevus formation, mongolian spots, or ink (tattoos).

T ABLE   2 – 1 Physical Level of Lesion Types

Flat Lesions (Same plane as skin)	Elevated Lesions (Above plane of skin)	Depressed Lesions (Below plane of skin)
Infarct	Abscess	Atrophy
Macule	Burrow	Erosion
Purpura	Cyst	Excoriation
Sclerosis	Exudate (crusts)	Gangrene
Telangiectasia	Lichenification	Scar
	Nodule	Sclerosis
	Papule	Sinus
	Plaque	Ulcer
	Pustule	
	Scales	
	Vesicle and bulla	
	Wheal	

Brown macules may be café-au-lait spots, freckles, fixed drug reactions (ie, macular rashes that appear on the same body area each time a particular drug reaction occurs), nevi, stasis dermatitis, or erythrasma. Hypopigmented macules may be seen in nevus formation,

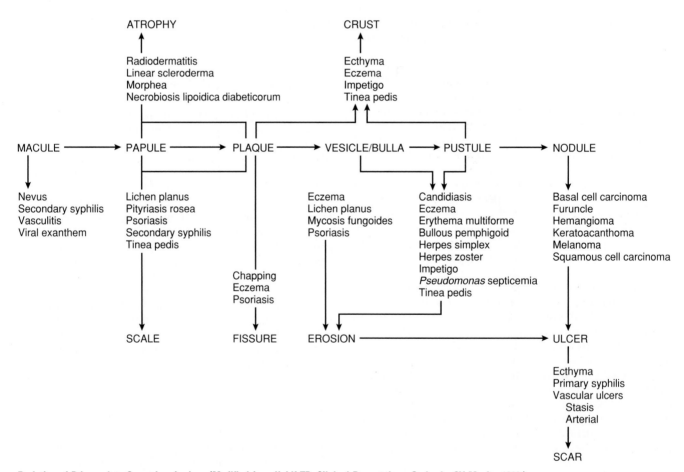

Evolution of Primary into Secondary Lesions (Modified from Habif TP: Clinical Dermatology. St. Louis, CV Mosby, 1990.)

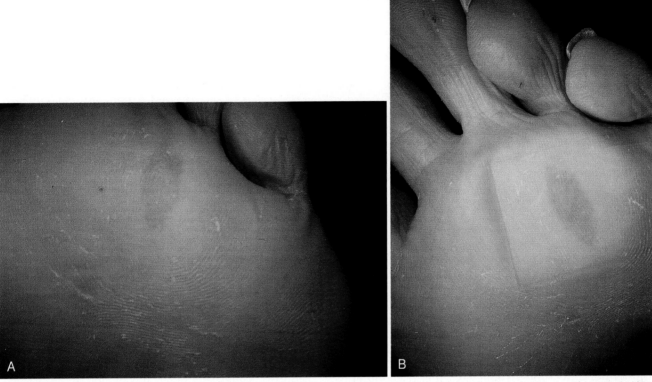

Figure 2 – 2   Diascopy. *A,* A discolored macular lesion may be difficult to classify as erythema or purpura. *B,* Using a glass slide to apply pressure to the lesion helps to differentiate these lesions. If the redness stays visible through the glass after pressure is applied, the lesion is purpuric.

postinflammatory dermatosis, tinea versicolor, tuberous sclerosis, leukoderma, and vitiligo.

PAPULES. A papule is a solid lesion that is elevated above, rather than within, the plane of the surrounding skin and can be felt. It may vary in size from 1.0 mm to 0.5 cm. Smaller papules may be identified by using oblique lighting with a flashlight in a dimmed room. Papules may have a variety of shapes and presentations. They may be flat topped, as in lichen planus; pointed, as in milia; dome shaped, as in molluscum contagiosum; or defined with sharp borders and irregular tops, as in verruca. Papules may vary considerably in color. Red papules may represent atopic dermatitis, eczema, folliculitis, insect bites, psoriasis, pyogenic granuloma, scabies, or urticaria. Yellow or white papules may be flat warts, lichen nitidus, basal cell epithelioma, molluscum contagiosum, neurofibroma, skin tags, or xanthomatosis. Brown papules are typical of dermatofibroma, keratosis follicularis, melanoma, nevi, seborrheic keratosis, and warts. Violaceous or blue papules may suggest a blue nevus, nodular melanoma, angiokeratoma, lichen planus, lymphoma, venous lake, or Kaposi's sarcoma.

PLAQUES. Confluence of papules leads to the development of larger, usually flat-topped, circumscribed elevations known as plaques. This mesa-like elevation may occupy a relatively large area in comparison with its height above the surface of the skin. Plaques are solid lesions more than 0.5 cm in diameter. This entity is also sometimes referred to as vegetation, which may be covered with thick dry scales. Examples include eczema, lichen planus, psoriasis, tinea pedis, pityriasis rosea, and seborrheic dermatitis.

NODULES. A nodule is a solid, palpable, round or ellipsoidal lesion larger than a papule (greater than 0.5 cm) and is in the epidermis, dermis, or subcutaneous layer or mixed layers of the skin. Epidermal nodules include keratoacanthoma, warts, and basal cell carcinoma. Epidermodermal lesions include melanoma, squamous cell carcinoma, and compound nevi. Dermal nodules are dermatofibromas and granuloma annulare. Dermosubdermal nodules include erythema nodosum and foreign-body reactions. Another example of a subcutaneous nodule is the lipoma.

WHEALS. A wheal is a plate-like, rounded, or flat-topped elevation produced by edema in the upper corium (dermis) and the extravasation of blood plasma through the vessel walls. Wheals may be round, oval, gyrate, or irregular with outreaching branches. The lesion may change rapidly in size, color, and shape as a result of edema within the skin. The epidermis is not involved, and no scaling is present. These lesions are also known as hives or urticaria. Wheals may be seen as a result of two general factors: external or internal causes. Wheals secondary to external causes result as an allergic response to agents such as chemicals, topical medications, or insect bites. Thermal conditions such as burns or frostbite may produce wheals, as can mechanical factors such as friction or pressure. Internal factors secondary to drug or medication ingestion or food allergies may respond by producing urticarial lesions. Stroking the skin may produce wheals in some patients and is termed *dermatographism.*

VESICLES. A vesicle is a circumscribed epidermal elevation containing fluid (a blister). Often the vesicle walls are very thin and the fluid within (serum or blood) may be visible. The vesicle measures less than 0.5 cm in diameter and is characterized by the roof, contents, or base. On the plantar surface of the foot they may be neither raised nor palpable. Vesicles may be seen in impetigo, *Rhus* dermatitis, contact eczematous dermatitis, and dyshidrotic eczema (pompholyx).

BULLAE. A large vesicle (greater than 0.5 cm) is considered a bulla and represents a very marked reaction of the skin. The bulla is usually spherical and frequently tense with taut surfaces. Bullae arise as a result of edema, and the reaction is characterized as a vigorous effort to counteract the effects of physical trauma or noxious agents. Two main factors causing bullae, as with vesicles, include internal and external conditions. External factors involve chemical reactions such as those from cantharides or adhesives; thermal conditions from burns or cold injury; and mechanical problems from friction or pressure. Internal conditions include reactions to systemic medications and disorders such as erythema multiforme, pemphigus and pemphigoid, porphyria, bullous lichen planus, and epidermolysis bullosa simplex.

PUSTULES. A pustule is a circumscribed collection of cloudy exudate or free fluid greater than 0.5 cm in diameter that may start as either a vesicle or bulla. The pustule is usually filled with pus composed of leukocytes with or without cellular debris. These raised lesions may contain bacteria or they may be sterile, such as in pustular psoriasis. Pustules may coalesce or remain singular in presentation. They may be white, yellow, or greenish, depending on the exudate color. Pustules are characteristic of several conditions, including candidiasis, dermatophyte infections, dyshidrosis, folliculitis, impetigo, pustular psoriasis, pustulosis palmaris et plantaris, and pyoderma gangrenosum. These lesions may also form with viral diseases (herpes simplex and herpes zoster), as well as with some drug reactions (e.g., iodine, povidone-iodine [Betadine], bromide). The taut pustules may spontaneously rupture and generally heal without scarring. A culture and sensitivity test and a Gram's stain should always be performed on the exudate.

CYSTS. Cysts and pseudocysts are similar in general appearance. A cyst is a circumscribed lesion with a wall and a lumen. The lumen may contain liquid, semisolid, or solid material. These lesions may be spherical or oval and on palpation appear resilient. The most common cyst is the epidermoid cyst, which is lined with squamous epithelium and produces keratinous material. Another very common cyst is the epidermal inclusion cyst, which occurs secondary to traumatic or surgical implantation of epidermis within the dermis. The implanted epidermis then grows in the dermis with accumulation of keratin within a cyst cavity. The cyst wall is composed of stratified squamous epithelium with a well-formed granular layer. This is sometimes termed a *traumatic epidermoid cyst* and is frequently identified on the lower extremities and soles of the feet. The most common pseudocyst is the digital mucoid cyst, which is commonly found on the distal fingers and toes. This solitary cyst does not have an epithelial lining and is filled with a gelatinous mucin material that is histologically distinct. It may communicate with the joint space or tendon sheath.

TUMORS. The tumor is sometimes listed as a special lesion or secondary classification but is considered here as a primary lesion. The word *tumor* is a general term for any new growth or mass, whether benign or malignant, that is usually regarded as a large nodule. Skin tumors have a wide range of presentations, and benign skin tumors must be differentiated from malignant ones. In general, benign skin tumors are slow growing and expansile. They push aside a supporting stroma rather than invading it, and metastasis does not occur. Examples would include seborrheic keratosis, stucco keratosis, cutaneous horn, digital fibrokeratoma, skin tags, dermatofibroma, keratoacanthoma, and epidermal nevus. Malignant skin tumors usually show a disorganized structural pattern with rapid growth. They also show infiltrative growth with invasion and destruction of adjacent tissue. Metastases may occur. Examples of malignant and premalignant lesions include basal cell carcinoma, squamous cell carcinoma, Bowen's disease, verrucous carcinoma, arsenical keratoses, and cutaneous metastasis. For most lay persons the word "tumor" means malignancy. For this reason, the indiscriminant use of the term tumor should be limited.

Secondary Lesions

SCALES. The exfoliation of accumulated debris of dead stratum corneum presents as perceptible flakes, and this condition is termed *scaling* or *desquamation.* The normal turnover of skin cells of the epidermis is 27 days. When the normal keratinocyte production occurs at an increased rate, immature cells reach the skin surface early (parakeratosis), and these parakeratotic cells may pile up and form scales. Scales are usually classified by their color or general appearance. Scales may appear as either thin, mica-like sheets (micaceous scales) in exfoliative dermatitis and ichthyosis or thick in layers suggesting an oyster shell (ostraceous scale) as in actinic keratoses. Scales with a silvery appearance may be seen in psoriasis, and brawny scales might suggest fungal infections or pityriasis rubra pilaris. Conditions that consist of macules with scaling are termed *maculosquamous* (e.g., erythrasma and tinea versicolor), and lesions with papules and scales are called *papulosquamous* (e.g., psoriasis and lichen planus).

CRUSTS. A crust results from the drying of fluid, serum, or blood in combination with scales, dirt, or bacteria and is sometimes referred to as a scab. This condition frequently occurs after breakage of pustules, bullae, or vesicles. Crusts may be thin and loosely connected, thick and adherent, or bloody or necrotic. They may be differentiated by their color. Yellow crusts may be due to dried serum (eczematous exudate). Golden or honey-colored crusts occur in impetigo. Yellow-green or green crusts are evident from purulent exudate; brown or dark red crusts are from blood or serosanguineous fluid. When the crust is thick and adherent and involves the entire epidermal layer with ulceration below the crust, it is termed *ecthyma*. A small, cup-shaped crust with a yellow coloration is termed a *scutula*.

EXCORIATION. The loss of superficial substance of the skin (superficial excavations of the epidermis) as the result of scratching or digging of the skin with the fingernails is termed *excoriation*. Exposure of the dermis and bleeding result from the mechanical removal of the overlying epidermis. These lesions may be linear or punctate and usually result from scratching of pruritic skin lesions. No primary lesion is identified. The condition is also seen in different forms of psychocutaneous disorders such as neurotic excoriations and delusions of parasitosis or infestations.

FISSURES. Fissures are cracks or linear cleavages in the skin that may be painful. Normal fissures are preformed on the soles of the feet. Acquired fissures represent the loss of elasticity secondary to inflammation or loss of normal hydration of the skin. This condition may be seen when the skin thickens excessively (hyperkeratosis), around eczematous dermatoses, and in areas in which therapy has caused excessive drying of the skin. Other conditions that commonly show fissures include chronic tinea pedis, keratoderma climactericum, plantar psoriasis, and candidiasis.

ULCERS. Ulcers are produced by a destruction of skin with focal loss of the epidermis and dermis with resultant scar formation at the time of healing. Ulcers are described by size, depth, number, and induration, and by the presence of underlying disease. They may be caused by vascular conditions such as stasis dermatitis, ischemic or hypertensive ulcers, atrophie blanche, and vasospastic disorders; systemic conditions such as diabetes mellitus (diabetic dermopathy or necrobiosis lipoidica), ulcerative colitis, and medications (corticosteroid injections); external factors such as solar exposure, topical corticosteroids, and x-ray dermatitis; mechanical injury such as trauma, burns, decubiti, and self-induced factitial lesions; or infectious processes such as ecthyma or pyoderma gangrenosum.

EROSIONS. Erosions are denuded, moist, depressed, and circumscribed lesions, resulting from a focal loss of all or a portion of the epidermis. Erosions do not penetrate below the dermoepidermal junction, and they are, therefore, more superficial or shallower than ulcerations. They often occur after the breakage of vesicles, bullae, or papules. Erosions usually heal without scarring unless they become secondarily infected and convert to an ulcer. Conditions that cause erosions include candidiasis, fungal infections, eczematous dermatitis, and vesiculobullous diseases.

SCARS. Scars are an abnormal formation of connective tissue indicative of dermal damage. They may be hard, or sclerotic, if there is excessive collagen proliferation. The scarred epidermis is usually thin with total disruption of the normal skin lines. Scars usually form after trauma or surgery and may be initially pink and thick but will become white and atrophic with time. They may be normal, hypertrophic, or keloidal. Other causes of scars include burns, herpes zosters, and ulcerations.

ATROPHY. Atrophy represents a depression in the skin resulting from thinning of the epidermis or dermis, or it may simultaneously occur in both layers. Epidermal atrophy is manifested by a thin, transparent-like epidermis. Dermal atrophy results from a decrease in papillary or reticular dermal connective tissue and manifests as a depression of the skin. Subcutaneous atrophy may also occur as a depression of the skin surface. Epidermal atrophy is frequently associated with dermal alterations such as inflammation or trauma with or without ulceration. The skin may show no loss of color or show markings with dermal atrophy alone. When atrophy occurs in both layers, there is often a loss of normal skin lines, wrinkling, and increased translucence along with the localized depression of the skin. Atrophy may be seen with normal aging, excessive sunlight exposure, dermatomyositis, necrobiosis lipoidica diabeticorum, radiodermatitis, topical and intralesional corticosteroid use, and scleroderma.

Elementary Lesions

Lesions that do not fit well into the primary or secondary categories are sometimes labeled elementary lesions.

COMEDO. In this noninflammatory lesion there is a plug of sebaceous and keratinous material lodged in the opening of a hair follicle. The most common form of comedo occurs in acne.

BURROW. A burrow is a narrow, elevated and tortuous channel or tunnel caused by a burrowing organism. The most common presentation of burrows on the lower extremity is caused by scabies and cutaneous larva migrans.

LICHENIFICATION. Lichenification generally refers to thickening of the epidermis. Hyperpigmentation usually follows and may extend to the surrounding tissue. The skin markings are usually greatly accentuated, and the skin feels thick and hard. Histologically, the accentuated skin markings and epidermal thickening are clearly seen. Repeated rubbing or scratching of the skin leads to lichenification. Proliferation of keratinocytes and stratum corneum, along with collagen changes in the dermis, causes lichenified skin to appear as thick plaques. This accentuation of the skin markings may resemble tree bark. The most common cause of lichenification is lichen simplex chronicus.

PURPURA. Purpura is a circumscribed deposit of blood in the skin greater than 0.5 cm. It results from leakage of blood into the skin and may be classified as either palpable or nonpalpable. The palpable forms of purpura are considered as inflammatory vasculopathies, whereas the nonpalpable forms are associated with trauma or coagulopathies. Small purpuric lesions are petechiae and larger lesions are ecchymotic. Purpuric conditions include idiopathic thrombocytopenic purpura, drug-induced thrombocytopenia, progressive pigmented purpura of Schamberg, senile (traumatic) purpura, scurvy, Majocchi's disease, talon noir (hemorrhage into the heel), Kaposi's sarcoma, trauma, and chemical burns.

TELANGIECTASIA. Telangiectasia is visible, small, and localized superficial dilatation of blood vessels. Primary telangiectasia includes generalized essential telangiectasia, spider telangiectases, hereditary hemorrhagic telangiectasia, and angioma serpiginosum. Cases of secondary telangiectasia include chronic graft-versus-host disease, corticosteroid-induced lesions, hepatic cirrhosis, lupus erythematosus, radiation-induced lesions, varicose veins, systemic sclerosis, and trauma.

BIBLIOGRAPHY

Bodmer EJ, Evancho G, Sweeney JM: Dermatoglyphics: A study and its significance to podiatry. J Am Podiatr Assoc 69:665–669, 1979.

Callen JP, Greer KE, Hood AF, Paller AS, Swinyer LJ: Color Atlas of Dermatology, pp 3–25. Philadelphia, WB Saunders, 1993.

Caplan RM: Medical uses of Wood's lamp. JAMA 202:123–125, 1967.

Dockery GL: Dermatology flow sheet. Clin Podiatr Med Surg 3:391–397, 1986.

Dockery GL: An algorithmic approach for the diagnosis of common lower extremity skin conditions. Lower Extremity 2:253–261, 1995.

Fitzpatrick TB, Walker SA: Dermatologic Differential Diagnosis. Chicago, Year Book Medical Publishers, 1962.

Fitzpatrick TB, Bernhard JD: The structure of skin lesions and fundamentals of diagnosis. In Fitzpatrick TB, Eisen AZ, Wolff K, Freedberg IM, Austen KF (eds): Dermatology in General Medicine, 3rd ed, pp 20–49. New York, McGraw-Hill, 1987.

Fitzpatrick TB, Johnson RA, Polano MK, Suurmond D, Wolff K: Color Atlas and Synopsis of Clinical Dermatology, 2nd ed. New York, McGraw-Hill, 1992.

Graff GE: General cutaneous examination of the podiatric patient. Clin Podiatr Med Surg 3:385–389, 1986.

Greaves MW: Pathophysiology of pruritus. In Fitzpatrick TB, Eisen AZ, Wolff K, Freeberg IM, Austen KF (eds): Dermatology in General Medicine, 3rd ed, pp 74–78. New York, McGraw-Hill, 1987.

Koh HK, Bhawan J: Tumors of the skin. In Moschella SL, Hurley HJ (editors): Dermatology, 3rd ed, pp 1721–1808. Philadelphia, WB Saunders, 1992.

Lazarus GS, Goldsmith LA: Diagnosis of Skin Disease. Philadelphia, FA Davis, 1980.

Lookingbill DP: Yield from a complete skin examination: Findings in 1157 new dermatology patients. J Am Acad Dermatol, 18:31–35, 1988.

Moschella SL, Hurley HJ: Dermatology, 3rd ed, pp 206–207. Philadelphia, WB Saunders, 1992.

3

LABORATORY TESTS AND DIAGNOSTIC STUDIES

INTRODUCTION

An accurate dermatological diagnosis requires an understanding of the anatomy and presentation of skin diseases, a careful patient examination and historical review, along with categorization of the findings. Important information may also be obtained from laboratory tests and diagnostic studies. This information may be essential to confirmation of a final diagnosis. In most cases of dermatological conditions, the collection of additional information is simple and reliable. A number of these tests and studies may be performed in the office; others are performed in clinical laboratories. It is highly recommended that specimens collected be sent to an accredited pathology laboratory, preferably one that specializes in dermatopathology. Although there are a number of tests and studies available for diagnosis of skin conditions, the most commonly employed ones for the lower extremities include microscopic evaluation of scrapings, cultures, and skin or lesion biopsy specimens and patch tests.

MICROSCOPIC EVALUATION

POTASSIUM HYDROXIDE MOUNT. This test may be performed for the identification of hyphae, mycelium, and spores in dermatophyte or candidal infections. To begin with, a No. 15 scalpel blade is used to vigorously scrap the edge of a scaling lesion. Vesicles and pustules may also be scraped by deroofing the lesion and collecting the underlying material. The scrapings are then collected and placed onto a microscopic collection slide and covered with one or two drops of 10% to 20% aqueous potassium hydroxide (KOH) solution. The coverslip is then placed on top of the collected specimen and solution, and the slide is carefully heated until warm to the touch to dissolve the keratinous materials. The surplus KOH solution is blotted out by pressing a paper towel or absorbent cloth to the edge of the coverslip and slide. Immediate examination is recommended. Overheating or boiling the KOH solution also dissolves the hyphae and mycelial elements and invalidates the end results. The slide is then mounted on a microscope and examined using both the low-power and the high-power lenses on low illumination. The entire slide is scanned under low power and, if elements are seen, the high-power objective is used for further examination.

SCABIES SCRAPING. In lesions suspected of being infected by the scabies mite the diagnosis may be confirmed with light microscopic evaluation of the scrapings. A No. 15 scalpel blade is held perpendicular to the skin surface, and the burrow or small papules are scraped vigorously. The contents may be collected dry for examination. To improve the collection rate, the blade should be moistened with oil so that the scrapings adhere to the blade. The specimen is transferred to the microscopic slide, and an additional drop of oil is added. This preparation is covered with a coverslip and examined. The specimen should not be warmed or heated as with the potassium hydroxide cultures. Frequently, mites and eggs may be identified within the scrapings and provide an impressive visual confirmation of the condition (see Chapter 8).

CULTURES. The Gram stain is a very common and useful examination in the evaluation of skin disorders, especially vesicles, pustules, and other "wet" lesions. Because ruptured vesicles and pustules may be contaminated with surface bacteria, the examination of fluid from an intact lesion is more valuable. This test is designed to identify bacterial elements and determine their negativity or positivity. Crystal violet or one of the triphenylmethane dyes is used to stain the heat-fixed smear of the specimen, and then it is counterstained with a dilute solution of iodine. Decolorization then takes place using acetone or alcohol. Gram-positive organisms resist the decolorization process and retain the dye stain coloration. Alternately, gram-negative organisms decolorize rapidly and the differentiation is easily made. In many cases, the results of the Gram stain allow the early intervention of appropriate antibiotic therapy in infections.

TZANCK'S STAIN. Specimen collection for the Tzanck preparation is the same as that for KOH mounts but is more practical in fluid identification. Fluid from vesicles and bullae is collected and placed on the microscopic glass slide, air dried, and fixed with methanol. The fixed slide is then stained with Giemsa blue (or similar blue stain) and examined. This test is useful for fluids from possible herpes simplex infections and varicella-zoster viral infections.

BACTERIAL AND FUNGAL CULTURES. Obtaining fluid or tissue specimens from suspected infected areas is usually straightforward. Care must be taken not to procure materials or contaminants from the adjacent area of the infection because this might lead to misinformation and delay accurate diagnosis. Culture specimens may be obtained using standard culture swabs and collecting tubes in sterile envelopes. The cotton-tipped applicator is used to obtain the exudate or specimen, and the swab is then returned to the culture tube. The lid or cap is replaced securely. These culture tubes contain a transport medium within a breakable ampule. The ampule is then broken, and the medium stabilizes the specimen. The entire collection tube is replaced in the paper envelope and properly labeled with the patient information. It is delivered to the microbiology laboratory for testing. It is helpful to provide information regarding the location of the problem, the type of fluid collected, whether the patient has been or is currently on any antibiotics, the date of collection, and any other information that is pertinent to the case. A specific request to the laboratory to evaluate for bacteria, fungus, or tissue cells may be made at this time.

BIOPSY. The collection of tissue specimen by biopsy along with the subsequent evaluation of the collected material is another important diagnostic procedure. Several types of biopsies are recognized and include shave, punch, and excisional.

Shave biopsy, or scissors biopsy, is reserved for elevated lesions or those in which a more complex technique is not warranted. The specimen in simply shaved with a surgical scalpel or sharp scissors. The bleeding is stopped with compression, topical hemostatic agent, or light electrocoagulation. The specimen is placed in 10% formalin for fixation and sent to the dermatopathology laboratory for identification. This is usually not the preferred method of obtaining a specimen, and the other types described are favored.

The *punch* biopsy is frequently employed for the examination and identification of skin lesions (Fig. 3–1). This technique provides more information than that from the shave biopsy. Dermal punches are available in reusable sets or individual sterile disposable units. The preferred size is between 2- and 6-mm diameter, depending on the size of the lesion being tested. In some cases it is advisable to take several punch biopsy samples from different areas of the questionable lesion so that a broader base of information might be obtained from the tissues collected. The 4-mm punch biopsy is used most often since it provides enough material for adequate pathological examination and is very easy to use (Fig. 3–2). The procedure is simple and quick to learn. For most lesions the center of the area is used. The exception is for dermatoses that are clear in the central portion with spreading or advancing edges and for bullous lesions in which the specimen should be collected from the leading edge. The lesion area is blocked with local anesthetic, the skin is painted with an antiseptic or antimicrobial agent, and the biopsy tool is placed in a representative area (Fig. 3–3). The skin surrounding the lesion is then stretched taut perpendicular to the relaxed skin tension lines before the punch is made. Once the biopsy tool is situated it is rotated back and forth or drilled like a screw through the upper lay-

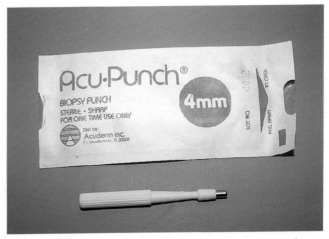

Figure 3–2   The 4-mm punch biopsy tool is the size used most commonly in clinical practice. (Courtesy of Acuderm inc., Ft. Lauderdale, FL 3309.)

ers of the skin lesion into the underlying subcutaneous layers (Fig. 3–4). The specimen is then gently lifted without damage and cut at the deep subcutaneous level (Fig. 3–5). The resultant opening may be sutured or stapled closed, packed with absorbable gelatin, compressed, and painted with hemostatic solution (Fig. 3–6). Handling of the collected specimen should continue to be gentle to prevent damage to the tissues. The specimen is then placed in 10% neutral buffered aqueous formalin for transportation to the laboratory. However, if electron microscopy is to be performed, the specimen should be fixed in a special buffered transport medium or buffered glutaraldehyde.

Excisional biopsies are those in which a portion of a larger lesion is excised (Fig. 3–7) or the entire specimen area is removed completely (Fig. 3–8), and the remaining skin is closed with suture, sterile tape strips, or staples. For smaller lesions or in cases of questionable conditions, the excisional biopsy is preferred and pro-

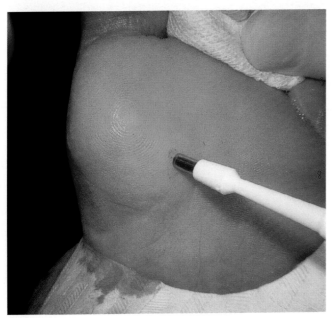

Figure 3–1   Use of the punch biopsy tool for specimen collection.

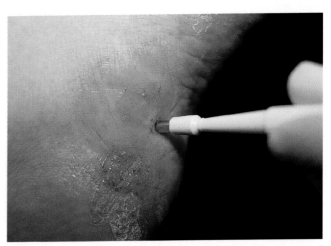

Figure 3–3   The skin area is injected with local anesthetic and prepped with skin antimicrobial paint. The biopsy tool is centered squarely over the lesion.

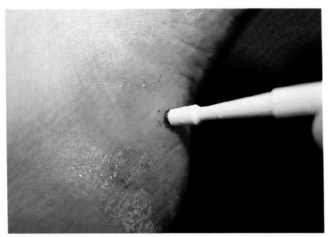

Figure 3–4   The biopsy tool is twisted firmly as pressure is slightly increased until the cutting edge penetrates the dermis.

vides the dermatopathologist with the entire specimen along with adjacent normal tissue for comparison and evaluation. There is much less chance that the lesion will be too shallow, cut too thin, or damaged during the collection phase with the excision technique. The specimen is fixed and handled in the same manner as described for other biopsy specimens. It is important that additional information is provided along with the specimen. Location of the lesion, history of its presence, prior treatment, patient age and sex, and other conditions are part of the necessary information that may assist the pathologist in the evaluation of the tissue submitted.

PHYSICAL TESTS

DIASCOPY. The test for blanchability is termed *diascopy.* This simple examination is performed by applying pressure with a finger or a glass slide. Once the finger is re-

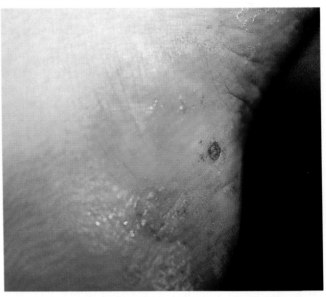

Figure 3–6   The biopsy site is then painted with Monsel's solution or closed with a Steri-Strip or suture.

moved (or while looking through the pressed glass), the area is observed for color changes. If redness in the lesion or area is secondary to erythema (increased blood in the dermal skin within dilated vessels), the skin will blanch when compressed (Fig. 3–9). Alternately, if the redness is due to purpura (extravasation of blood from disrupted vessels), the dermis will be nonblanchable.

DARIER'S TEST. When a brown macule or papular lesion becomes elevated or becomes a palpable wheal af-

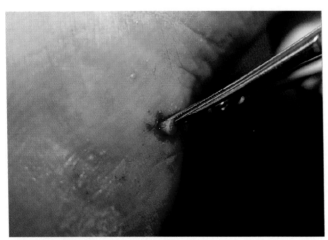

Figure 3–5   The biopsy tool is removed, and the specimen is gently elevated without damaging the tissue and cut at the deep subcutaneous layer.

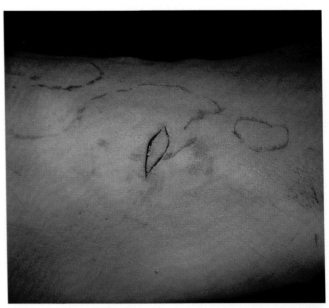

Figure 3–7   Excisional biopsy of a large area of dermatitis with excision of an active border of the area along with a portion of adjacent normal tissue.

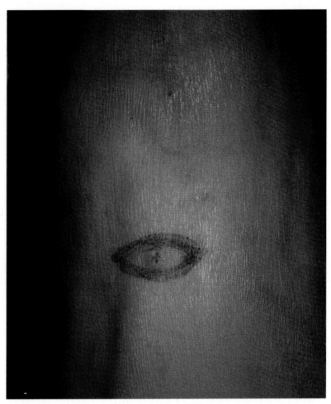

Figure 3 – 8 Excisional biopsy of a small lesion with complete removal of the lesion along with adjacent normal tissue.

ter being rubbed with a smooth instrument, the test produces a "positive sign." This finding is common in urticaria pigmentosa.

NIKOLSKY'S SIGN. Gentle traction causes sheet-like removal of the epidermis, as is seen in systemic drug reactions, toxic epidermal necrolysis, and pemphigus vulgaris. The test is performed by rubbing off the epidermis between the bullae with slight friction or by pulling the ruptured wall of the blister back into the apparently normal skin, producing a moist surface (Fig. 3–10).

DERMATOFIBROMA DIMPLE SIGN. This test is useful in differentiating a dermatofibroma (histiocytoma) from basal cell or malignant nodular melanoma. The test is performed by lateral squeezing pressure on the lesion (Fig. 3–11). A dermatofibroma will indent or dimple in the center, whereas other lesions will protrude above the plane of the adjacent skin.

WOOD'S LIGHT. Wood's lamp contains a filter that transmits ultraviolet light at a wavelength of 365 nm. It may be a small hand-held lamp or a large floor or wall-mounted unit. This light produces fluorescence of the skin in darkened rooms. The technique is helpful in the identification of tinea versicolor (golden fluorescence), erythrasma (coral red fluorescence), and vitiligo (reflection of the purple ultraviolet light). Contrary to much misinformation, Wood's light does not confirm the diagnosis of most fungal or candidal infections and does not detect the presence of bacteria on the skin. Even though the indications for the use of the Wood's lamp are limited, it is still an appropriate and inexpensive tool for the office setting.

PATCH TESTING. Patch tests are extremely valuable in the identification of the etiological agents in contact dermatitis. The patch test is used to detect a delayed hypersensitivity response to an allergen that contacts the skin. The test may be used in two ways. One is to apply a series of the most common sensitizers with the expectation that one will produce a positive response. The second method is to perform a patch test for a specific suspected agent, such as bits of lining from the shoe, to demonstrate that this particular allergy does indeed exist. Compounds generally used in patch test kits

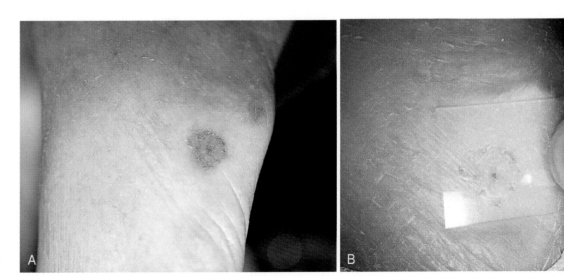

Figure 3 – 9 *A*, Erythematous plantar foot lesion. *B*, Diascopy test with application of pressure using a glass slide. If the lesion blanches, it indicates a vascular lesion rather than a purpuric lesion.

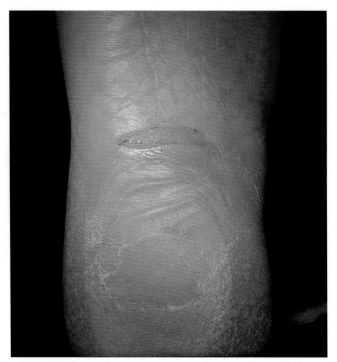

Figure 3–10   Nikolsky's sign. Gentle traction on a bulla causes separation and sheet-like removal of the epidermis.

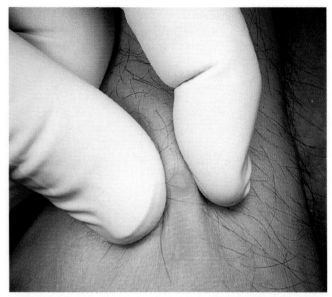

Figure 3–11   Dermatofibroma dimple sign. The test is performed by lateral squeezing pressure on the lesion. A dermatofibroma indents or dimples in the center.

for allergens in shoes include many stabilizers, glues, perfumes, dyes, and other chemicals commonly found in leather and vinyl. For either the entire battery of allergens or the specific allergen tests, standardized test trays of common sensitizing chemicals are available, each diluted and ready to apply in solution or petrolatum. These materials are then applied directly to exposed (usually glabrous) skin under occlusion. The patient is instructed to keep the area dry and intact, and in 48 hours the region is reinspected. If the allergen test result is positive, the involved area will show a response and the agent is then identified. False-positive results are possible with topical allergens placed under occlusion, with the use of improper concentrations, or with improper amounts of pressure, or in highly sensitive patients. Clinical correlation is advised.

BIBLIOGRAPHY

Adams RM: Occupational Skin Disease, 2nd ed. Philadelphia, WB Saunders, 1990.

Barr RJ: Cutaneous cytology. J Am Acad Dermatol 10:163–165, 1984.

Brooks NA: Curettage and shave excision. J Am Acad Dermatol 10:279–284, 1984.

Dockery GL: Scabies: A case report. J Am Podiatr Assoc 70:177–181, 1980.

Epstein E: Simplified patch test screening with mixtures. Arch Dermatol 95:269–271, 1967.

Fitzpatrick TB, Gilchrest BA: Dimple sign to differentiate benign from malignant pigmented cutaneous lesions. N Engl J Med 296:1518–1519, 1977.

Kuwada GT, Dockery GL: Contact dermatitis: A review. Clin Podiatr Med Surg 3:551–561, 1986.

Lookingbill DP, Marks JG: Principles of clinical diagnosis. In Moschella SL, Hurley HJ (eds): Dermatology, 3rd ed, pp 165–205. Philadelphia, WB Saunders, 1992.

Lookingbill DP: Yield from a complete skin examination: Findings in 1157 new dermatology patients. J Am Acad Dermatol 18:31–35, 1988.

McCarthy DJ: Dermatologic diagnostic techniques. In McCarthy DJ, Montgomery R (eds): Podiatric Dermatology, pp 39–52. Baltimore, Williams & Wilkins, 1986.

DERMATOLOGY
FLOW SHEETS

INTRODUCTION

One of the basic problems of most dermatology text-books is that they require knowledge of the proper diagnosis before the disease can be looked up (much like using the dictionary), or the physician is faced with flipping through the pages of clinical illustrations, hoping to find a match with a patient's lesion. If the particular lesion is not illustrated or if the patient presents differently, the physician may not be able to make a diagnosis at all. By not recognizing the lesion, the physician at worst may admit complete ignorance of the diagnosis and possibly not treat it; may attempt to diagnose the problem based not on rational thought but on the two or three diagnoses he or she knows or has heard of; or may refer the patient to the dermatologist, which is the best of these choices.

Reading about skin disease is probably not all that is needed to make an accurate diagnosis. However, once you have seen a disease that has been properly diagnosed, you will be able to recognize it much more easily the next time. Even though each disease has its own specific characteristics, there are many variations that tend to confuse the observer. Several mechanisms to evaluate lesions using morphological charts, configuration sheets, algorithms, and class-ification schemes are discussed in this chapter. Learning these will be extremely helpful in accurately classifying and identifying skin lesions. This system is not foolproof but is an excellent guide that is more reliable than comparing illustrations in a book. I spend a great deal of time studying and observing skin diseases of the lower extremities, and I still encounter exceptions and unusual presentations of well-known conditions.

Many physicians still believe that treatment of dermatoses with a corticosteroid cream is sufficient. If the patient's problem persists, the physician will then prescribe an antifungal cream or a stronger preparation. This practice may stem from the misconception by many physicians that skin problems on the feet must be either fungal infections or contact dermatitis. I do not believe that this approach is suitable, and I strongly recommend that the physician who is treating a nonresponsive skin problem refer the patient to a dermatologist.

Why is it not possible to recognize skin disease in the same way that we recognize and diagnose fractures or the way we classify ankle sprains? Professors of dermatology at medical schools and dermatology clinics have been using a problem-oriented approach to teach their art to students for many years. Learning and understanding these problem-oriented flow sheets takes practice and persistence, and some say it is difficult. However, after using these flow sheets on specific cases, numerous physicians have told me that they have correctly identified and successfully treated previously undiagnosed skin diseases.

PROBLEM-ORIENTED ALGORITHM

Some of the techniques to work through the problem of diagnosing unknown lesions are presented in this chapter. One type of approach is use of the problem-oriented algorithm. This approach to the diagnosis of skin disease along with the proper use of a dermatology flow chart is an extracted, shortened, and slightly modified teaching version of Lynch[1] and Sams.[2]

The method is relatively simple and frequently provides the practitioner with an answer when questioning a diagnosis relative to skin disease. First, use the accompanying algorithm to obtain the proper grouping from the Major Diagnostic Group, then go to the list of diseases for that group (Table 4–1) to further clarify the basic characteristics. Finally, select the most likely diagnosis from the corresponding group categories listed in Table 4–2.

For example, suppose that your patient presents with several small, elevated, whitish papules on the ankle. Begin at the top of the algorithm. The first question is whether or not blisters are present? Answering "no" leads us to the next question. Are the lesions red? Again, answering "no" to this question leads us to follow the path to noncolored lesions, which, in turn,

T A B L E   4 – 1 Problem-Oriented Groups: Major Characteristics

Group 1:	The Vesiculobullous Diseases Characterized by clear fluid-filled blisters
Group 2:	The Pustular Diseases Characterized by yellow pus-filled blisters
Group 3:	The Skin-Colored Papules and Nodules Characterized by skin-colored (the color of that individual patient) lesions that may have a rough (keratotic) or smooth surface
Group 4:	The White Lesions Characterized by white macular patches or by white papules
Group 5:	The Brown-Black Lesions Characterized by brown macules or patches or by brown papules
Group 6:	The Yellow Lesions Characterized by either a smooth surface or by crusted yellow lesions
Group 7:	The Inflammatory Papules and Nodules Characterized by red, elevated lesions
Group 8:	The Vascular Reactions Characterized by a combination of vasodilation, edema, and purpura
Group 9:	The Papulosquamous Diseases Characterized by papules and plaques with sharp margins
Group 10:	The Eczematous Diseases Characterized by papules and plaques that have poor margins and may or may not have excoriations. Acute eczema is weeping and crusted, whereas chronic eczema is dry and scaling.

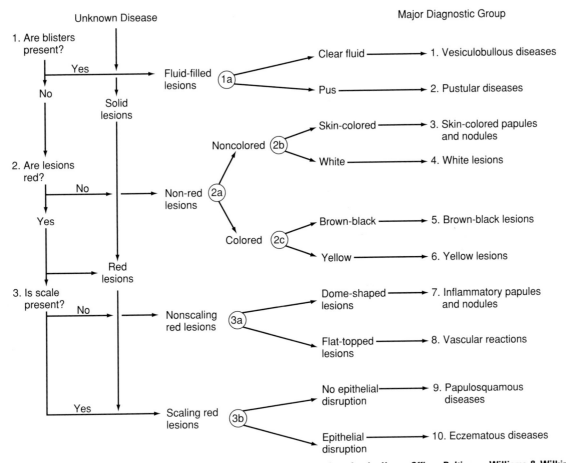

Algorithm for Unknown Skin Diseases (Modified from Lynch PJ: *Dermatology for the House Officer.* Baltimore, Williams & Wilkins, 1982.)

takes us to the category of white lesions. This step puts us at Major Diagnostic Group 4. Going to Table 4–1 provides additional information and, in this case, a review of Diagnostic Group 4 confirms that our white papules are located here. Finally, by using Table 4–2, the review of Group 4: The White Lesions includes milia, keratosis pilaris, and molluscum contagiosum. This part now allows us to evaluate these topics specifically and to more easily confirm the diagnosis.

The majority of common dermatological lesions fit into this diagnostic scheme. Failure to arrive at the correct final diagnosis may mean that the condition is not very common or that the algorithm was not followed precisely. If the algorithm flow was done improperly, it is best to go back over the questions asked and retrace the flow chart branches. If questions can be answered slightly differently from the last attempt, a new group of diagnoses may be made available. This will allow for additional consideration of the lesions presented.

One difficult area with the flow-chart type of algorithm is the case in which the presenting lesion has erosions with no intact vesicles. This finding may be due to excoriations or late-stage presentations and may mislead the examiner away from the vesiculobullous disease group. Another problem exists when two or more conditions are present simultaneously. This case may cause difficulty in following the proper branches of the algorithm and lead to an erroneous diagnosis.

All algorithms have an inherent flaw of being arbitrary. In other words, the algorithm is simply a tool or guideline to be used to help direct the pathway in difficult or confusing issues. For this reason it is much more useful to beginners and less experienced practitioners. Once additional diagnostic skills are acquired the algorithm becomes less useful and may, in fact, lead to complacency in diagnosis and treatment.

SCHEMATIC PRESENTATION ALGORITHM

Most skin conditions can be classified into neoplasms or eruptions. A few other conditions might fit into a third miscellaneous classification that would include ulcers, nail disorders, hair disorders, and mucous membrane conditions.

Neoplasms

Neoplasms or "growths" are subdivided into epidermal, pigmented, dermal, or subcutaneous lesions (Table 4–3).

TABLE 4–2 Problem-Oriented Groups: Outline of Specific Lesion

Group 1: Vesiculobullous Diseases
Vesicular Diseases
Herpes simplex
Varicella (chickenpox)
Herpes zoster (shingles)
Vesicular tinea pedis
Dyshidrosis
Scabies
Dermatitis herpetiformis
Bullous Diseases
Pemphigus
Pemphigoid
Erythema multiforme bullosum
Poison ivy–type contact dermatitis
Bullous impetigo

Group 2:   Pustular Diseases
Pustules
Rosacea
Bacterial folliculitis
Fungal folliculitis
Candidiasis or intertriginous skin
Pseudopustules
Keratosis pilaris
Milia

Group 3:   Skin-Colored Papules and Nodules
Keratotic (Rough) Papules and Nodules
Warts (verruca vulgaris, plantar, mosaic)
Actinic keratoses
Corns and calluses
Nonkeratotic (Smooth) Papules and Nodules
Warts (condylomata acuminata, flat warts)
Basal cell carcinomas
Squamous cell carcinomas
Epidermoid (sebaceous) cysts
Lipomas
Molluscum contagiosum
Skin tags
Nonpigmented dermal nevi

Group 4:   The White Lesions
White Patches and Plaques
Pityriasis alba
Pityriasis (tinea) versicolor
Vitiligo
Postinflammatory hypopigmentation
Morphea
White Papules
Milia
Keratosis pilaris
Molluscum contagiosum

Group 5:   Brown-Black Lesions
Brown Macules
Freckles
Lentigines
Junctional nevi
Brown-Black Papules and Nodules
Compound and intradermal nevi
Seborrheic keratosis
Melanomas
Dermatofibromas
Skin tags
Brown Patches and Plaques
Tinea versicolor
Postinflammatory hyperpigmentation
Chloasma
Giant hairy pigmented nevus
Café-au-lait patches

Group 6:   Yellow Lesions
Smooth-Surfaced Yellow Lesions
Xanthelasma
Necrobiosis lipoidica diabeticorum
Xanthomas
Crusted Yellow Lesions
Actinic keratosis
Impetigo
Seborrheic dermatitis

Group 7:   Inflammatory Papules and Nodules
Inflammatory Papules
Insect bites
Cherry angiomas
Pyogenic granulomas
Granuloma annulare
Pityriasis rosea
Secondary syphilis
Lichen planus
Inflammatory Nodules
Furuncles
Cellulitis
Hidradenitis suppurativa
Inflamed epidermoid cysts
Erythema nodosum

Group 8:   Vascular Reactions
Nonpurpuric (Blanchable) Lesions
Macular and diffuse erythemas
Urticaria (hives)
Erythema multiforme
Erythema nodosum
Fixed-drug reaction
Gyrate erythemas
Cellulitis
Purpuric Lesions
Palpable purpura (vasculitis)
Petechial and ecchymotic diseases

Group 9:   Papulosquamous Lesions
Prominent Plaque Formation
Psoriasis
Tinea corporis
Lupus erythematosus
Cutaneous T-cell lymphoma
Parapsoriasis
Prominent Papular Formation
Pityriasis rosea
Lichen planus
Secondary syphilis
Guttate psoriasis
Rubella
Rubeola

Group 10:   Eczematous Lesions
Eczema with Prominent Excoriations
Atopic dermatitis (neurodermatitis)
Dyshidrotic eczema
Stasis dermatitis
Fungal eczema
Candidiasis
Scabetic eczema
Eczema without Prominent Excoriations
Seborrheic dermatitis
Contact dermatitis
Xerotic eczema

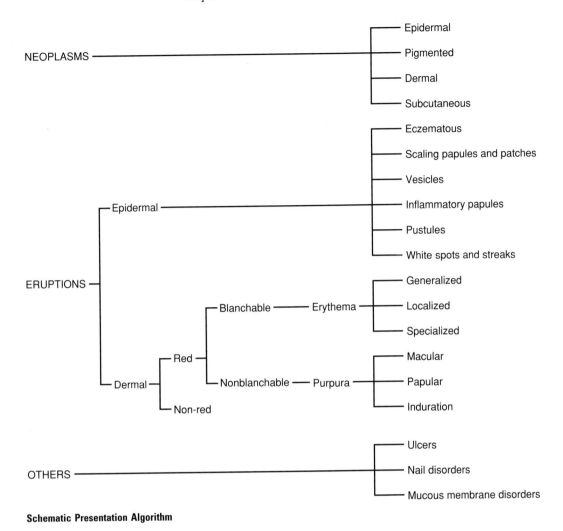

Schematic Presentation Algorithm

EPIDERMAL LESIONS. The epidermal lesions follow keratinocytic hyperplasia, and many have scales as a result of this activity. Examples include actinic keratosis, corns, calluses, molluscum contagiosum, verrucae, seborrheic keratosis, and basal and squamous cell carcinoma.

PIGMENTED LESIONS. The pigmented conditions arise from an increased production of melanin or an increased production of melanocytes. The lesions may be either macular or papular. Freckles, lentigo, café-au-lait spots, nevi, and malignant melanomas are in this classification.

DERMAL LESIONS. Dermal growths result from proliferation of dermal elements and are not usually accompanied by epidermal changes, except in the case of keloid formation. Examples include dermatofibroma, inclusion cyst, keloid, neurofibroma, malignant tumor, and xanthoma formation.

SUBCUTANEOUS LESIONS. Fat tumors or growths usually do not involve the dermal or epidermal layers, but there may be some overlapping involvement. Subcutaneous hemangioma, lipoma, and angiolipoma represent conditions in this category.

Eruptions

These inflammatory rashes may be predominantly epidermal or may occur as only dermal involvement.

EPIDERMAL ERUPTIONS. Eruptions with epidermal participation include several types: eczematous lesions, scaling papules and patches, vesicles and bullae, inflammatory papules, pustules, and white spots and streaks. Several specific skin conditions may be grouped into these epidermal types for generalized classification (Table 4–4). Eczematous eruptions are characterized by vesicles, wet papules, or lichenification secondary to intercellular spongiosis (edema). Scaling as a result of thickening of the stratum corneum may be seen with many different conditions, but frequently the papulosquamous lesions. When fluid accumulates within or beneath the epidermis, vesicles and bullae occur. The inflammatory papules are frequently the result of external factors such as insect or parasite activity or temperature changes. These lesions may occur as purely epidermal or may be combined epidermodermal inflammatory processes. When inflammatory cells accumulate within the epidermis, pustules may occur.

TABLE 4-3 Neoplasms

Type	Common	Less Common
Epidermal	Actinic keratosis Basal cell carcinoma Corn Callus Molluscum contagiosum Seborrheic keratosis Verruca	Squamous cell carcinoma
Pigmented	Café-au-lait spots Freckle Lentigo Nevus	Malignant melanoma
Dermal	Dermatofibroma Inclusion cyst Keloid	Malignant tumor Neurofibroma Xanthoma
Subcutaneous	Hemangioma Lipoma	Angiolipoma

White spots result from melanin pigment loss from the epidermis.

DERMAL ERUPTIONS. Dermal rashes are either inflammatory (red) or infiltrative (indurated). Redness is either secondary to purpura or erythema. In purpura, the blood has extravasated from the blood vessels into the surrounding dermis and is nonblanchable on diascopy. With erythema, there is increased blood in the dermis within the dilated blood vessels. Accordingly, erythema is blanchable on diascopic examination. Erythematous eruptions are classified in generalized, localized, and

TABLE 4-4 Epidermal Eruptions

Type	Common	Less Common
Eczematous	Atopic dermatitis Contact dermatitis Dyshidrotic eczema Nummular eczema Seborrheic dermatitis Stasis dermatitis	
Scaling papules and patches	Dermatophytosis Lichen planus Psoriasis Seborrheic dermatitis	Secondary syphilis
Vesicles and bullae	Bullous impetigo Contact dermatitis Dyshidrotic eczema Herpes simplex Herpes zoster	Bullous pemphigoid Epidermolysis bullosa Dermatitis herpetiformis
Inflammatory papules	Insect bites Miliaria Scabies	Lichen planus
Pustules	Candidiasis Folliculitis Impetigo Pustular psoriasis	Miliaria pustulosis
White spots and streaks	Postinflammatory Tinea versicolor Pityriasis alba Perilymphatic atrophy Vitiligo	Tuberous sclerosis

specialized subgroups (Table 4–5). Purpuric eruptions are either macular or papular. Eruptions resulting from infiltrative processes in the dermis are less common and occur as induration.

Generalized erythema may be present in patients with drug reactions (urticaria, maculopapular eruption, pruritus) and viral exanthems (symmetrical erythematous maculopapular eruption) due to echovirus and coxsackievirus infections. Less common conditions presenting with generalized cutaneous erythema include erythroderma, lupus erythematosus, scarlet fever, and toxic erythema. Localized erythema is seen in cases of dermal abscesses and cellulitis and less commonly in erythema nodosum, which may also be a local expression of a drug reaction. Specialized erythema is seen in urticaria and erythema multiforme.

Purpuric dermal eruptions are either macular or papular. The macular lesions include senile purpura, progressive pigmented purpura of Schamberg, and traumatic purpura. Less common forms of dermal macular purpura include those secondary to scurvy and thrombocytopenia purpura. The papular purpuric lesions may be due to vasculitis. Scleroderma is an example of indurated rashes resulting from infiltrative processes within the dermis.

The miscellaneous category contains epidermodermal ulcers, nail diseases, and mucous membrane disorders. These conditions are usually not difficult to recognize and classify. Ulcerations may be seen in vascular disorders and occur as arterial or stasis ulcers; infected ulcers such as found in sporotrichosis and ecthyma; traumatic ulcers; self-induced ulcers of neurotic excoriations; and neoplastic ulcers such as found in squamous and basal cell carcinoma. Nail diseases include fungal infections, psoriasis, and paronychia. Mucous membrane disorders include lichen planus, leukoplakia, and thrush.

Patterns and Configurations

Once the type, color, location, and presentation of the lesion have been identified, it is necessary to consider

TABLE 4-5 Dermal Eruptions

Type	Subtype	Common	Less Common
Erythema	Generalized	Drug eruption Viral exanthem	Erythroderma Lupus erythematosus Scarlet fever Toxic erythema
	Localized	Abscess Cellulitis	Erythema nodosum
	Specialized	Urticaria	Erythema multiforme
Purpura	Macular	Progressive pigmented purpura Senile purpura	Scurvy Thrombocytopenic purpura
	Papular		Vasculitis
Induration			Scleroderma

the pattern or configuration (arrangement) of lesions in relation to each other. The pattern, arrangement, and general distribution of lesions are helpful in finalizing the diagnosis. The following descriptions of the pattern and configuration of lesions can apply to single or multiple lesions. A list of the patterns and configurations is found in Table 4–6. A configuration is not completely specific for a given disease, although there are common presentations for many conditions. The conditions with more characteristic patterns are listed as "more common," and the conditions that show a pattern less frequently are listed as "less common." The isomorphic reaction (Koebner's phenomenon) occurs in certain conditions, especially lichen planus and psoriasis, and may create a linear pattern of the condition secondary to trauma or scratching.

The *annular configuration* is the most common configuration and consists of lesions that are round or oval with central clearing in most cases. Annular lesions are created in two distinct ways: by the pathological process of the condition spreading peripherally into new areas while receding centrally or by the formation of a ring-shaped pattern by individual lesions.

Several different subcategories of annular lesions exist, and they have separate morphological presentations. Annular scaling shows fine scales at the active peripheral border of the lesion. Tinea corporis, psoriasis, and pityriasis rosea represent this type of lesion. Annular dermal lesions are chronic and more indurated lesions of the dermal layer and include granuloma annulare and erythema marginatum. Annular crusts show crusting of the peripheral border seen in conditions such as impetigo and ecthyma. Annular erythematous lesions are characteristic of erythema multiforme and urticaria. The terms *annular* and *nummular* should not be used to describe the same lesions. Nummular (coin-shaped) lesions are distinctive lesions that are raised and active in the central core and occur in eczema. Discoid (disk-like) is used to describe those flat lesions of cutaneous lupus erythematosus. *Arciform* and *polycyclic lesions* are variations of the annular lesion and represent incomplete, broken, or contiguous rings.

Geographical lesions show a very irregular border suggesting a winding coastline. This presentation is frequently seen in urticaria and drug reactions. Lesions with bizarre, extremely irregular borders with no other

T ABLE 4–6 Patterns and Configurations

Pattern	Morphology	Common	Less Common
Annular: epidermal change	Scales	Tinea corporis Drug reactions Dermatophytosis	Psoriasis Nummular eczema Pityriasis rosea Lichen planus Epidermal nevus
Annular: without epidermal change	Erythema	Erythema marginatum	Urticaria Erythema multiforme
	Induration	Granuloma annulare	Sarcoid Lupus vulgaris
Annular: with epidermal change	Crusts	Impetigo	Ecthyma Hailey-Hailey disease
Arciform-polycyclic	Scales Macules Papules Plaques	Erythema annulare	Mycosis fungoides
Geographic	Wheals Plaques	Urticaria Drug reaction Psychocutaneous	Mycosis fungoides
Grouped	Vesicles	Herpes simplex Herpes zoster Dermatitis herpetiformis	Contact dermatitis
	Papules	Insect bites	Verrucae
Gyrate-serpiginous	Vesicles Wheals	Larva migrans	Scabies
Linear	Vesicles	Contact dermatitis Herpes zoster	
	Papules	Dermatographism Lichen striatus	Lichen planus Psoriasis Verrucae Epidermal nevus
	Induration	Linear scleroderma	Keloids
Reticular	Macules Erythema	Livedo reticularis	

findings consistent with dermatosis may represent factitial or self-induced lesions.

Grouped lesions may occur with papules, nodules, wheals, or vesicles. Clusters or groups of vesicles may occur anywhere on the skin and are sometimes referred to as "herpetiform" because of the characteristic findings in herpes simplex and herpes zoster. The term *corymbiform* is used to describe a grouped arrangement of lesions with scattered peripheral individual lesions. This condition is seen in verruca vulgaris, plantaris, and tinea versicolor. Indurated grouped lesions may represent linear scleroderma or keloid scars.

Gyrate and *serpiginous* lesions are variations of the linear pattern with snake-like patterns winding around through the skin. This arrangement of vesicles or wheals is a common finding in cutaneous larva migrans (creeping eruption).

Linear lesions are usually vesicles or papules. Linear vesicles are seen characteristically in contact dermatitis (especially *Rhus* dermatitis), herpes zoster, and warts. Lichen planus and psoriatic lesions usually form linear patterns owing to the Koebner effect.

Reticular patterns are those that have a net-like appearance, and they occur in several conditions, the most common being livedo reticularis. Individual lesions may also have a reticular (fine lacy) pattern, such as in Wickham's striae in lichen planus.

Use of patterns and configurations is helpful in the diagnosis of skin conditions, but the morphological classification is more important and consistent. If there is any confusion or disagreement between the pattern and the morphology of the lesion, the morphology always takes precedence.

REFERENCES

1. Lynch PM: Dermatology for the House Officer, pp 55–62. Baltimore, Williams & Wilkins, 1982.
2. Sams WM: A problem-oriented approach to clinical dermatology. Contin Ed 8:73–89, 1983.

BIBLIOGRAPHY

Dockery GL: Dermatology flow sheet. Clin Podiatr Med Surg 3:391–397, 1986.

Dockery GL: An algorithmic approach for the diagnosis of common lower extremity skin conditions. Lower Extremity. 2:253–261, 1995.

Graff GE: General cutaneous examination of the podiatric patient. Clin Podiatr Med Surg 3:385–389, 1986.

Lookingbill DP, Marks JG Jr: Principles of Dermatology, 2nd ed. Philadelphia, WB Saunders, 1992.

Lookingbill DP, Marks JG Jr: Principles of clinical diagnosis. In Moschella SL, Hurley HJ (eds): Dermatology, 3rd ed, pp 165–239. Philadelphia, WB Saunders, 1992.

5

BACTERIAL SKIN INFECTIONS

INTRODUCTION

Bacterial skin infections may be manifested in several different ways, but, in general, they may be divided into *primary infections* and *secondary infections*. Primary cutaneous infections are initiated by a single organism and may arise in normal skin. These infections are most likely caused by coagulase-positive staphylococci or beta-hemolytic streptococci. Secondary cutaneous infections originate in damaged skin as a superimposed condition. The causative agents include those found in primary infections as well as *Proteus, Pseudomonas,* and *Escherichia coli.* These gram-negative organisms frequently colonize dermal lesions and may cause secondary infection in ulcers and open wounds on the lower extremities. The cutaneous changes noted with skin infections are not always suppurative and may occur as a hypersensitivity response or as a vasculitis.

There are many systemic bacterial infections for which the skin is the portal of entry. The normal skin is highly resistant to most bacteria to which it is exposed on a constant basis. It is difficult to create a localized primary infection in healthy intact skin. Because bacteria are unable to penetrate the keratinized layers of normal skin, the numbers of bacteria quickly diminish when in contact with the intact skin. If there is a disruption of the integument by any means, such as injury, insect bite, abrasion, or foreign-body penetration, pathogenic organisms, such as *Streptococcus pyogenes* or *Staphylococcus aureus,* may quickly produce primary infections.

The distinction between primary and secondary infections is not absolute but, in general, for a secondary infection to occur a preexisting local or systemic condition must be present. In most cases it is not difficult to distinguish the secondary infection because a lesion such as a burn, a cut, an ulcer, or open skin dermatitis is already present. The colonization of lesions, especially ulcers, by pathogenic organisms, however, is not always indicative of an active secondary infection. Secondary infections cannot be diagnosed by positive laboratory cultures alone. In fact, all ulcers contain bacteria and without secondary findings (cellulitis or pus) or systemic changes (fever or leukocytosis) they are not true infections. This does not mean that they should not be treated but that topical cleansing is usually all that is necessary.

The primary infections that are discussed in this chapter include impetigo (superficial and bullous), ecthyma, cellulitis, erysipelas, cutaneous abscesses, folliculitis, furunculosis, paronychia, pyogenic granuloma, pitted keratolysis, and interdigital erythrasma. A comparison of topical and systemic treatments of various etiological agents is presented in Table 5–1. Discussions of secondary infections include infected ulcerations, infected eccrine sweat apparatus (miliaria), intertrigo, pustular bacterid, eczema of the feet and legs, and postsurgical wound infections.

PRIMARY SKIN INFECTIONS

Impetigo

Impetigo contagiosa is one of the most common skin infections in childhood, although it may occur at any age. In adults, it occurs more frequently in those groups with increased chances of bruising injuries (military personnel and athletes). It is also seen in elderly patients living in close quarters or under poor hygienic conditions.

This contagious superficial skin infection usually begins as a vesicular or pustular lesion that develops into exudative and crusting stages. Unless there is trauma or excoriation to the lesions, they usually heal without scarring. *Staphylococcus aureus* is the predominant organism isolated from impetiginous lesions. *S. aureus* combined with group A streptococci is the next most common culture isolate. *Streptococcus pyogenes* can be the causative agent in some cases of impetigo. The two classic forms of impetigo are superficial and bullous impetigo.

Superficial vesiculopurulent pyoderma, or common impetigo, is more prevalent during the summer months and in areas with high humidity. Lack of hygiene and crowding are also predisposing factors. The typical lesion of superficial impetigo usually starts as an erythematous vesicle or papule in a traumatized area (scratch or insect bite). Small vesicles may then form, and the lesion rapidly evolves to a thick, crusted lesion. The adherent crust is classically honey colored, and when the crust is removed the base of the lesion excretes a serous amber exudate and rapidly becomes encrusted again (Fig. 5–1).

These lesions are rarely painful and may be neglected for an extended time before medical attention is sought. Impetigo may be slowly progressive but tends to be relatively stable for several weeks. Regional lymphadenopathy is common, but other systemic signs such as malaise, fever, and toxic appearance are usually absent.

Cleanliness and proper treatment of superficial skin injury may help prevent impetigo. In cases of impetigo, the family should be instructed to bathe any areas of skin irritation or abrasion regularly with antibacterial soaps and to apply topical antiseptics or antibiotics to cuts, abrasions, insect bites, and scratches immediately after the incident occurs. Prompt treatment is important for the prevention of spreading the infection within families and to reduce any complications.

Beta-lactamase–resistant drugs (erythromycin, oxacillin, cloxacillin) are given orally for 10 days. Erythromycin should be avoided if there is widespread erythromycin resistance in the community. Topical erythromycin 2% solution and Neosporin ointment are beneficial. Neosporin may have a potential for causing a contact dermatitis if used long term. Mupirocin 2% ointment, a topical antibiotic agent, is highly active against gram-positive pathogens, especially *S. aureus*

T A B L E 5–1 Treatment of Primary Bacterial Infections

Condition	Bacteria	Antibiotic Agent	
		Topical	*Systemic*
Impetigo, superficial	*Staphylococcus aureus,* group A streptococci	Erythromycin Neomycin Mupirocin	Erythromycin Penicillin Dicloxacillin
Impetigo, bullous	*S. aureus*	Erythromycin Neosporin Mupirocin	Cloxacillin Dicloxacillin Erythromycin
Ecthyma	Group A streptococci	Erythromycin Neosporin Mupirocin	Erythromycin Dicloxacillin
Cellulitis	Group A streptococci, *S. aureus*	Cool wet dressings	Penicillin Cephalosporin
Erysipelas	Group A streptococci	Cool wet dressings	Penicillin Erythromycin Cephalosporin
Abscess	*S. aureus,* others	Erythromycin Mupirocin	Cloxacillin Dicloxacillin
Folliculitis	*S. aureus*	Bacitracin Neomycin Mupirocin	Cloxacillin Dicloxacillin Erythromycin
Furunculosis	*S. aureus*	Warm wet compresses	Erythromycin Cloxacillin Dicloxacillin Methicillin Cephalexin
Paronychia	Staphylococci, streptococci	Epsom salts soaks Erythromycin Neosporin	Erythromycin Cephalosporin
Pyogenic granuloma	*S. aureus*	Erythromycin Polysporin cream	
Pitted keratolysis	*Corynebacterium* sp., others	Epsom salts soaks Erythromycin Clindamycin	Erythromycin
Erythrasma	*Corynebacterium minutissimum*	Antibacterial soaps Erythromycin	Erythromycin

and group A streptococci. In milder infections the topical mupirocin ointment may be all that is necessary for complete healing. If after a week of treatment the lesions have not resolved, antibiotic resistance or poor compliance should be suspected. At this point, a new culture should be obtained from the base of the lesion below the crust. Antibiotic therapy should be adjusted accordingly. If the patient is noncompliant, ceftriaxone may be started. This agent is very effective against both *S. aureus* and group A streptococci but is not to be considered a primary treatment for impetigo (see Table 5–1 and flow chart).

Bullous impetigo is much less common than superficial impetigo. The characteristic lesions are thin-walled bullae usually less than 3 cm in diameter that are easily ruptured (Fig. 5–2). Unlike superficial impetigo, the blister of bullous impetigo may form on previously untraumatized skin. The fluid may be a thin amber liquid or opaque pus of white or yellow. Once the blister ruptures the erythematous base dries quickly, forming a

thin and shiny surface classically referred to as a varnish-like crust (Fig. 5–3). The causative bacteria is usually *S. aureus* (phage group II). Regional lymphadenopathy is usually absent. Severe bullous impetigo is treated with oral antistaphylococcal agents (erythromycin, cloxacillin, dicloxacillin) rather than topical antibiotics. Because of increasing erythromycin-resistant bacteria, the use of cloxacillin is recommended over erythromycin. As in superficial impetigo, topical erythromycin 2% solution and Neosporin ointment may be used in mild cases. Mupirocin 2% ointment may also be indicated for the treatment of bullous impetigo when small areas of infection are present.

Ecthyma

Ecthyma is similar to superficial impetigo. It begins in a similar fashion but proceeds to deep erosion through the epidermis, producing a shallow ulceration. Group

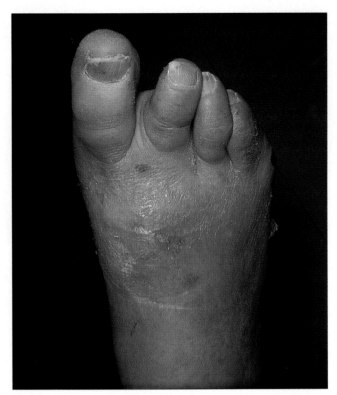

Figure 5–1   Superficial impetigo. The honey-colored crust has been removed, exposing a moist base with serous amber exudate.

A streptococci characteristically initiates the condition, although in the later stages the ulcer may be infected by several different organisms. In the early stages, ecthyma may not be differentiated from superficial impetigo. It starts with a vesicle or vesiculopustule arising on an inflamed base. The lesion enlarges over several days to a maximum diameter of 3 cm and then starts to crust over. The early crust is hard, thick, dry, and firmly adherent to the base (Fig. 5–4). In general, the crust is much thicker and harder than that seen in impetigo. Removal of the crust shows underlying ulceration with the granulating base extending deeply into the dermis. The lesions of ecthyma are usually on the lower extremities (recurrent traumatic infected ulcers), and extension of the condition into new areas is common. The lesions are very slow to heal and frequently produce scarring. Topical cleansing of the area with removal of the crust followed by soap and water washing will remove much of the debris. Topical antibiotic ointments along with oral erythromycin or dicloxacillin is effective in clearing the condition. Parenteral antibiotics are usually only necessary in widespread infections. Lesions having the same ultimate appearance may be seen in *Pseudomonas* septicemia, and this condition is termed *ecthyma gangrenosum* (Fig. 5–5). This very serious condition must be recognized and diagnosed early, so that appropriate systemic antibiotic therapy can be initiated. In patients with systemic symptoms of sepsis, a suspicion of ecthyma gangrenosum should be raised with the appearance of

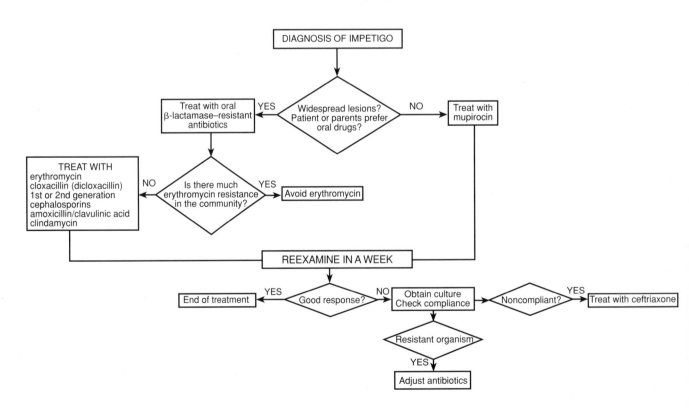

Impetigo Treatment Guidelines (From Dagan R: Impetigo in childhood: Changing epidemiology and new treatments. Pediatr Ann 22:235–240, 1993.)

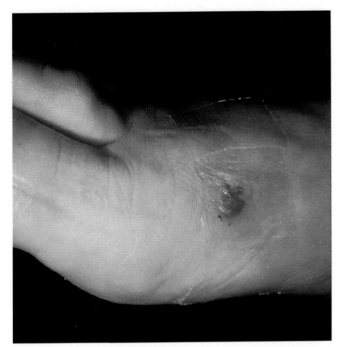

Figure 5 – 2 Bullous impetigo. A thin-walled bulla has formed on previously untraumatized skin of the foot. The surrounding tissue is erythematous, and the bulla fluid is amber.

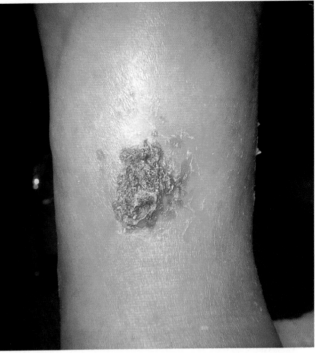

Figure 5 – 4 Ecthyma. A large, hard, thick, dry, and firmly adherent crust forms over several days. The crust is usually much thicker and harder than that seen in impetigo.

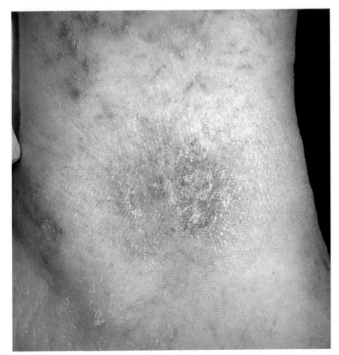

Figure 5 – 3 Impetigo. The classic formation of varnish-like crust may be seen once the blister ruptures and the erythematous base dries.

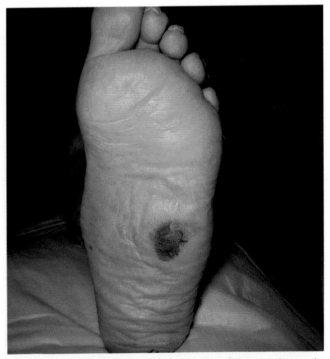

Figure 5 – 5 Ecthyma gangrenosum. This lesion is frequently seen in patients with pseudomonal septicemia and must be recognized, diagnosed, and treated early.

vesicles, pustules, and necrotic or gangrenous ulcers on the skin.

Cellulitis

Cellulitis is a subcutaneous and dermal tissue infection that is usually caused by group A streptococci and *Staphylococcus aureus*. It may also be caused by non–group A streptococci, *Pseudomonas aeruginosa*, or other organisms. Cellulitis typically occurs when there has been a previous break in the skin but may occur at times in seemingly normal tissue. The presentation is distinctive and includes erythema, edema, pain, and increased warmth. Systemic and laboratory changes may include fever, chills, mild leukocytosis with a left shift, elevated erythrocyte sedimentation rate, and, in more involved cases, malaise. Tender regional lymphadenopathy is common and may include lymphangitis, which extends proximally. On the feet and legs there is usually a portal of entry for the bacteria secondary to fissures, cracks, puncture wounds, other trauma, insect bites, or other minor damage to the intact skin (Fig. 5–6).

Cultures from open areas may provide evidence of the infective bacteria. Treatment consists of topical applications of cool wet compresses and oral administration of a penicillinase-resistant penicillin or cephalosporin. Pain may be reduced with cool compresses. The response to treatment is usually very rapid. If there has been no change in the cellulitis within 24 hours of treatment, additional diagnostic and laboratory studies

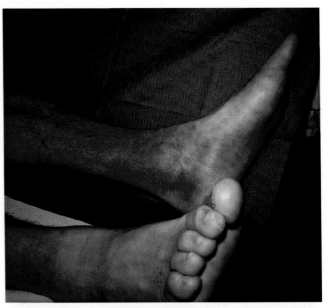

Figure 5–7　Erysipelas. Rapidly spreading, bright erythematous, and fiery hot superficial cellulitis is secondary to a primary pyogenic infection often called St. Anthony's fire.

are indicated to rule out a deep abscess or deep space infection.

Erysipelas

Erysipelas, also known historically as *St. Anthony's fire*, is a primary pyogenic infection that is characterized by a superficial cellulitis involving the skin. The affected area becomes edematous, fiery hot, and indurated, and a bright erythematous, sharply marginated, elevated plaque develops that rapidly spreads peripherally with the progression of the infection. The spreading peripheral inflammation is sometimes characterized by bright red to deep red or even brown coloration of the skin (Fig. 5–7).

The lower extremities are a common site for this infection, along with the face and ears. In the legs, erysipelas is noted to occur and recur in areas of chronic lymphatic obstruction. The disease is noted for its acute initial systemic symptoms, which frequently include chills, headache, fever, anorexia, leukocytosis, regional lymphadenopathy, and generalized malaise.

The skin lesion may be uncomfortably pruritic and may reach its maximum size in several days to a week. Vesicles and bullae may also occur on the inflammatory surface of the skin and are typical in severe infections. In recurrent erysipelas of the lower extremity the chronic edema, cellulitis, thrombophlebitis, and lymphedema can lead to a morbid condition known as elephantiasis nostras verrucosa (Fig. 5–8).

Erysipelas is most often caused by group A beta-hemolytic streptococci, specifically, *Streptococcus pyogenes*. This is the etiological bacteria in over 90% of erysipelas cases; however, other streptococcal species

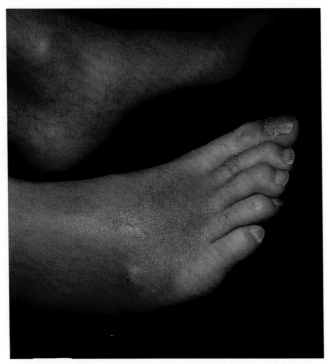

Figure 5–6　Cellulitis. Erythema, edema, pain, and increased warmth are characteristic of cellulitis.

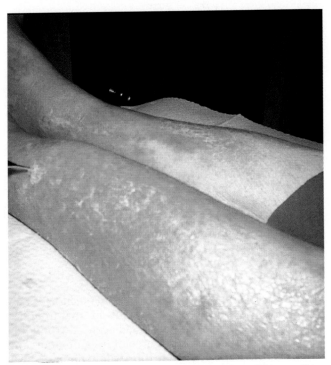

Figure 5–8 Elephantiasis nostras verrucosa. This condition is secondary to recurrent episodes of erysipelas of the lower extremities with chronic edema, cellulitis, and lymphedema.

(group B or G) and other organisms have been implicated.

Erysipelas can be accompanied by bacteremia and high fever and was a disease of historical significance because of the high mortality during the preantibiotic era. Fatalities still occur among young, elderly (especially Jewish males), debilitated, and immunosuppressed individuals. Treatment begins with complete bed rest, elevation of the extremity, application of cool, wet dressings, and appropriate antibiotic therapy. If severe edema is present, a compression Unna boot dressing may be applied. Penicillinase-resistant penicillin is the drug of choice. Cephalosporins may also be indicated, and erythromycin may be used in patients allergic to penicillin. In debilitated patients and patients with recurrent infections, systemic antibiotics should be provided on a long-term maintenance basis to prevent some of the sequelae of recurrent erysipelas. Patients should be followed for evaluation on a regular basis to prevent recurrence.

Cutaneous Abscess

An abscess is a localized subcutaneous or dermal accumulation of purulent material that is so deep that the pus is usually not visible. The lesion is usually erythematous, tender, and hot to the touch (Fig. 5–9). An abscess frequently begins as a folliculitis. The condition is a primary infection due to streptococci or *Staphylococcus aureus*. Other bacteria isolated from ab-

scesses include *Bacteroides fragilis, B. corrodens, Peptococcus,* and *Peptostreptococcus.* Incision along with drainage is the primary treatment of choice in the otherwise healthy patient. In patients with compromised immune system or with systemic infection, incision and drainage should be combined with antibiotic treatment. Results of a Gram's stain and culture and sensitivity test dictate the appropriate antibiotic drug.

Folliculitis

Folliculitis is inflammation of the hair follicle caused by infection or physical injury. The inflammation may be superficial or deep within the hair follicle. In superficial folliculitis, the erythema and swelling are limited to the shallow part of the hair follicle.

Clinically, the infection is represented by a red, elevated, and slightly tender pustule (Fig. 5–10). The hair shaft in the center of the pustule is not always visible. When pathogenic bacteria cannot be recovered from the pustule the lesion may be classified as pseudofolliculitis. Deeper infections involving the entire follicle usually have larger areas of erythema and are more painful. This condition is usually initiated by coagulase-positive staphylococci. Most of these lesions heal without scarring with simple evacuation and cleansing of the skin with antiseptic soap and warm water.

Spreading staphylococcal folliculitis occurs after abrasion injury or surgical incisions, or after other areas are covered with occlusive wraps. It may also be seen in

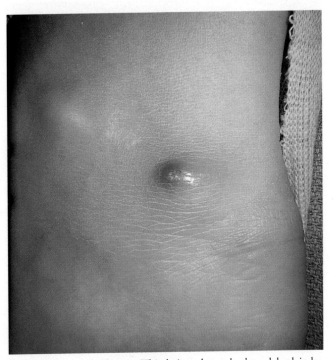

Figure 5–9 Abscess. This lesion above the lateral heel is localized, erythematous, tender, and hot to the touch. Incision and drainage is the primary treatment of choice.

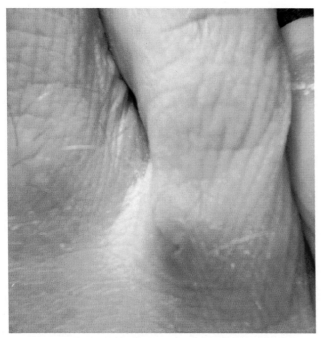

Figure 5–10   Folliculitis. Inflammation with redness, elevation, and tenderness of the hair follicle on the toe is caused by an infection or a physical injury.

areas covered with occlusive topical corticosteroid tape. Follicular pustules may actually coalesce, forming a pattern that is somewhat difficult to recognize in the later stages (Fig. 5–11). Cultures are obtained by scraping the entire top and contents of the pustule with a surgical scalpel blade and transferring the material to a culture medium. Topical applications of bacitracin, Neosporin, or mupirocin may reduce the skin count of bacteria. A 7-day treatment with appropriate oral antibiotic will alleviate the condition completely.

Pseudomonal folliculitis (hot tub dermatitis) is a distinct type of folliculitis seen several hours to days after exposure to a contaminated hot tub. Lesions usually involve the legs, buttocks, and arms (Fig. 5–12). *Pseudomonas aeruginosa* may be cultured from the water and from the pustules of the lesions. The course of pseudomonal folliculitis is usually benign, and no treatment is necessary in most cases when the source of the infection is corrected. Repeated exposure may cause a severe superficial case of folliculitis.

Furunculosis

Furunculosis is an acute staphylococcal infection of hair follicles that differs from folliculitis in that there is spread of the cellulitis into the adjacent surrounding dermis and a much greater degree of inflammation and pain. Pus may extrude from the lesion spontaneously or with slight side-to-side pressure (Fig. 5–13). Single lesions are common on the lower extremities in athletes, especially football players and wrestlers, as a result of knee and ankle padding. Warm, wet compresses will relieve much of the discomfort about the furuncle. Incision and drainage, followed by appropriate antibiotic therapy, is curative.

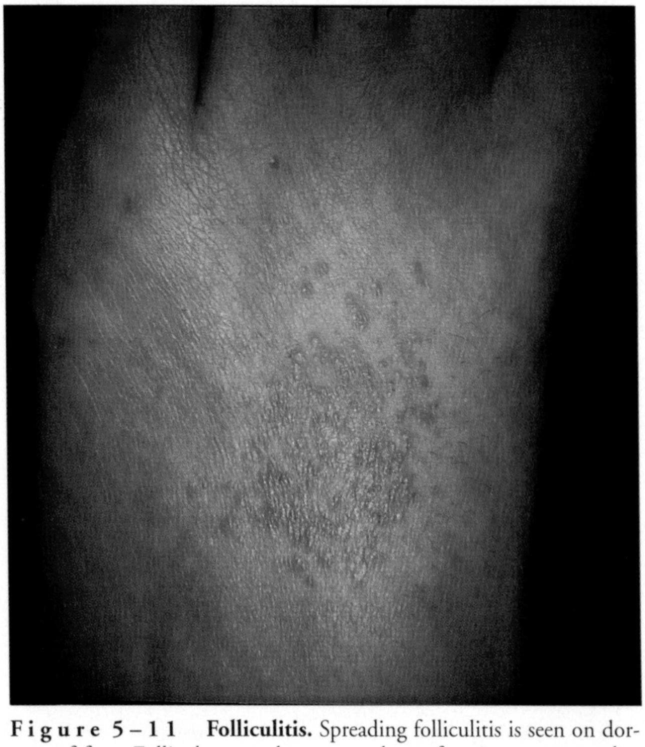

Figure 5–11   Folliculitis. Spreading folliculitis is seen on dorsum of foot. Follicular pustules may coalesce, forming a pattern that is difficult to recognize.

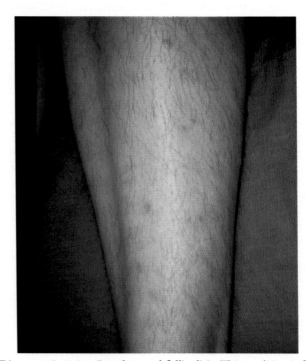

Figure 5–12   Pseudomonal folliculitis. This condition is frequently seen after exposure to a contaminated hot tub.

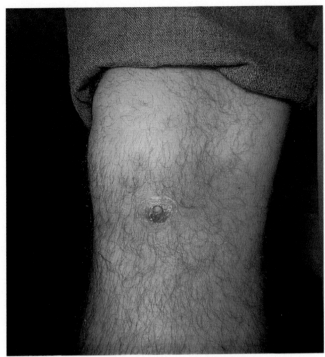

Figure 5–13 **Furunculosis.** An acute staphylococcal infection of the hair follicle appears as spreading cellulitis into the adjacent dermis. Pus may extrude from the lesion spontaneously.

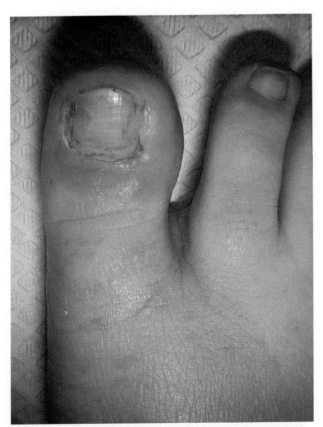

Figure 5–14 **Paronychia.** Typical appearance of staphylococcal infection with localized, swollen, erythematous, and draining at toenail border.

Paronychia

Paronychia is inflammation of the toenail folds initiated by infection by pathogenic staphylococci or streptococci. Other bacteria such as *Escherichia coli* and *Pseudomonas aeruginosa* have been isolated from paronychial infections. This condition is more correctly termed pyonychia, but this term seems to be used infrequently by most specialists.

Bacterial infections usually involve the skin surrounding the toenail rather than infecting the toenail itself. Generally, staphylococcal infections appear as chronic, localized, slightly erythematous and draining borders of the involved toenail (Fig. 5–14). Streptococcal infections, however, appear as acute, hot, bright red toenail borders with a large amount of purulent drainage and considerable tenderness (Fig. 5–15).

Incision and drainage may be needed to alleviate the pressure along the nail border. In some cases it will be necessary to remove the offending ingrown nail edge in the area of the paronychia. Antiseptic astringent wet dressings or foot soaks are helpful. Topical antibiotics are helpful but when used alone are usually insufficient to clear the infection. Oral antibiotics may be necessary in some cases that do not respond to incision and drainage or partial nail avulsion combined with foot soaks.

Pyogenic Granuloma

Pyogenic granulomas (granuloma pyogenicum) are usually small, rapidly growing, pink to bright red vascular tumors. They may arise rapidly in areas of minor trauma, especially next to an ingrown toenail, and may be very tender (Fig. 5–16). The brain-like lesion is friable, bleeds easily, and can grow from a small stalk to

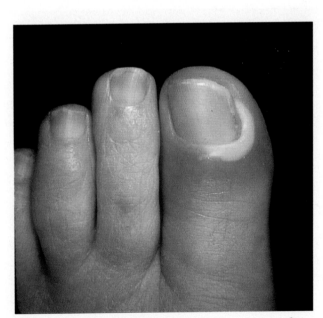

Figure 5–15 **Paronychia.** Characteristic appearance of streptococcal infection with acute, hot, bright-red toenail border with large amount of purulent drainage.

reach a centimeter or more in diameter (Fig. 5–17). The base of the pyogenic granuloma may have a collar of scales or a thick epidermal shell.

Histologically, the lesion consists of long muscular vascular trunks from which numerous tortuous capillary vessels arise. The tumors are frequently initiated by exuberant formation of granulation tissue in a response to minor trauma with superficial infection. *Staphylococcus aureus* is occasionally isolated from cultures. In many cases, however, no direct pathogenic bacteria can be identified, indicating that these vascular tumors may not always be primarily due to infection.

Treatment consists of tissue debridement or thorough curettage of the base and border followed by desiccation of the base with electrocoagulation, silver nitrate, or ferric subsulfate (Monsel's solution). Pyogenic granuloma may recur if all of the involved tissue is not removed. Topical application of erythromycin 2% solution, Polysporin cream or mupirocin 2% ointment may be helpful. Oral antibiotics are usually not necessary.

Pitted Keratolysis

Pitted keratolysis is a superficial infection that occurs as an asymptomatic eruption on the weight-bearing surface of the soles. The characteristic lesions are many small circular or longitudinal punched-out pits found in the stratum corneum (Fig. 5–18). The pits may coalesce to form irregularly shaped, superficial erosions or large craters. In some cases, the craters may show a brownish discoloration, secondary to chromhidrosis, giving the area a dirty appearance (Fig. 5–19). The disorder is often found in association with hyperhidrosis or in pa-

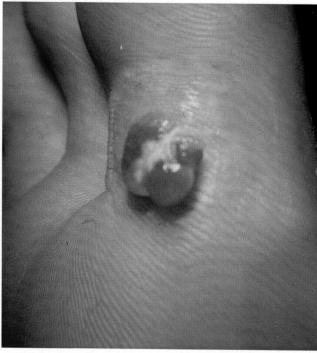

F i g u r e   5 – 1 7   Pyogenic granuloma. This brain-like lesion is friable, bleeds easily, and can grow from a small stalk to reach a centimeter or more in diameter.

tients whose occupations involve their feet getting wet daily. Even though most cases are asymptomatic, in severe involvement and when there is excessive erythema on the sole, patients may complain of an in-

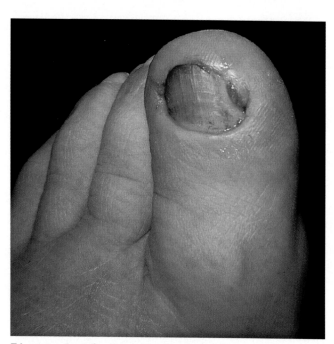

F i g u r e   5 – 1 6   Pyogenic granuloma. A common location of this lesion is on the hallux toenail border.

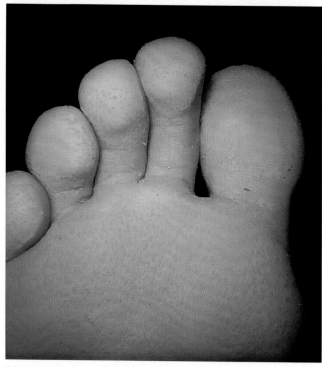

F i g u r e   5 – 1 8   Pitted keratolysis. The characteristic lesions are small circular or punched-out pits found in the stratum corneum.

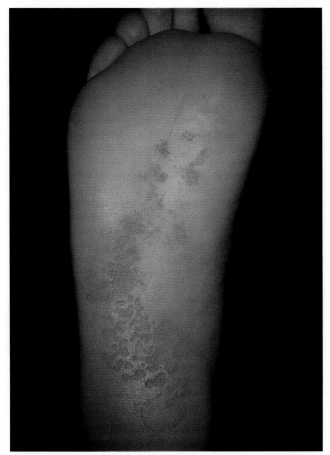

Figure 5–19 Pitted keratolysis. The crater may show a brownish discoloration that is secondary to chromhidrosis, making the area appear dirty.

tense burning sensation. The cause of the tenderness in symptomatic cases is not known.

The primary isolate in pitted keratolysis with no odor is *Corynebacterium* species. The primary isolate in pitted keratolysis with odor is *Micrococcus sedentarius*. Other causative bacteria include species of *Streptomyces* as well as *Dermatophilus congolensis*. These organisms are not easily cultured, but Gram's stain of the ground-up stratum corneum from an involved area may demonstrate the filamentous and coccoid microorganisms. The clinical appearance is so characteristic and dramatic that laboratory confirmation is not necessary.

Treatment begins with removing the patient from the moist environment and controlling the hyperhidrosis with astringent foot soaks. Topical treatment of the involved areas with 2% erythromycin or 1% clindamycin solution leads to rapid and complete resolution in almost all cases. For the severe symptomatic cases, the addition of oral erythromycin, 1 g daily, for 7 to 10 days is very beneficial.

Interdigital Erythrasma

Erythrasma is a bacterial infection involving the toe web area and other body folds such as the groin. This

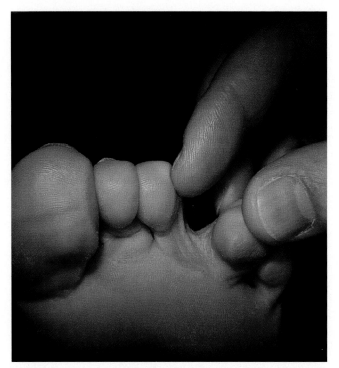

Figure 5–20 Erythrasma. This chronic condition frequently involves the web spaces of the third and fourth toes.

condition is frequently confused with fungal and candidal infections. The invading organism is *Corynebacterium minutissimum*. Predisposing factors include humidity, hyperhidrosis, heat, obesity, and poor foot hygiene. This chronic condition frequently involves the third and fourth toe web spaces of the foot (Fig. 5–20). The condition may be seen in all web spaces. Painful, longitudinal fissures may occur in advanced cases (Fig. 5–21).

Erythrasma differs from fungal infections in that it has no advancing borders, is uniformly reddish brown and scaly, and fluoresces bright coral-red with Wood's light. Diagnosis is based primarily on clinical presentation. Potassium hydroxide preparations are usually

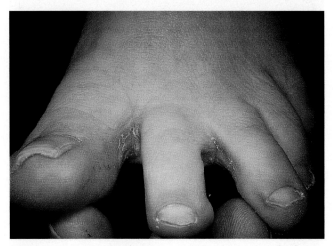

Figure 5–21 Erythrasma. In advanced cases, painful fissures are evident in all toe web spaces.

negative. Gram's stains of ground-up stratum corneum examined under oil immersion may show gram-positive filamentous and coccoid rods. The filamentous forms are predominantly from the groin, and the bacillary forms are found mostly on the toe webs.

Treatment involves extensive washing of the involved area with antibacterial soap with thorough drying after each wash. Topical 2% erythromycin solution is curative when applied daily. In severe cases, oral erythromycin taken 1 g daily for 7 days may be necessary.

SECONDARY SKIN INFECTIONS

Infected Ulcerations

There are a large number of causes for ulcerations of the lower extremities, including trauma, metabolic disease, vascular disease, granulomatous disease, hematological disease, and a variety of miscellaneous causes. In all of these conditions there is damage to the dermal layers, which can predispose the patient to secondary infection of the wound.

Only a few ulcerative conditions have bacteria as the primary causative agent. It is generally accepted that all open ulcers are colonized to some extent by bacteria but not all of them are frankly infected. However, when the ulcer is complicated with infection, the treatment goal must include resolution of the infection, as well as de-

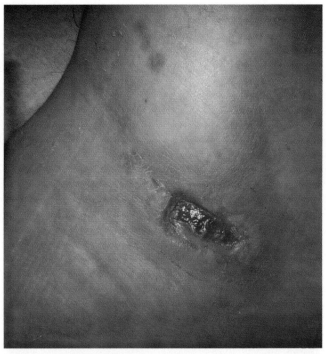

Figure 5–23 Ulceration. Traumatically induced ulceration with secondary infection on lateral ankle.

termining the cause of the ulcer. Almost any bacteria can colonize an open wound, but *Staphylococcus aureus* and beta-hemolytic streptococci are the usual offenders. Older ulcers are frequently contaminated by mixed

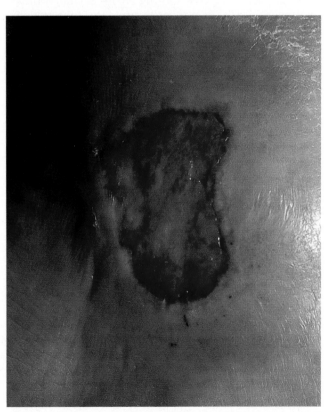

Figure 5–22 Ulceration. Varicose or stasis ulcer associated with secondary infection on medial ankle.

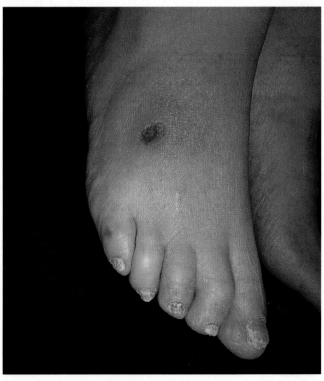

Figure 5–24 Ulceration. Infected factitial or self-induced ulceration on dorsum of foot.

aerobic and anaerobic pathogens. Common ulcers that become secondarily infected are varicose or stasis ulcers (Fig. 5–22), traumatic ulcers (Fig. 5–23), factitial or self-induced ulcers (Fig. 5–24), and ulcers from mechanical injury (Fig. 5–25). Ulcers that are secondarily infected usually show a yellow to yellow-brown crusting with peripheral erythema of the adjacent skin (Fig. 5–26). There may also be severe swelling, erythema, and pain, especially in streptococcal infections (Fig. 5–27).

Treatment involves regular wound care with gentle cleansing of the wound to remove debris and the establishment of a good granulation tissue bed. Obtaining culture and sensitivity results from any drainage with appropriate antibiotic coverage follows. The significance of the isolation of the organisms in infections of the foot depends on the manner in which the organisms are obtained. Superficial culture swabs of ulcerative lesions will yield numerous organisms that may be insignificant. Deep tissue cultures obtained by curettage or needle aspiration have much greater correlation with the true pathogens causing an infection. Once the infection is treated appropriately, the diagnosis and treatment of the underlying cause of the ulcer is absolutely essential to prevent recurrence.

Miliaria

Infection of the eccrine sweat gland apparatus produces a skin disorder characterized by a vesicular dermatitis secondary to trapping of sweat at some point in the skin. This condition is not common on the feet but does occur. Two main types of miliaria are miliaria crystallina and miliaria rubra.

Miliaria crystallina occurs as a number of small, asymptomatic, discrete vesicular lesions of about 1 mm on the sole of the foot, ankle, or lower leg region (Fig.

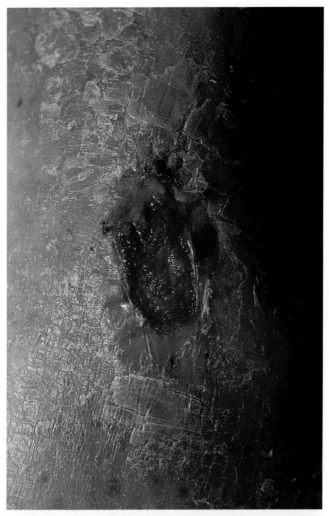

Figure 5–26 Ulceration. Chronic, infected ulcer with yellow-brown crusting and peripheral erythema and scaling of the adjacent skin on lower leg.

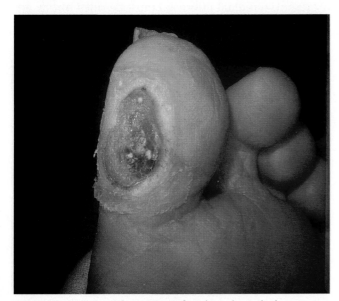

Figure 5–25 Ulceration. Infected mechanical ulcer on medial hallux in patient with neuropathy.

5–28). They resemble tiny drops of water on the skin and may be firm to light touch. The condition is caused by obstruction of the sweat pore within the stratum corneum. The lesions of miliaria crystallina are common in intertriginous areas, on the dorsum of the foot and ankle, and on the forehead of some individuals. It is seen clinically after mild sunburn, during humid weather conditions, and in occluded areas. No secondary erythema or swelling is present. The process is usually self-limiting.

Miliaria rubra is characterized by blockage of the sweat pore at a deeper level within the epidermis. The lesions are erythematous and vesiculopapular and are usually symptomatic with pruritus, burning, or stinging reported by the patient (Fig. 5–29). These red and inflamed lesions are usually secondarily infected by staphylococci and are seen more often on the legs and plantar non–weight-bearing surface of the foot. Small pustules may also be seen in the central area of several lesions. This condition can be differentiated from folliculitis in that miliaria is extrafollicular.

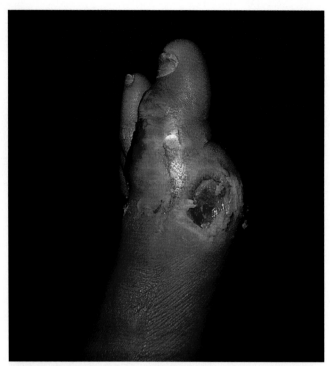

Figure 5–27   Streptococcal infection. Appears with intense erythema, swelling, and pain.

Treatment involves drying and cooling the affected areas. Cool water and Epsom salts foot soaks followed by topical 2% erythromycin solution may be curative. The use of topical anhydrous lanolin is helpful. Absor-

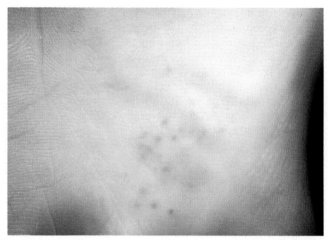

Figure 5–29   Miliaria rubra. Erythematous vesiculopapular lesions on the lower extremities may be symptomatic with pruritus, burning, or stinging.

bent and drying foot powders are also helpful in relieving some of the itching.

Intertrigo

Intertrigo is a mechanical abrasion of skin that becomes secondarily infected with bacteria or fungus. Favored areas are occluded skin folds such as the groin, axillae, below the breast, and between the toes. In many instances the condition is initiated by maceration of the web spaces with closed footgear. The condition is characterized by web space skin that is red, macerated, and tender (Fig. 5–30). In later stages, this may progress to complete denudation and erosion with weeping of the area (Fig. 5–31). Staphylococci and beta-hemolytic streptococci are most commonly involved. Unlike erythrasma and tinea pedis, usually no crusts or scaling is present. Candidal intertrigo must be ruled out by appropriate laboratory tests.

Treatment centers on drying of the maceration with

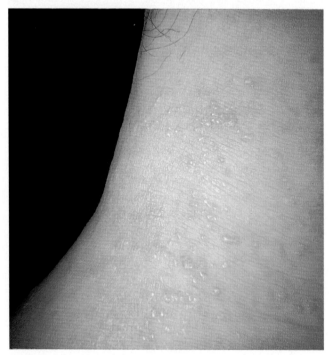

Figure 5–28   Miliaria crystallina. Small, asymptomatic, discrete vesicular lesions of around 1 mm are evident on the ankle secondary to trapped sweat in the skin.

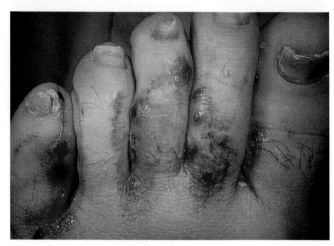

Figure 5–30   Intertrigo. Web space infection with red, macerated, and tender skin changes.

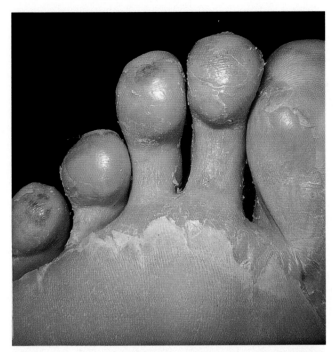

Figure 5–31 Intertrigo. Later stages may progress to complete denudation and erosion with weeping between and under the toes.

Epsom salts foot soaks. Wearing better ventilated or open footgear and regular dusting with medicated talcum powders to the affected areas help to prevent recurrence of the condition. Topical gentian violet and topical antibiotics may be useful in moderate conditions; in more severe cases, oral antibiotics may be necessary.

Pustular Bacterid

Also known as persistent palmoplantar pustulosis, pustular bacterid is similar in general appearance to pustular psoriasis but it does not have the histological characteristics of psoriasis. The condition is characterized clinically by erythematous and vesiculopustular eruptions of the soles or palms or both. This eruption is marked by short periods of remission followed by prolonged severe exacerbations.

The basic lesions are pustules that erupt when fully developed leaving a hemorrhagic base (Fig. 5–32). Multiple areas of tiny hemorrhagic puncta may be intermingled with the pustules. The condition usually begins in the midportion of the arch but may extend to the lateral aspects of the foot. It may start on the ends of the toes or on the heels. No cases have been reported affecting the web spaces or flexor creases of the toes.

The onset is usually in young to middle-aged adults with no history of psoriasis or eczema. Patients may report a long history of the recurrent condition with times of almost complete healing. Pruritus is often severe, and in some cases swelling, pain, or burning sensations are reported by the patients. Skin tests with *Streptococcus* and *Staphylococcus* toxins are strongly positive. Leukocytosis is often present, especially during severe outcrops of pustules. The disease is initiated as a result of focal infections of the gums, tonsils, sinuses, or some other part of the body. When the source of infection is localized and successfully treated, the pustular bacterid resolves.

Treatment consists of wet dressings, topical antibiotics, and systemic antibacterial agents. Removal of the causative focus of infection is necessary for complete subsidence of lesions.

Infected Eczema and Infectious Eczematous Dermatitis

Infected eczema exists in any case in which a preexisting persistent eczema becomes secondarily infected with bacteria (Fig. 5–33). *Staphylococcus aureus* and hemolytic streptococci are the most commonly cultured isolates. This condition must be differentiated from infectious eczematous dermatitis that arises from a primary lesion that is the source of infectious exudate (Fig. 5–34). This may be an ulcer, an infected abscess, a surgical incision, or any infected process that is a source of drainage.

The surrounding skin that comes into contact with the exudate or purulent drainage ultimately establishes an area of acute dermatitis, which becomes eczematous.

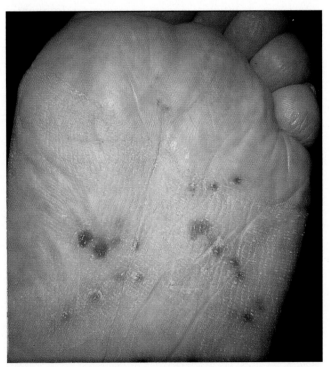

Figure 5–32 Pustular bacterid. This chronic condition is characterized by erythematous and vesiculopustular eruptions of the soles. Multiple areas of hemorrhagic puncta may be mixed with pustules.

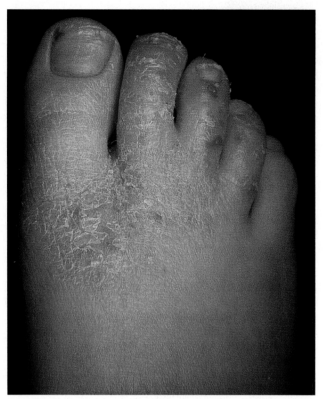

Figure 5–33   Infected eczema. Secondary bacterial infection of preexisting eczema on the foot secondary to rubbing and scratching.

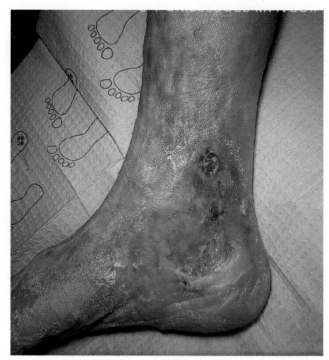

Figure 5–34   Infectious eczematous dermatitis. This condition arose from an existing ulcer that became infected. The lesion began draining, and the surrounding skin reacted to the exudate with an area of acute dermatitis that became eczematous.

Coagulase-positive staphylococci are most frequently isolated from these cases. In the case of infected eczema, the infection is purely secondary and clearing of the infection leaves the dermatitis still present. Treatment of the bacterial infection in infectious eczematous dermatitis will usually result in clearing of the infection as well as the dermatitis. In both conditions, the primary treatment is directed toward identification of the infective source followed by appropriate antibacterial therapy. Cool compresses may be helpful when combined with either topical or parenteral antibiotic treatment. Once the infection has been cleared, in cases of infected eczema, the remaining dermatitis may be treated with topical corticosteroids.

Infected Postsurgical Incisions

One of the most common complications of lower extremity surgery is postsurgical infection of the incision (Fig. 5–35). This secondary infection may be superficial or deep, and immediate recognition and attention to the condition are necessary. The most common infective agent in postsurgical incisions is *Staphylococcus aureus*. Symptoms may include erythema, swelling, drainage, and pain.

The results of culture and sensitivity of the drainage dictate the appropriate antibiotic drug. However, before the final results of the culture and sensitivity of the drainage are obtained, the most effective initial antibiotic is a penicillinase-resistant penicillin. If the patient is allergic to penicillin, a cephalosporin can be selected. Erythromycin and tetracycline are not alternative drugs

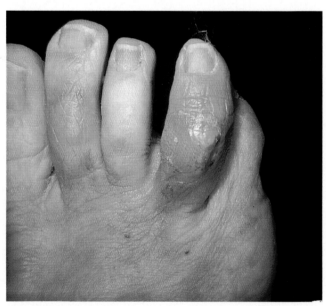

Figure 5–35   Secondary bacterial infection. Erythema, swelling, drainage, and increased pain in the fourth toe occurred after surgery and secondary to *Staphylococcus aureus*.

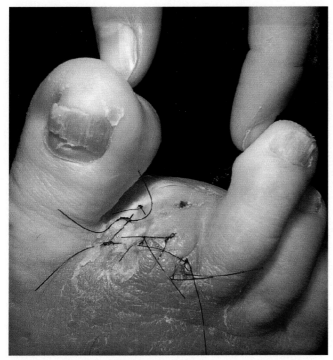

Figure 5–36 Streptococcal infection. When the surgical site becomes intensely red, hot, painful, and swollen without drainage, the infection is frequently caused by *Streptococcus.*

and are not recommended in the treatment of postsurgical infections, even when shown to be effective by culture and sensitivity tests. When the surgical site shows intense erythema, heat, pain, and swelling without drainage, the causative bacteria may be *Streptococcus* (Fig. 5–36). Once there is confirmation that the infection is caused by *Streptococcus pyogenes*, erythromycin is the first alternative drug. A variety of other organisms have been isolated from surgical wounds, and they may all be pathogens at some point. Once the cultures and sensitivity tests have been completed the appropriate antibiotic drug may be selected. This drug should be the drug of choice for the condition. It should also be bactericidal, show a low bacterial resistance potential, produce high tissue levels, and have the least amount of toxicity.

BIBLIOGRAPHY

Andres GC, Machacek GF: Pustular bacterid of the hands and feet. Arch Derm Syph 32:837–840, 1935.

Brenner MA: Pyodermas. In McCarthy DJ, Montgomery R (eds): Podiatric Dermatology, pp 122–132. Baltimore, Williams & Wilkins, 1986.

Burkhart CG: Pitted keratolysis: A new form of treatment (letter). Arch Dermatol 116:1104, 1980.

Christensen JC: Surgical complications of the forefoot. In Butterworth R, Dockery GL (eds): Color Atlas and Text of Forefoot Surgery, pp 237–258. St. Louis, Mosby–Year Book, 1992.

Dagan R, Bar-David Y: Double-blind study comparing erythromycin and mupirocin for treatment of impetigo in children: Implications of a high prevalence of erythromycin-resistant *Staphylococcus aureus* strains. Antimicrob Agents Chemother 36:287–290, 1992.

Dagan R: Impetigo in childhood: Changing epidemiology and new treatments. Pediatr Ann 22:235–240, 1993.

Dockery GL: Nails. In McGlamry ED, Banks AS, Downey MS (eds): Comprehensive Textbook of Foot Surgery, 2nd ed, pp 277–303. Baltimore, Williams & Wilkins, 1992.

Greene SL, Su WPD, Muller SA: Ecthyma gangrenosum: Report of clinical, histopathologic, and bacteriologic aspects of eight cases. J Am Acad Dermatol 11:781–787, 1984.

Hodson SB, Henslee TM, Tachibana DK, Harvey CK: Interdigital erythrasma: I. A review of the literature. J Am Podiatr Med Assoc 78:551–558, 1988.

Hugo-Persson M, Norlin K: Erysipelas and group G streptococci. Infection 15:36–39, 1987.

Maiback HI, Aly R: Bacterial infections of the skin. In Moschella SL, Hurley HJ (eds): Dermatology, 3rd ed, pp 710–750. Philadelphia, WB Saunders, 1992.

Miller SJ: The diagnosis and treatment of infections of the pedal integument. Clin Podiatr Med Surg 3:505–513, 1986.

O'Keefe RG, Pikscher I: Ulcers of the lower Extremity. In McCarthy DL, Montgomery R (eds): Podiatric Dermatology, pp 198–209. Baltimore, Williams & Wilkins, 1986.

Pruksachatkunakorn D, Vaniyapongs T, Pruksakorn S: Impetigo: An assessment of etiology and appropriate therapy in infants and children. J Med Assoc Thai 76:222–229, 1993.

Richman B, Young G: Chronic elephantiasis: A case report. J Am Podiatr Med Assoc 85:268–270, 1995.

Saccoman S, Rifleman GT: Elephantiasis nostras verrucosa: A case report. J Am Podiatr Med Assoc 85:265–267, 1995.

Shah AS, Kamino H, Prose NS: Painful, plaque-like, pitted keratolysis occurring in childhood. Pediatric Dermatol 9:251–254, 1992.

Weinberg AN, Swartz MN: General considerations of bacterial diseases. In Fitzpatrick TB, Eisen AZ, Wolff K, Freedbery IM, Austen KF (eds): Dermatology in General Medicine, 3rd ed, pp 2089–2100. New York, McGraw-Hill, 1987.

Woodridge WE: Managing skin infections in children. Postgrad Med 89:109–112, 1991.

Zaias N: Pitted and ringed keratolysis. J Am Acad Dermatol 7:787–791, 1982.

6

FUNGAL SKIN AND NAIL INFECTIONS

INTRODUCTION

The dermatophytes include a group of fungi that have the ability to infect the keratin layer of the skin or the stratum corneum. They cannot survive on mucosal surfaces and only very rarely penetrate into the deep layers. Dermatophytes are responsible for the majority of fungal infections of the skin and toenails of the lower extremities. Laboratory confirmation is usually necessary because many of the clinical presentations of fungal infections mimic other dermatological conditions.

Dermatophytes are classified in three groups: *Microsporum, Trichophyton,* and *Epidermophyton*. The anthropophilic fungi grow on human skin and nails. The zoophilic fungi grow on animals and the geophilic fungi live in soil, but both of these dermatophytes may infect humans. The yeast-like fungus *Candida albicans* and a few other *Candida* species are also capable of producing superficial skin, mucosal, nail, and deep fungal infections. Additionally, a lipophilic yeast, *Malassezia furfur (Pityrosporum orbiculare)*, causes a common fungal skin infection called tinea versicolor. All of these conditions are considered and discussed with reference to their appearance on the lower extremities.

Tinea literally means "worm," from ringworm, and has been applied for centuries to indicate the presence of superficial fungal infections of the skin. The site of infection is usually designated by a modifying term, such as *tinea pedis* for fungal infection of the feet. Lower extremity presentations of superficial fungal infections

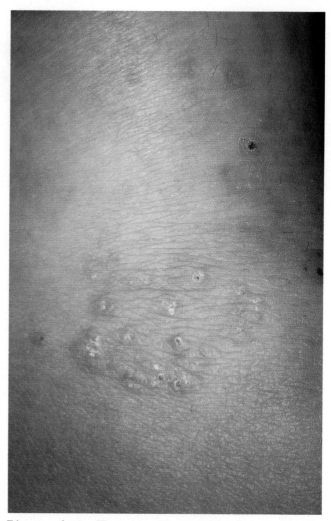

Figure 6–2   Tinea corporis variant. Vesiculation and crusting are not limited to the peripheral rim of the lesion.

include tinea corporis, tinea pedis, interdigital tinea pedis, and tinea unguium (onychomycosis). Superficial infections including candidal infections and tinea versicolor are also reviewed. For most superficial fungal infections, topical treatment with one of the imidazoles (miconazole, clotrimazole, econazole, or sulconazole) is sufficient to eliminate the condition. Finally, the deeper, subcutaneous fungal infections include a condition referred to as Majocchi's granuloma, sporotrichosis, and chromoblastomycosis.

SUPERFICIAL FUNGAL INFECTIONS

Tinea Corporis

Tinea corporis involves superficial fungal infections of the glabrous skin. This condition is frequently called ringworm of the skin. The characteristic fungal infection occurs with an expanding circular or patterned designed scale, in which the fungal elements can be demonstrated on potassium hydroxide (KOH) examination.

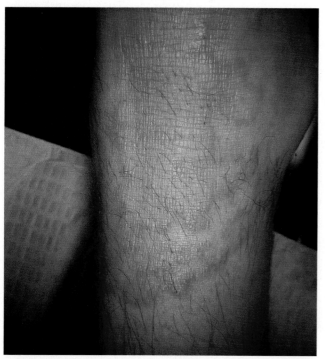

Figure 6–1   Tinea corporis. Lesions on the lower extremity show characteristic expanding circular and patterned scale. The active margins tend to migrate outward, and the lesions are red, scaly, and asymmetrically placed.

It is caused by a number of different anthropophilic fungi, especially *Trichophyton rubrum, Epidermophyton floccosum,* and *Trichophyton mentagrophytes.*

The lesions have a tendency toward active margins with a healing central area that is usually hyperpigmented brown but occasionally shows hypopigmented changes (Fig. 6–1). The fungus tends to migrate outward, and the lesions are red, scaly, and asymmetrical. There is a broad range of presentations from just one ring that grows to a few centimeters in diameter to several annular or irregular lesions that enlarge and coalesce to cover large areas of the body. A variant of tinea corporis shows an area of vesiculation and crusting not limited to the peripheral rim of the lesion that is uniformly elevated (Fig. 6–2). There may be visible central clearing as the lesion enlarges. Tinea corporis is usually self-limiting, but it is easily treated with topical antifungal creams applied twice daily for 1 week.

Tinea Pedis

The single most important test for the diagnosis of tinea pedis, and all other dermatophyte infections, is direct visualization under the microscope of branching hyphae in keratinized material on the KOH wet mount preparation slide. Fungal infections of the feet are much more common in adolescent and adult men than in women. Although once considered uncommon, tinea pedis does occur frequently in young children (Fig. 6–3). Four distinct types or variants of tinea pedis are recognized: the acute vesicular type (or vesiculobullous), the chronic papulosquamous pattern, the chronic interdigital form, and the acute ulcerative variant.

ACUTE VESICULAR TYPE. Acute vesicular tinea pedis usually begins in the instep of the arch, leading to inflammation, which may be severe. Vesicles and blisters are common and may spread from the arch to the sides of the foot (Fig. 6–4). This condition does not usually infect the weight-bearing surfaces of the sole. This variant may be inactive during the cooler months with severe exacerbation during warmer or wetter months. The most common fungus cultured is *T. mentagrophytes* and, occasionally, *E. floccosum.* In the vesiculobullous form of tinea pedis it may be difficult to obtain a positive KOH mount identification, and fungal agar plate cultures may be necessary for a positive identification. Treatment with most topical antifungal creams is usually quickly effective.

CHRONIC, PAPULOSQUAMOUS PATTERN. Chronic papulosquamous tinea pedis is the most common variant of dermatophyte infection of the foot. A moccasin-type distribution on the foot consisting of a dry, thick scale on the sole and sides of the foot is characteristic of this chronic infection caused primarily by *T. rubrum* (Fig. 6–5). The hands may be similarly infected, but it is very uncommon for both hands and both feet to show involvement (Fig. 6-6). The common pattern is for both feet and one hand to be infected. Occasionally, *T. mentagrophytes* is the causative fungus, and in this case it is more common for both hands to be infected (Fig. 6–7). A variant of the thick, dry squamous tinea pedis occurs as an erythematous or pink base of skin on the plantar foot with fissuring and thin, flaky scales (Fig. 6–8).

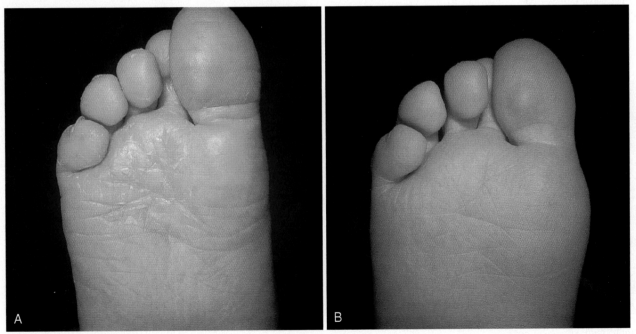

F i g u r e   6 – 3   **Tinea pedis.** *A,* Chronic fungal infection in a 2-year-old boy was confirmed by potassium hydroxide preparation. *B,* Clearing occurred within 2 weeks of topical therapy with antifungal cream. This condition had previously been misdiagnosed as atopic eczema.

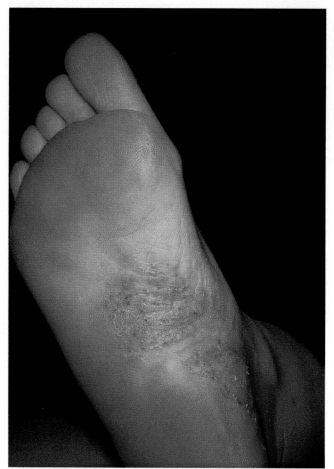

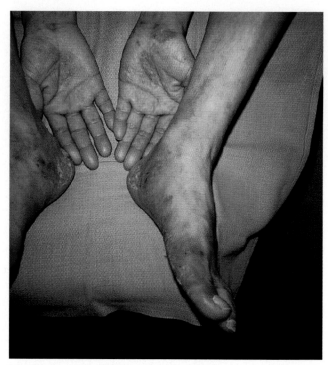

Figure 6 – 6   Tinea pedis. Involvement of two feet and two hands with chronic papulosquamous tinea pedis.

Figure 6 – 4   Acute vesicular tinea pedis. Vesicles and blisters are common at the inner arch area of the foot. This condition does not usually involve the weight-bearing areas and is more active in the warmer and wetter months.

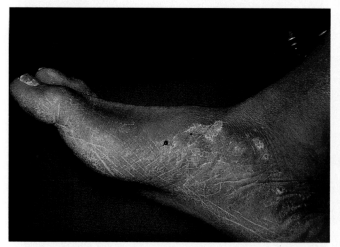

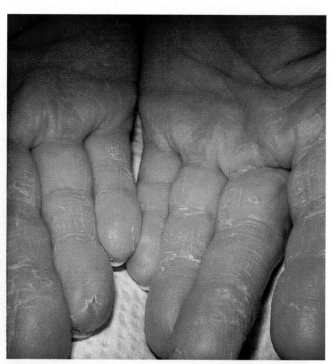

Figure 6 – 5   Tinea pedis. Chronic papulosquamous moccasin distribution is evident secondary to *Trichophyton rubrum.*

Figure 6 – 7   Tinea manuum. Both hands are involved secondary to *Trichophyton mentagrophytes* infection.

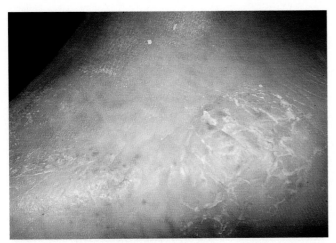

Figure 6–8 **Tinea pedis.** Chronic infection with an erythematous or pink base of skin on the plantar foot with fissuring and thin, flaky scales secondary to *Trichophyton rubrum*.

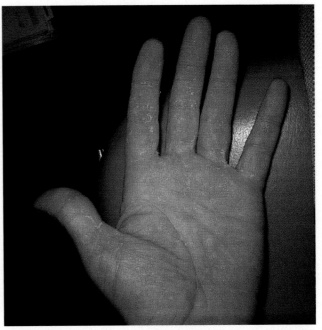

Figure 6–9 **Vesicular dermatophytid or id reaction.** This dyshidrotic eczema of one or both hands may appear after widespread fungal foot infections.

When there is a widespread chronic infection or significant inflammatory reaction in the feet there may be an inflammatory reaction in one or both hands. This condition is referred to as *vesicular dermatophytid* or, more frequently, an *id reaction* (Fig. 6–9). This dyshidrotic eczema of the hands appears at some time after the appearance of the foot infection. The fungus cannot be cultured from the lesions on the hand and does not respond to topical antifungal therapy. When the foot condition is brought under control the eruption on the hands gradually clears. In some cases, topical corticosteroids are necessary to resolve the hand eczema.

Tinea pedis is frequently associated with hereditary palmoplantar keratoderma. The condition presents as a thick, boggy hyperkeratosis that appears yellow to brown and may show peripheral scaling or fissuring (Fig. 6–10). There may be a ring of erythema surrounding the areas of hyperkeratosis. *T. rubrum* is commonly isolated from the keratin, but it is not the primary cause of the hereditary keratoderma. Treatment of this condition is with topical econazole in 50% propylene glycol applied twice daily.

Topical treatment of chronic tinea pedis, in general, is not very successful alone. A combination of local skin care, topical antifungal agents, and systemic antifungal agents is necessary to eradicate the condition. Unfortunately, reappearance of the infection is common after stopping the therapy program.

CHRONIC, INTERDIGITAL FORM. Chronic interdigital tinea pedis usually starts in the toe web spaces and is characterized by scaling, maceration, and itching (Fig. 6–11). Intertriginous involvement of the third and fourth interdigital web spaces with spread across the subdigital areas is most common (Fig. 6–12). From here the condition may spread to the sole of the foot but seldom involves the dorsal aspect of the foot. *T. mentagrophytes* is commonly isolated from cultures from the in-

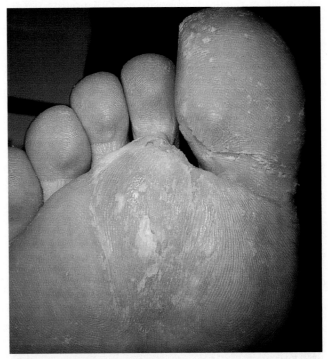

Figure 6–10 **Tinea pedis.** Infection associated with hereditary palmoplantar keratoderma occurs as a thick, boggy hyperkeratosis that appears yellow to brown and may show peripheral scaling or fissuring.

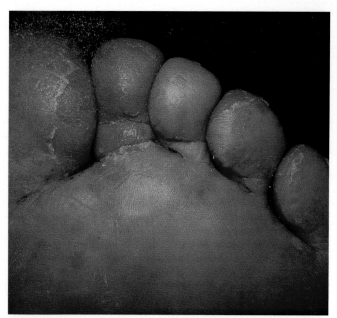

Figure 6–11   Chronic interdigital tinea pedis. This condition usually starts in the toe web spaces and is characterized by scaling, maceration, and itching.

terdigital web spaces. *E. floccosum* and *T. rubrum* may also be isolated. A single variant of this condition involves scaling and maceration between the fourth and fifth toes only (Fig. 6–13). Identification of the fungus is by cultures of web scrapings, positive dermatophyte test medium results, and positive KOH mounts. Treat-

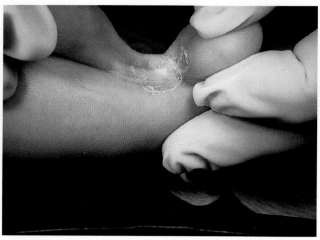

Figure 6–13   Chronic interdigital tinea pedis. A single variant involves scaling and maceration only between the fourth and fifth toes.

ment of the interdigital tinea pedis is very successful with topical antifungal creams applied twice daily.

ACUTE ULCERATIVE VARIANT. Acute ulcerative tinea pedis occurs as a very distinct clinical condition with maceration, weeping denuded tissue, and ulcerations of the epidermal skin layers (Fig. 6–14). This infection spreads rapidly with considerable areas of the foot involved. *T. mentagrophytes* is the most common isolate in this con-

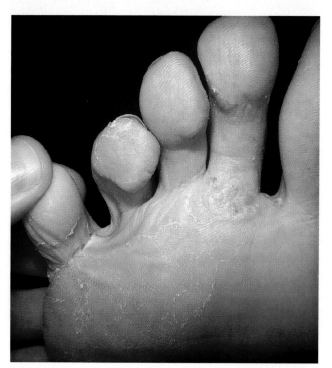

Figure 6–12   Chronic interdigital tinea pedis. Intertriginous involvement with spread across the subdigital areas is common.

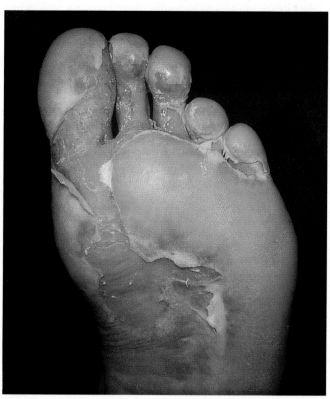

Figure 6–14   Acute ulcerative tinea pedis. Clinical presentation is distinctive with macerated, weeping, and denuded tissue on the feet.

dition. A pungent or fetid odor is usually present, and the area is frequently complicated by a gram-negative bacterial overgrowth (usually *Pseudomonas* or *Proteus* species). An id reaction may follow on one or both hands.

When a patient with this condition presents, the physician must rule out the secondary infection first by cultures and Gram's stains. Dicloxacillin should be started while waiting for the results. Appropriate systemic antibiotics should be started as soon as confirmation of infection is made. Adjunctive topical treatment with antibacterial soaks is helpful. Stainless or colorless Castellani's paint may be applied to start drying the denuded areas. Once the bacterial infection is under control the involved area may be treated with topical antifungal creams. In many cases there is underlying hyperhidrosis, and this condition should be treated as well to try to prevent recurrence of the infection. In more severe cases the patient may have symptoms of fever, chills, cellulitis, lymphangitis, and malaise. In these patients hospitalization may be advised; the limbs should be elevated and parenteral antibiotic therapy begun. This condition is referred to as dermatophytosis complex-severe.

NONANTHROPOPHILIC TINEA PEDIS. Although less common, nonanthropophilic tinea pedis may be seen with presentations that are similar to those of other dermatophytic lesions. The zoophilic fungus *Microsporum canis* is known to cause a form of tinea pedis (Fig. 6–15). The clinical lesion is characterized by well-marginated, raised borders that are composed of several coalescing small erythematous papulovesicles with central clear-

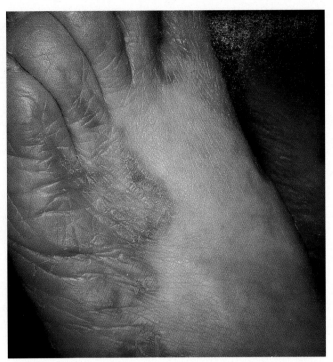

Figure 6–16   Tinea pedis. Infection is secondary to the geophilic organism *Microsporum gypseum.* Note increased erythema, thickening of the skin, and accentuation of the skin lines with a very active leading border.

ing. It is very common for patients so infected to have pets that are similarly infected. Other cases of tinea pedis may be caused by geophilic organisms such as *M. gypseum* (Fig. 6–16). The clinical lesion shows much more erythema than in most anthropophilic tinea pedis. There is thickening of the skin with accentuation of the skin lines and a very active leading border. These infections do not usually respond easily to the standard topical antifungal agents. Treatment with oral antifungal agents is considered to be more effective in eradicating these infections.

Tinea Unguium (Onychomycosis)

Tinea unguium is secondary to infection of the nail plate by dermatophytes. Onychomycosis includes all infections of the nail whether caused by dermatophytes, nondermatophytes, or yeast. It is uncommon for most foot specialists, however, to use the term *tinea unguium.* Nail infections may occur simultaneously in the hand and foot, but toenail infections are much more common than fingernail infections. The confirmation of fungal infection is important before instituting therapy. Fragments of the nail plate and nail bed may be placed on Sabouraud's medium or sent to a mycology pathology laboratory for confirmation.

Even though nail infections secondary to fungi are still considered superficial, they are usually chronic and more recalcitrant to therapy than similar skin infections. The occlusive nature of footgear, trauma to the

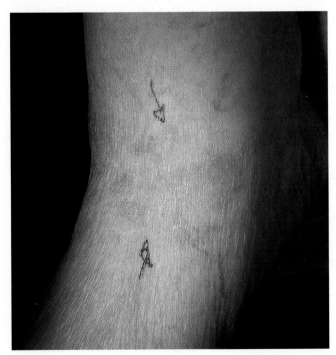

Figure 6–15   Tinea pedis. Infection is secondary to the zoophilic fungus *Microsporum canis.* The lesion is characterized by well-marginated, raised borders with central clearing.

T A B L E 6–1 Tinea Unguium

Clinical Type	Causative Agent	Appearance
Type I: Distal subungual infections	**Dermatophytes** *Trichophyton rubrum, T. mentagrophytes,* and, occasionally, *Epidermophyton floccosum* **Molds** *Scopulariopsis, Cephalosporium, Aspergillus niger, Fusarium* **Yeasts** *Candida albicans, C. parapsilosis*	Infection starts distally or laterally. It spreads under the nail, and the nail bed keratinizes. Nail bed thickens, and nail plate loses transparency and becomes thick and friable. Continued progress shows increased thickening (ram's horn) of nails with total dystrophic changes. Color is yellow, brown, or blue-green.
Type II: Proximal subungual infections	**Dermatophytes** *Trichophyton rubrum, T. schoenleinii, T. tonsurans, T. mentagrophytes* (var. *interdigitale*)	Fungi enter from posterior nail fold migrating to matrix and nail plate. Infection occurs within the substance of the nail plate, but surface of nail remains intact. Nail plate may loosen. Infection may extend distally to involve entire nail.
Type III: White superficial infections	**Dermatophytes** *Trichophyton mentagrophytes* (var. *interdigitale*), rarely *T. rubrum* **Molds** *Aspergillus, Cephalosporium, Fusarium*	Fungus infects the superficial nail plate, causing the nail to turn white and become dry, soft, and powdery brittle. Small opacities may coalesce and cover the entire nail. Old lesions turn yellow.
Type IV: Candidal infections	**Yeasts** *Candida albicans* and other species	Nails start to thicken and turn yellow or yellow-brown. The entire nail plate is invaded by the organisms with marked destruction of the nail plate. Paronychia and bulbous formation of the toetip may occur.

toenails, decreased circulation to the toenail bed, and the fact that toenail infections provide an endogenous source of reinfection may account for the chronicity of the condition. The most common dermatophytes isolated from toenails are *Trichophyton rubrum, T. mentagrophytes* (var. *interdigitale*), and *E. floccosum*. Several forms of tinea unguium are seen: distal subungual, proximal subungual, white superficial, and candidal (Table 6–1). Each of these forms of fungal infection is established according to the site of fungal attack of the nail (Fig. 6–17). Treatment with oral antifungal agents (itraconazole, terbinafine, fluconazole) may be necessary.

DISTAL SUBUNGUAL. Distal subungual infection is the most common form of tinea unguium, and it is sometimes referred to as distal lateral subungual onychomycosis. *T. rubrum* and *T. mentagrophytes* (var. *interdigitale*) are usually isolated from cultures, although *E. floccosum* is found with some frequency. The fungus penetrates

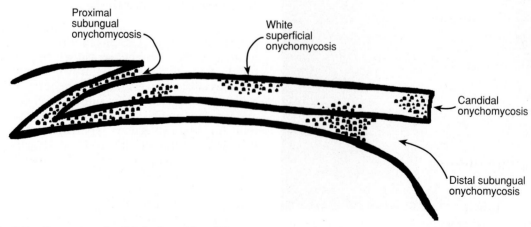

F i g u r e 6 – 1 7   **Four types of nail infections.** Note different entry points by infecting organisms. (Modified from Zaias N: Onychomycosis. Arch Dermatol 10:263–274, 1972. Copyright 1972, American Medical Association.)

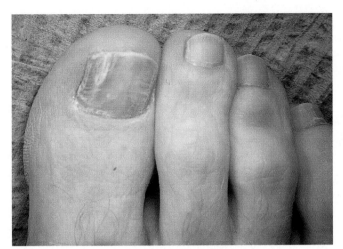

Figure 6–18   Distal subungual infection. Yellowing, onycholysis, and subungual debris are characteristic.

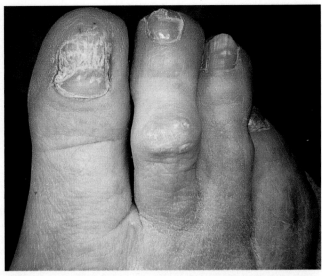

Figure 6–20   Chronic distal subungual infection. Note large, round, and smooth proximal nail plate.

the distal hyponychium or lateral nail fold region. Yellowing, onycholysis, and subungual debris form. In the early stages, the nail may show distinct borders as the infected nail starts to separate from the normal nail (Fig. 6–18). Nail debridement and topical antifungal creams may be beneficial in the early stages.

If the infection has been present for many years there is usually keratinization of the distal nail bed and the nail bed tends to cornify (Fig. 6–19). With time the nail grooves lose their normal contour. The proximal nail plate is susceptible to the formation of a large, smooth, thickened mound (Fig. 6–20). When there is no nail care given in the chronic form of distal subungual infection, the nails may overgrow the nail plate and large deformed (ram's horn) toenails may occur (Fig. 6–21).

In these cases, the nails should be avulsed (chemically or manually) and the nail bed treated with topical antifungal agents. There may be a good response to oral antifungal agents, but the recurrence rate is high. Other nondermatophytes or molds such as *Scopulariopsis*, *Cephalosporium*, and *Aspergillus niger* may cause pigmented forms of distal subungual onychomycosis that may be confused with infections of *Pseudomonas* species (Fig. 6–22).

PROXIMAL SUBUNGUAL. Proximal subungual infection is secondary to fungi entering the proximal (posterior) nail fold and then migrating to the underlying matrix and nail plate. The infection occurs within the substance of the nail plate, but the surface of the nail re-

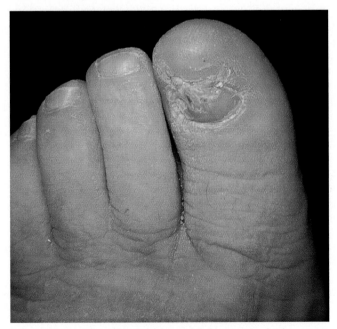

Figure 6–19   Distal subungual infection. In the late stages there is keratinization of the distal nail bed.

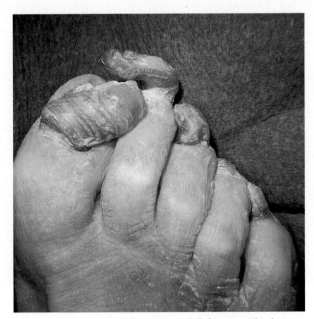

Figure 6–21   Ram's horn toenail deformity. This lesion was the result of chronic infection and lack of proper care.

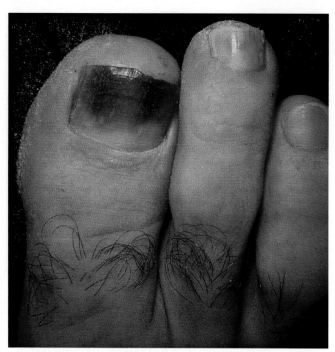

F i g u r e 6 – 2 2   Subungual infection with *Aspergillus niger.* A distal onychomycosis may be created that may be difficult to diagnose without cultures.

mains intact. Hyperkeratotic debris accumulates under the nail plate and causes the toenail to loosen and separate from the nail bed (Fig. 6–23). Once separation occurs, the nail may appear white and clear fluid may accumulate under the nail. *T. rubrum* is frequently the causative fungus.

WHITE SUPERFICIAL. White superficial fungal nails (also

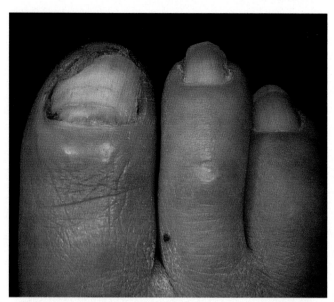

F i g u r e 6 – 2 3   Proximal subungual infection of hallux toenail. The nail has loosened and separated from the nail bed. Once separation occurs, the nail may appear white or pale. Fluid may accumulate under the nail.

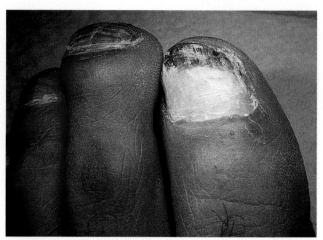

F i g u r e 6 – 2 4   White superficial fungal nails (leukonychia mycotica). Toenails are dry, soft, brittle with a powdery consistency, and white.

termed *leukonychia mycotica*) are most often caused by *T. mentagrophytes.* The fungi infect the superficial nail plate, and the nails are dry, soft, and powdery brittle. The nail plate is usually not thickened and remains firmly adherent to the nail bed (Fig. 6–24). Topical treatment with haloprogin, sulconazole, clotrimazole, and miconazole creams applied twice daily may be useful in early cases. Oral antifungal agents may be very effective. New oral antifungal agents, terbinafine (UK, Canada) and itraconazole (US), have been approved for the systemic treatment of onychomycosis. They have shown promising results.

CANDIDAL. Candidal infections of toenails are caused by *Candida albicans.* Clinically, the nails thicken and turn whitish yellow or yellow-brown (Fig. 6–25). There is frequently involvement of the fingernails in chronic mucocutaneous candidiasis. Unlike distal subungual infections, the entire nail plate is invaded by the candidal organisms and marked destruction is present. Often there is surrounding paronychial inflammation and bulbous formation at the toe tip. Topical antifungal or anti-

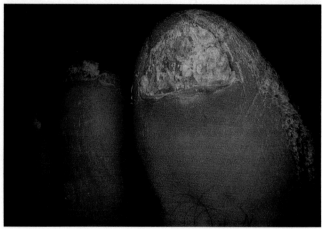

F i g u r e 6 – 2 5   Candidal infection. Thickening results with crumbling whitish yellow or yellow-brown color changes.

yeast creams (e.g., nystatin) will eradicate individual toenail conditions after avulsion. In more severe involvement with chronic mucocutaneous candidiasis, consultation and referral for systemic therapy are advised.

OTHER SUPERFICIAL SKIN INFECTIONS

Candidiasis

Candidiasis is also known as candidosis and moniliasis and is caused by the yeast-like fungus *Candida albicans* and occasionally by other *Candida* species. This fungus is not considered to be part of the normal flora of the skin, although it may be recovered from the intertriginous toe areas and occasionally from mucosal membranes. Cutaneous candidiasis may be contracted through several pathways but most involve an abnormal epithelium secondary to predisposing local, systemic, or environmental factors. Factors that predispose a patient to candidiasis include local occlusion resulting in heat, moisture, and maceration; cutaneous trauma; suppressed immune system; endocrinopathy, such as diabetes mellitus; and preexisting ulcerations or fissures. *C. albicans* is, therefore, frequently a saprophyte that becomes an opportunist when the host has diminished defenses. Candidiasis is differentiated from other fungal skin infections with laboratory test confirmation. The clinical manifestations of cutaneous candidiasis include intertrigo, paronychia, onychomycosis, folliculitis, and localized tinea pedis.

Intertrigo of the interdigital spaces of the feet secondarily infected by *C. albicans* is thought to be due to the warmth, moisture, and maceration in this area. This may be an acute condition with a thin, soft, white, and boggy area with peripheral erythema seen between the

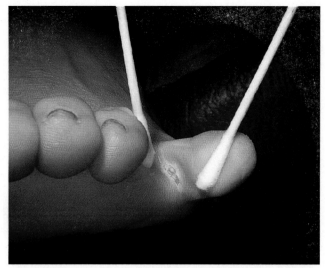

Figure 6–27 **Erosio interdigitalis blastomycetica.** This candidal infection is seen between the fourth and fifth toes and is characterized by maceration, desquamation, and deep fissuring with a white rim of tissue.

toes (Fig. 6–26). A variant of the acute form is observed between the fourth and fifth toes and characterized by maceration, desquamation, and deep fissuring with a white rim of tissue (Fig. 6–27). This condition is also found in the hand and is termed *erosio interdigitalis blastomycetica*.

In the chronic form of interdigital candidiasis, there is a thick, white, overhydrated layer of stratum corneum overlying the epidermis (Fig. 6–28). In all forms of intertrigo the patients may complain of intense itching and burning. Warm water and Epsom salt foot soaks followed by thorough drying help to relieve the maceration. Topical treatment of the web spaces with nystatin cream usually provides rapid clearing of the infection.

Paronychia secondary to *C. albicans* is characterized by swelling and erythema around the edges of the toenails. There is frequently prominent retraction of the cuticle toward the proximal nail fold with increased erythema of the overlying skin (Fig. 6–29). Occasionally, mild pressure in this area will express a creamy, white exudate rich with *C. albicans*. Topical treatment of the nail bed and skin folds with clotrimazole solution usually clears the condition in 4 to 6 weeks.

Onychomycosis, with or without paronychia, is relatively common and results in marked destruction of the nail. This condition has been discussed earlier.

Folliculitis due to *C. albicans* is characterized by erythematous perifollicular pustular lesions (Fig. 6–30). This form of infectious folliculitis is difficult to differentiate from other similar conditions without positive culture results. Topical clotrimazole solution applied daily after bathing will clear the condition.

Localized cutaneous tinea pedis is not as common as the other forms of candidiasis. *C. albicans* has a predilection for moist, macerated skin folds and mucous

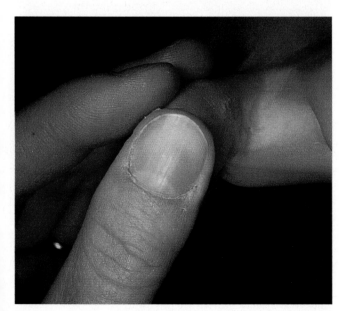

Figure 6–26 **Candidal intertrigo.** A thin, soft, white, and boggy area with peripheral erythema is seen between the toes.

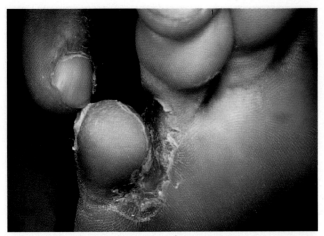

Figure 6–28   Chronic interdigital candidiasis. Thick, white, scaling is associated with intense itching and burning.

Figure 6–30   Candidal folliculitis. Note erythematous perifollicular pustular lesions. This form of infectious folliculitis is difficult to differentiate from other similar conditions without positive culture results.

membranes. On some occasions it may infect glabrous areas outside skin folds. Small areas of candidiasis have a characteristic appearance of pruritic, erythematous, macerated areas with satellite vesicopustules. When the vesicles or pustules break, they leave a red macular base with a collar of elevated epidermis (Fig. 6–31). In chronic candidiasis of the foot the characteristic presentation is a widespread red, denuded, glistening surface with long, cigarette paper—like scaling and advancing borders (Fig. 6–32). Both of these foot infections are thought to be extensions of interdigital candidiasis. Treatment with topical clotrimazole, nystatin, or am-

photericin B cream or lotion is applied two or three times daily.

Tinea Versicolor

Tinea versicolor (pityriasis versicolor) is a chronically recurring, superficial fungal infection of the skin characterized by hypopigmented or hyperpigmented, irregular macular lesions. The infection is usually limited to the trunk and upper legs and is caused by *Malassezia furfur* (*Pityrosporum orbiculare*) (Fig. 6–33). The organism invades the hair follicles and spreads from the fol-

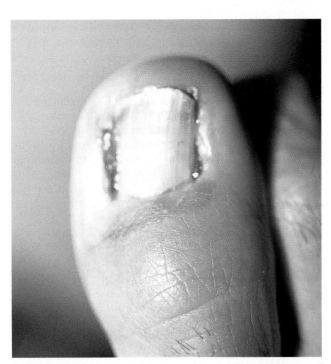

Figure 6–29   Candidal paronychia. Swelling, erythema, and pain occur around the edge of the hallux toenail. Note the prominent retraction of the proximal nail fold with erythema of the skin.

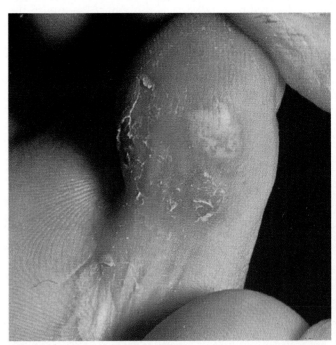

Figure 6–31   Localized cutaneous tinea pedis. This condition is secondary to candidal infection and is characterized by pruritic, erythematous, macerated blisters with satellite vesicopustules. When the vesicles or pustules break, they leave a red macular base with a collar of elevated epidermis.

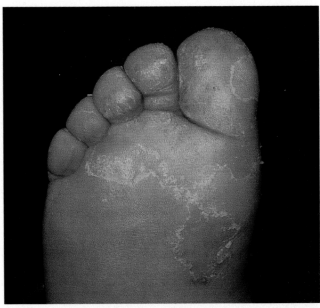

Figure 6–32 Chronic candidiasis. Red, denuded, glistening surfaces with cigarette paper–like scaling and advancing borders are characteristic.

licle to produce fine scales, which are darker than the patient's normal skin color. The small circular macules enlarge outward in irregular patterns. When the affected area is exposed to ultraviolet sunlight it will not tan, leaving the involved area lighter than the adjacent normal skin. Confirmation of the condition is with KOH examination, which shows short hyphae and clumps of spores classically referred to as "spaghetti and meatballs" or "grapes on a vine." Treatment is with selenium sulfide 2.5% solution daily for 2 weeks. The imidazoles are also effective topically but may be more difficult to apply in widespread infections. Reinfection or recurrence is common.

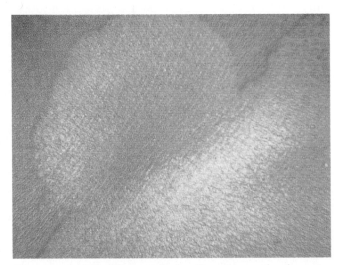

Figure 6–33 Tinea versicolor. Hypopigmented or hyperpigmented, irregular macular lesions enlarge outward. The infected areas do not tan when exposed to ultraviolet light.

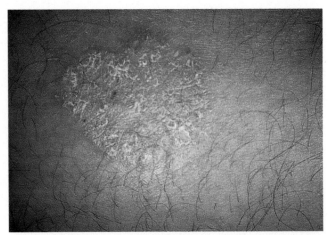

Figure 6–34 Majocchi's granuloma. This erythematous, scaly, elevated lesion has an irregular border and no central clearing. The causative agent is *Trichophyton rubrum.*

DEEP FUNGAL SKIN INFECTIONS

Majocchi's Granuloma

Majocchi's granuloma usually begins as a fungal folliculitis. The fungus spreads from the hair follicle into the dermis. The lesion may be either a follicular or an inflammatory nodule. Clinically, the characteristic lesion is erythematous and scaly with an indistinct border (Fig. 6–34). In dark-skinned persons this lesion is usually darker than the surrounding skin (Fig. 6–35). Pustules may be present, and the lesion usually does not show central clearing. The causative agent is *T. rubrum.* Skin

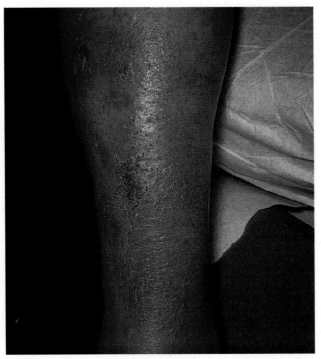

Figure 6–35 Majocchi's granuloma. In dark-skinned individuals this lesion is usually darker than surrounding normal skin.

biopsy with special stains for fungi is necessary for accurate diagnosis. Because the fungal elements are deep within the dermis, topical treatment is not successful. Oral antifungal therapy is recommended.

Sporotrichosis

Sporotrichosis is a deep fungal infection secondary to the dermal implantation of *Sporothrix schenckii*. The organism is usually introduced into the deep tissue layers from trauma from thorns, splinters, or other materials covered with the conidia of *S. schenckii*. The infection begins with an indurated papule that enlarges until it breaks, and the area becomes ulcerated. Frequently, adjacent lymph nodes are infected. Several nodular lesions may form in a linear fashion along the lymphatics. On the lower extremities a gummatous form of the disease may be present. Once the lesion ulcerates it has a ragged undermined atrophic border with an erythematous edge (Fig. 6–36). The lesions are usually painless unless they become secondarily infected with bacteria. The usual course of cutaneous lower extremity sporotrichosis is chronic progression. The organism is difficult to isolate but stains with periodic acid–Schiff and is gram positive. Cultures with Sabouraud's media are slow growing. Treatment is with potassium iodide, 10 drops of the saturated solution in juice or water three times a day after meals, until the lesions have cleared. Amphotericin B may be given intravenously. Topical and oral antifungal agents are generally not effective for this condition.

Chromoblastomycosis

Chromoblastomycosis (chromomycosis, verrucous dermatitis) is a chronic subcutaneous and cutaneous infection caused by species of *Phialophora, Fonsecaea,* and *Cladosporium.* This infection is seen in the United States, but many of the reported cases are in patients from

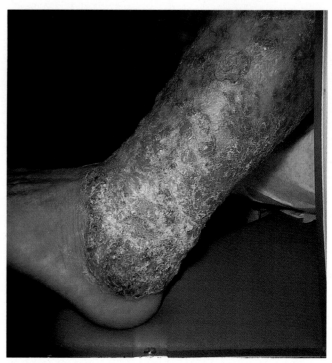

Figure 6–37 Chromoblastomycosis. This chronic infection with widespread involvement with nodules, ulcers, scaling, and crust formation occurs as a verrucous lesion. Secondary scarring and keloid formation are common as the ulcers heal.

the tropics or subtropics who have relocated to the United States. The characteristic lesion begins on the feet or legs in an area of previous injury to the skin. A nodule appears and quickly ulcerates, and the infection gradually spreads. Scales and crusts appear, and a verrucous lesion emerges (Fig. 6–37). The ulcerations heal with scarring and keloid formation. A suppurative granulomatous reaction occurs. The deep fungal infection is usually asymptomatic unless it becomes secondarily infected. It is not contagious from human to human. Diagnosis is characteristically based on the distinct clinical presentation, but KOH examination will confirm sclerotic bodies or brown, branching hyphae. Microbiology laboratory results of cultures will identify the causative organisms in most cases. Treatment is with locally applied heat and with intralesional amphotericin B. Current therapy also includes 5-fluorocytosine, 200 mg/kg/day.

BIBLIOGRAPHY

Bodman MA, Brlan MR: Superficial white onychomycosis. J Am Podiatr Med Assoc 85:205–208, 1995.

Brenner M: Efficacy of twice-daily dosing of econazole nitrate 1% cream for tinea pedis. J Am Podiatr Med Assoc 80:583–587, 1990.

Broberg A, Faergemann J: Scaly lesions on the feet in children: Tinea or eczema? Acta Paediatr Scand 79:349–351, 1990.

Burks JB, Wakabongo M, McGinnis MR: Chromoblastomycosis: A fungal infection primarily observed in the lower extremity. J Am Podiatr Med Assoc 85:260–264, 1995.

Chapel TA, Gagliardi C, Nichols W: Congenital cutaneous candidiasis. J Am Acad Dermatol 6:926–928, 1982.

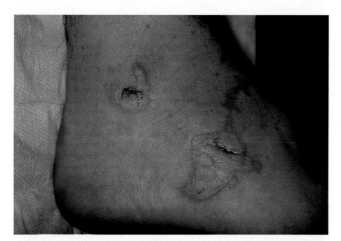

Figure 6–36 Sporotrichosis. This deep fungal infection is characterized by deep tissue breakdown and ulceration with ragged, undermined, atrophic erythematous borders.

Dockery GL: Common skin conditions of the foot. Today's Jogger 2:54–56, 1978.

Dockery GL: Common toenail conditions. Today's Jogger 2:57–59, 1978.

Dockery GL: Lower extremity skin problems related to sports. In Rinaldi RR, Sabia ML (eds): Sports Medicine '80, part 1, pp 57–94. Mt. Kisco, NY, Futura Publishing, 1980.

Dockery GL: Podiatric dermatologic therapeutics. In McCarthy DJ, Montgomery RM (eds): Podiatric Dermatology, pp 311–335. Baltimore, Williams & Wilkins, 1986.

Elgart ML, Warren NG: The Superficial and Subcutaneous Mycoses. In Moschella SL, Hurley HJ (eds): Dermatology, 3rd ed, pp 869–912. Philadelphia, WB Saunders, 1992.

Evans EGV, Dodman B, Williamson DM, Brown GJ, Bowen RG: Comparison of terbinafine and clotrimazole in treating tinea pedis. BMJ 307:645–647, 1993.

Goslen JB, Kobayashi GS: Mycologic infections. In Fitzpatrick TB, Eisen AZ, Wolff K, Freedberg IM, Austen KF (eds): Dermatology in General Medicine, 3rd ed, pp 2193–2248. New York, McGraw-Hill, 1987.

Haley L, Daniel CR: Fungal infections. In Scher RK, Daniel CR (eds): Nails: Therapy, Diagnosis, Surgery, pp 106–119. Philadelphia, WB Saunders, 1990.

Jaafar R, Pettit JHS: *Candida albicans*—saprophyte or pathogen? Int J Dermatol 31:783–785, 1992.

Leyden JJ, Kligman AM: Interdigital athlete's foot: The interaction of dermatophytes and resident bacteria. Arch Dermatol 114:1466–1472, 1978.

McBride A, Cohen BA: Tinea pedis in children. Am J Dis Child 146:844–847, 1992.

Montes LF: Candidiasis. In Moschella SL, Hurley HJ (eds): Dermatology, 3rd ed, pp 913–923. Philadelphia, WB Saunders, 1992.

O'Grady TC, Sahn EE: Investigation of asymptomatic tinea pedis in children. J Am Acad Dermatol 24:660–661, 1991.

Page JC, Abramson C, Lee W, McCarthy DJ, McGinley KJ, Williams D: Diagnosis and treatment of tinea pedis: A review and update. J Am Podiatr Med Assoc 81:304–316, 1991.

Prior TD, Patel S: The efficacy and side effects of terbinafine in the management of pedal mycotic infections. Br J Podiatr Med Surg 7:14–17, 1995.

Sperling LC, Read SI: Localized cutaneous sporotrichosis. Int J Dermatol 22:525–529, 1983.

Terragani L, Buzzetti I, Lasagni A, Oriani A: Tinea pedis in children. Mycoses 34:273–276, 1991.

Zaias N: Onychomycosis. Arch Dermatol 105:263–274, 1972.

7

VIRAL SKIN INFECTIONS

INTRODUCTION

Many viral infections have cutaneous manifestations. In some cases, the infection is strictly limited to the skin. In several viral infections the clinical presentation of the skin lesion may be sufficient to suggest a specific diagnosis. The physician must be aware of the common viral conditions of the lower extremities and be able to classify and treat each condition individually. Common viral infections of the lower extremities may occur as herpes simplex and herpes zoster, verrucae, molluscum contagiosum, and hand-foot-and-mouth disease. These viral conditions are described along with the current treatment recommendations.

HERPES SIMPLEX

Herpes simplex is a double-stranded DNA virus that causes a self-limiting eruption of the skin or mucous membrane. Herpes simplex virus (HSV) infections are caused by two different α-herpesviruses: herpes simplex-1 (HSV-1) and herpes simplex-2 (HSV-2). Other nonrelated viruses include the β-herpesviruses (cytomegaloviruses) and the γ-herpesviruses (Epstein-Barr virus). HSV-1 is usually associated with oral lesions, and HSV-2 is usually associated with genital lesions. Both types seem to produce identical patterns of infection, and they may both produce cutaneous lesions anywhere on the skin. Transmission is by skin-to-skin or mucus-to-skin contact.

Herpes simplex infections have two phases: primary infections and secondary infections. The primary phase involves individuals who have had no prior infection with a particular virus. The virus becomes established in a nerve ganglion, and lesions may occur over large areas, involving multiple or single dermatomes. The secondary or recurrent phase is characterized by a reinfection, producing a lesion at the same site. Recurrent

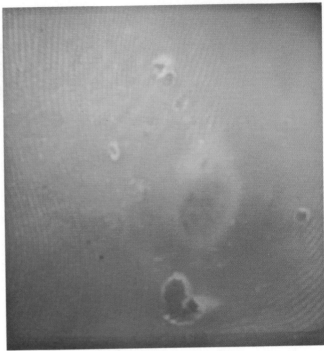

Figure 7–2   Herpes simplex viral infection. Coalescence is seen on plantar aspect of foot.

lesions are usually of brief duration and are less severe in clinical symptoms.

PRIMARY HERPES SIMPLEX VIRAL INFECTIONS. Primary HSV infection commonly occurs in individuals who have had no previous viral infections. Lesions may occur at any location and frequently begin with tingling or discomfort in the skin before the actual visual presentation of the lesion. Other "prodromal" symptoms may include burning, numbness, tenderness, mild paresthesias, or aching pain. Some patients report that they did not have any prodrome before the infection. Systemic complaints of fever, headache, malaise, or myalgia appear within 3 to 5 days after the lesions form. Regional lymph nodes may be enlarged and tender. The lesions usually begin as vesicles on an erythematous base (Fig. 7–1). These lesions may subsequently erode and crust over, or they may coalesce in the center and small peripheral lesions may erode and crust (Fig. 7–2). These eruptions may be very painful, and symptoms last from 3 to 10 days in most cases. The lesions may be present for 2 to 6 weeks before complete resolution is noted. Herpes simplex of the fingertip or distal toe is termed *herpetic whitlow,* and this condition may lead to a painful paronychium (Fig. 7–3).

During the primary stage of infection, the virus enters the skin nerve endings directly below the lesion and ascends through peripheral nerves to the dorsal root ganglia. When it reaches this level it apparently remains in a latent stage. The reasons for recurrence are obscure, but sunlight, fever, stress, trauma, and general illness have all been noted to cause a relapse. Diagnosis is

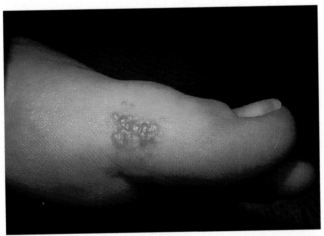

Figure 7–1   Primary herpes simplex viral infection. Multiple grouped vesicles on an erythematous base are present on the medial hallux.

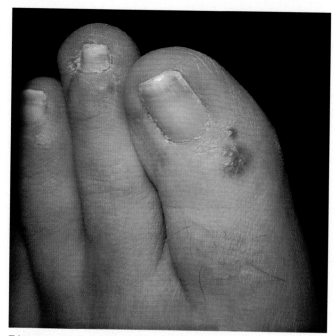

Figure 7-3 Herpes simplex viral infection. Note involvement of the first and second toes with paronychia of the second nail. A positive Tzanck's smear confirmed the diagnosis.

based on clinical evaluation confirmed by Tzanck's smear. Fluid from an intact vesicle is smeared on a glass microscope slide, dried, and stained with Giemsa's stain. Observation of giant acanthocytes (acantholytic giant cells) or multinucleated giant keratinocytes is a positive finding. This test is positive in 75% of early cases of primary or secondary HSV infections.

SECONDARY HERPES SIMPLEX VIRAL INFECTIONS. Secondary or recurrent herpes infections are poorly understood. HSV-1 is more antigenic than HSV-2, which is more frequently associated with recurrent herpetic infections. Because of this finding, reactivation of HSV infections may follow significant clinical events, as mentioned earlier. Recurrences average two or three events a year, and the length of the attack varies from 5 to 14 days. A prodrome of tingling, itching, or burning is common and usually precedes skin lesions by 24 hours. Systemic symptoms, as is noted in primary HSV infections, are usually absent. Recurrent HSV infections are typically not as severe as primary infections.

Treatment of cutaneous HSV infections is unsatisfactory. Acyclovir, an antiviral drug active against herpesviruses, reduces the length and severity of recurrent infections when applied topically but does not prevent recurrences. Oral acyclovir, 200 mg five times a day for 7 to 10 days, may be beneficial in more involved HSV infections. L-Lysine has anecdotally been claimed to be effective in the prevention of recurrent herpes infections when taken in 1-g doses daily. A cool tap water or Burow's compress will decrease symptoms and erythema. The astringent effect will aid in debriding crusts and promoting healing.

HERPES ZOSTER

Herpes zoster (commonly called shingles) is caused by the same virus that causes chickenpox (varicella). Primary infection with this varicella-zoster virus leads to chickenpox. The virus lies dormant in the dorsal root or nerve ganglion. Reactivation of the latent virus, in a previously exposed area, results in a more localized reaction, referred to as herpes zoster. Several years, or even decades, may pass between the primary infection and the reactivation. The condition is not contagious through personal contact. However, because the live virus is present in the zoster lesion, chickenpox may be contracted by an individual who has never had chickenpox from a person who has an active herpes zoster infection.

A prodrome of pain, itching, or burning, generally localized to an individual dermatome, precedes the infection by several days. There may also be headache, fever, and malaise before the eruption. Additionally, there may be intense segmental pain for 3 to 5 days during the preeruptive phase. The eruptions of herpes zoster usually involve the thoracic, cervical, sacral, and lumbar areas. Less common involvement is of one extremity with extension to the foot. The early lesions are usually macular areas that quickly convert to vesicular eruptions surrounded by erythema. The vesicles vary in size and development as compared with the vesicles of herpes simplex, which are of uniform size and character. The lesions of herpes zoster continue to evolve over several weeks, becoming hemorrhagic and pustular (Fig. 7-4). The vesicles may umbilicate or rupture, and in the later stages the lesions begin to crust and form scabs. As the scabs loosen and fall off there may be dermal scarring. Small satellite lesions away from the dermatome are common. Elderly or debilitated patients are more prone to severe zoster attacks and at higher risk for intractable post-herpetic neuralgia.

The diagnosis of herpes zoster is primarily based on

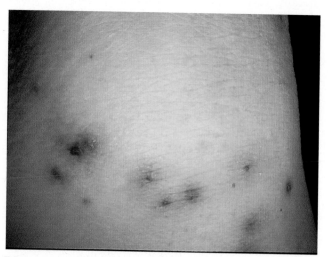

Figure 7-4 Herpes zoster. The lesions on the lower extremity become more hemorrhagic and turbid as they progress.

the clinical findings of clusters of vesicles, unilateral segmental dermatome distribution, and intense early pain. Laboratory tests are rarely required to confirm the diagnosis; however, the definitive test is a positive viral culture of fluid from an active vesicle. Tzanck's smear and the skin biopsy test findings are positive in up to 80% of cases. Electron microscopy produces the best analysis of zoster-varicella virus but is difficult and expensive in the average clinical setting.

Treatment of herpes zoster is limited. Because this painful dermatomic eruption is self-limiting, the decision to treat the condition must be individually based. Adequate analgesia is all that is required in the majority of lower extremity cases. In widespread or severe cases, intravenous acyclovir therapy may be necessary. Treatment must be started within 72 hours of the eruptions. Intravenous doses of acyclovir of 5 mg/kg every 8 hours for 7 days may significantly relieve pain, decrease viral shedding, and encourage early healing. Oral corticosteroids may decrease the incidence of postherpetic neuralgia, especially in the older patient. Prednisone, 60 mg, is given daily initially, with gradual tapering over 3 to 4 weeks. The recommended administration of prednisone is 30 mg twice a day for 1 week, 20 mg twice a day for 1 week, followed by 20 mg daily for the final week. Triamcinolone injection 2 g/ml, may be administered as an alternative to oral corticosteroid. This agent is administered with multiple sublesional injections along the affected dermatome site. Corticosteroid therapy has no effect on post-herpetic neuralgia when the lesions have healed and is contraindicated in immunocompromised patients. Topical capsaicin cream, a chemical that depletes the pain impulse transmitter substance P and prevents its resynthesis within the neuron, may be applied three to five times daily. Substantial pain relief may occur after continual application of capsaicin cream for 3 or 4 weeks. Maximal relief occurs with additional topical therapy for longer periods of time. Physical modalities such as ultrasound therapy, cryotherapy, and regional sympathetic nerve blocks may also assist in amelioration of the pain in post-herpetic neuralgia.

VERRUCAE

Verrucae are commonly termed *warts.* These benign epidermal neoplasms are caused by a variety of different viruses. Papillomaviruses belong to the family Papovaviridae and are species-specific double-stranded DNA viruses. There are approximately 46 different human papillomaviruses (HPV) that have been implicated in the formation of human warts. The HPV types are listed numerically by their DNA composition for identification purposes. Cutaneous warts may occur at any age but are more common in children and young adults. The course of warts is highly variable, with most lesions spontaneously resolving in a few weeks or months. Some warts may remain at the same location with no apparent change for many years, and others will continue to expand and enlarge with time. Warts are generally self-limiting and very harmless, but patients may undergo therapy because the warts are unsightly, cause embarrassment, become irritated, or cause pain.

Warts are transmitted by contact and may appear at sites of trauma or irritation. They may be contracted from other individuals, swimming pools, locker rooms, or other areas of public traffic. Individual variations in cell-mediated immunity may explain the differences in the size, severity, location, and duration of warts. Some warts respond readily to simple treatment, whereas others appear to be extremely resistant to most forms of therapy. Because warts are located in the epidermal layers of the skin they may be removed without scarring. All treatment forms should be approached with extreme care to prevent damage to the underlying dermis, thereby increasing the chances of scar formation.

Clinically, warts obscure the normal skin lines. This helps to differentiate them from other lesions with similar presentations. Warts vary in shape, size, location, and presentation. The HPV causes the keratinocytes to proliferate to form a mass within the epidermis. Contrary to popular misconception, there are no "roots" penetrating into the dermis. Thrombosed blood vessels may become entrapped in the cylindrical projections formed by the virus and are seen as small black dots on the surface of the some warts. The most common lower extremity warts are the common wart (verruca vulgaris), plane wart (verruca plana), cylindrical (or digitate) wart, periungual and subungual wart, plantar wart, and mosaic wart. There are numerous methods of treating warts with each method individualized for each patient.

The common wart, referred to as verruca vulgaris, starts as a smooth, flesh-colored papule. It eventually evolves into a dome-shaped, discolored, thickened growth with hemorrhagic or small thrombosed capillaries. Generally, these warts are few in number and are common on the non–weight-bearing surface of the lower extremities (Fig. 7–5). Verruca vulgaris is usually associated with HPV types 2 and 4. It may range in color from light brown to slightly erythematous to darkly pigmented. It varies from 1 mm to well over 1 cm in diameter and may coalesce to produce larger lesions.

Plane warts (verruca plana) are very small lesions with a slightly raised, smooth, skin-colored or slightly pigmented, flat surface (Fig. 7–6). These flat warts usually do not have the typical rough warty appearance of other warts. They may occur along a pressure area or an area that has been scratched (koebnerization) and are usually multiple and linear. They are commonly associated with HPV types 3 and 10. These flat warts are extremely likely to undergo spontaneous remission or involution but may be persistent and unresponsive to therapy. If these lesions are mistaken for inflammatory conditions and treated with topical corticosteroids, they will usually spread.

Cylindrical or digitate warts are uncommon on the foot but may be seen on the toes (Fig. 7–7). These warts are much more common on the face, neck, or anogeni-

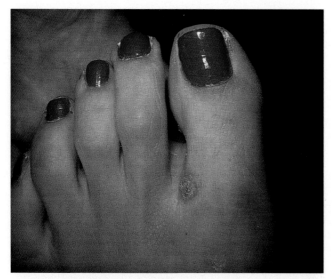

Figure 7–5 Verruca vulgaris. This discrete lesion of the dorsolateral base of the hallux is a raised, firm papule with a rough "warty" surface and small black streaks in the center.

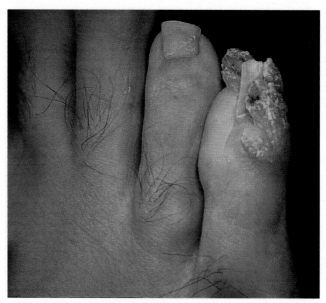

Figure 7–7 Filiform or digitate wart. Finger-like projections are observed around the fifth toenail.

tal region. They are commonly associated with HPV types 6 or 11. These growths consist of a few or many finger-like projections emanating from a single base. They may have visible capillaries within the cylinders that may bleed easily with trauma or trimming.

Periungual and subungual warts (Fig. 7–8) are sometimes more difficult to treat than free-standing warts because of the adjacent or overlying toenail. When the

wart is next to a nail, localized treatment may cause considerable pain and even paronychia. In younger patients a very simple treatment using adhesive tape to wrap and occlude the wart and nail area has been very successful. The tape should be allowed to remain in place for 1 week. It is then removed, and the skin is allowed to air dry for 1 day. The tape is reapplied for an additional week. Follow-up with the patient at 2

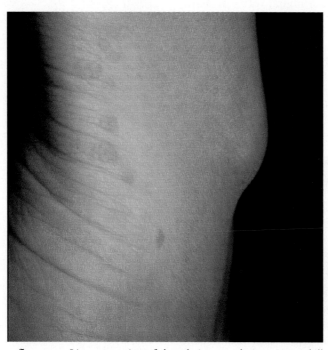

Figure 7–6 Plane or flat warts. Linear grouping of these lesions on the posterior Achilles tendon area is common.

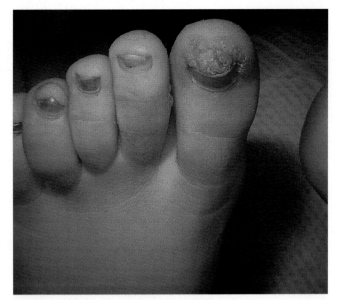

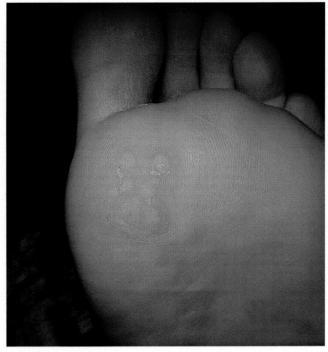

Figure 7 – 8   Subungual and periungual wart. This wart on the distal hallux caused discomfort and distortion of the nail plate. Nail avulsion may be necessary for adequate treatment.

weeks from the original office visit is recommended. If the wart is still present it is treated with a mild topical acid and retaped once again. This process is repeated until the wart is no longer present. Other types of treatment for periungual warts have produced variable results. The most consistent outcomes have been found with the conservative approach using topical salicylic acid and lactic acid paint, or with 40% salicylic acid plasters or the surgical approach using blunt dissection and curettage. Strong acids, cryotherapy, and surgery may cause permanent nail changes if the nail matrix is damaged during treatment. Subungual warts present a more difficult challenge because the conventional treatments usually do not work well. In some conditions the nail must be removed to provide adequate exposure to the wart. Topical acids and blunt dissection provide the best results, but once again care must be taken to prevent injury to the nail bed and nail matrix. Periungual and subungual warts are usually associated with HPV types 2 and 4.

Figure 7 – 10   Plantar warts. Grouped lesions occurred on the weight-bearing surface of the ball of the foot.

Plantar warts are frequently termed *verrucae* and are usually associated with HPV type 1. Any wart found on the weight-bearing surface or bottom of the foot may be called a plantar wart. These warts take on a different character because of the pressure and, in many

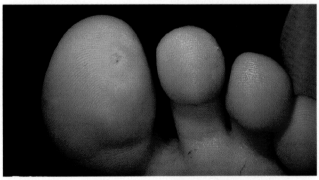

Figure 7 – 9   Plantar wart. This solitary lesion occurred on the weight-bearing surface of the hallux.

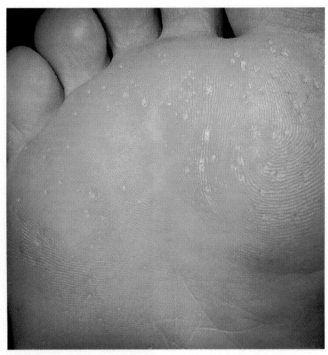

Figure 7 – 11 Multiple small "seed warts" on the plantar surface of the foot.

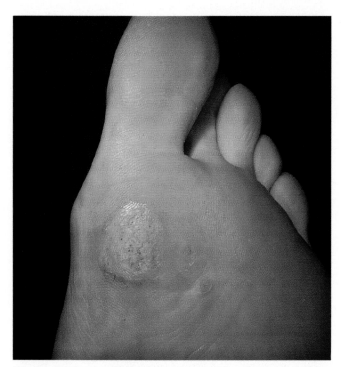

Figure 7–12   Mosaic wart. Large wart on the weight-bearing ball of the foot after debridement of the upper rough surface shows the uniform mosaic pattern that is unique to this lesion.

cases, the presence of overlying callus formation. The lesions may be solitary (Fig. 7–9), grouped (Fig. 7–10), or multiple (seed warts) (Fig. 7–11). They are often pale or yellow, due to the keratin levels or hyperkeratosis. The multiple or thrombosed capillaries are frequently visible in most of the larger lesions, and these will bleed on trimming of the wart.

Mosaic warts are generally a coalescence of several smaller warts or grouping of clusters to form a large plaque. They are usually associated with HPV type 2. These larger lesions may be found on any surface and are not necessarily found on weight-bearing surfaces (Figs. 7–12 through 7–14). When they are located on the direct pressure-bearing surfaces of the feet they may be painful and interfere with normal gait. Large crescentic mosaic warts may be seen in patients with acquired immunodeficiency syndrome. Mosaic warts are usually irregular and contain multiple cores that have coalesced. This effect results in variable depths of the lesions with one area usually very deep. This lesion bleeds freely when shaved or trimmed, owing to the multiple number of small looping capillaries. Treatment may be very difficult and require repeated attempts to resolve the lesion.

The primary goal of the treatment of warts is to rid the patient of visible lesions. Because the wart is in-

Figure 7–13   Mosaic wart. Plantar weight-bearing heel with mosaic wart shows the rough and highly organized mosaic pattern with light scales covering the surface of the lesion.

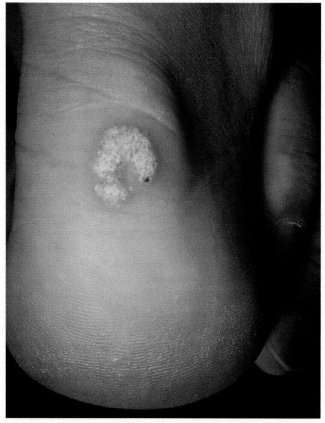

Figure 7–14   Mosaic wart. Large crescentic mosaic wart formed on the posterior aspect of the heel. This type of wart is termed a *summary wart* and may be seen in patients with acquired immunodeficiency syndrome.

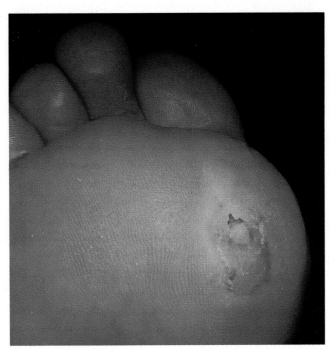

Figure 7–15 Appearance of the skin after topical salicylic acid (40%) has been applied under occlusion. There is a great deal of macerated tissue with elevation of the epidermis layer. At this point the loose tissue is debrided, and a decision is made whether to apply additional topical salicylic acid.

traepidermal, all methods of treatment must be of the type that will not penetrate or damage the dermal layer of the skin. Once patients have been infected with the human papillomavirus they are more likely to be reinfected again, implying that virological cure is not achieved by eliminating surface warts. There are many different types of treatments recommended for warts, which suggests that none of them are completely satisfactory for consistent usage. Selection of treatment depends on the type of wart present, its location and size, and the age of the patient. In children, the simplest and most innocuous treatments are recommended, owing to spontaneous regression of warts and the ease of resolution with treatment. In more resistant lesions in older patients the treatment may need to be more aggressive.

Posthypnotic suggestion or psychotherapy has been suggested as a method of ridding patients of warts. It may be that this technique simply relies on the spontaneous disappearance of warts. Many of these suggestive techniques have been passed along through families for years. One method involves tracing the body part on paper and drawing in the wart. The paper is then thrown away, burned, or buried. Another method involves painting the wart with a dye such as gentian violet or applying adhesive tape over the wart and asking the patient to absolutely refrain from looking at the wart for the next 2 or 3 weeks. A group of similar methods involves taping either a copper penny (Denver method), an eye of a potato (Idaho method), or a piece

of banana skin (tropical method) over the wart for 1 or 2 weeks. These techniques may have some added benefits over simple suggestion techniques because they may cause maceration, change of local tissue pH, ion transfer, or increased skin temperature. All of these treatments are very controversial and tend to work much better in children than adults.

Oral vitamin A compounds have been reported to cause an increase in the spontaneous remission of pedal warts. The usual dosage recommendation for vitamin A in water-soluble capsules is 50,000 IU daily. I found that the combined dosage of 10,000 IU vitamin A plus 15 mg zinc in tablet form taken orally twice a day for up to 2 months has been extremely successful in the treatment of lower extremity warts.

Keratolytic therapy is the principal treatment for warts. Topical acids are considered effective and relatively benign forms of treatment for most warts. This treatment relies on the chemical debridement of the epidermal layer of the skin, thereby removing the wart tissue. Salicylic acid in 20%, 40%, or 60% concentrations may be found in a variety of vehicles, including flexible collodion, polyacrylic solutions, or plaster pads. Liquid or ointment acid treatment requires persistent application and attention. Salicylic acid is applied over the debrided wart tissue and occluded with adhesive tape or moleskin (Fig. 7–15). The bandage is removed in 24 hours, and the white, macerated tissue is debrided to firm or pink underlying tissue (Fig. 7–16). The acid and a new cover are reapplied, and the process is repeated until the wart tissue resolves. The patient may experience tenderness or inflammation of the skin adjacent to the wart, and this may necessitate a periodic intermission from treatment. Because of the duration

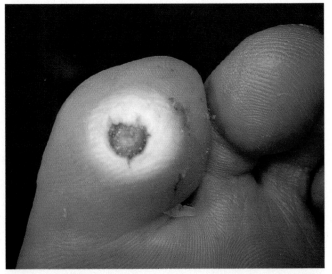

Figure 7–16 Local tissue reaction with wart treatment using topical salicylic acid (60%). The central lesion has been debrided to the underlying pink dermal layer, and the surrounding tissue is macerated. At this point no additional salicylic acid would be applied and the skin would be allowed to heal.

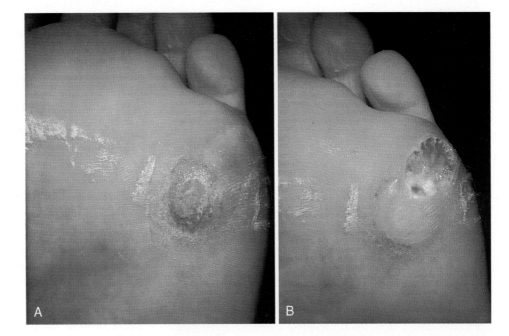

Figure 7–17 *A*, Treatment of a plantar wart with a 60% salicylic acid plaster that moved distally from the original treatment area causing a burn of the normal adjacent tissue. *B*, Debridement of blister over normal skin caused increased discomfort for the patient.

needed to remove wart tissue completely, some patients may not comply with this therapy.

The process of topical salicylic acid treatment is enhanced with the use of prepackaged plasters that may be in either 40% or 60% concentrations. This method is easier and cleaner for the patient to perform at home. The acid plaster sheet is simply cut to the size of the lesion, applied, and secured with tape or moleskin. It is important to ensure that the plaster remain over the wart and does not slip onto normal skin (Fig. 7–17). The plaster is then removed in 24 to 48 hours, and the process is repeated as described earlier. Similar treatment with other keratolytic liquids and creams containing lactic acid and salicylic acid produces a slightly more intense reaction and may need to be watched closely with occasional visits to the office.

Chemotherapy is similar to keratolytic therapy, and it has also been successfully used for treating warts. Several applications may be necessary, and because of the intense reactions it is advisable to see the patients regularly. Monochloroacetic acid, bichloroacetic acid, cantharidin, podophyllin, formalin, and phenol have all been used in the past.

Monochloroacetic and bichloroacetic acids work in a similar fashion. The wart is trimmed or shaved, the surrounding normal tissue is protected with petrolatum, and the entire surface of the wart is painted with the acid. The area is then covered with a protective bandage or moleskin and examined in 5 to 7 days. The process is repeated as needed.

Cantharidin, 0.7% to 1.0%, is a strong vesicant extracted from the tropical green blister beetle. The acid produces a local epidermal tissue necrosis and intense blister formation (Fig. 7–18). Cantharidin is most effective for the treatment of small warts and periungual warts. With cantharidin, as well as other blistering

treatments, a ring-shaped recurrence of wart may result where the virus has floated to the edge of the blister and reestablished itself.

Podophyllin resin, extracted from two species of may apples, causes necrosis of the tissue and is limited in use by low efficacy, unpredictable, and sometimes extremely severe local reactions (Fig. 7–19). Because of systemic absorption leading to neuropathy, seizures, and renal failure and systemic toxicity leading to death,

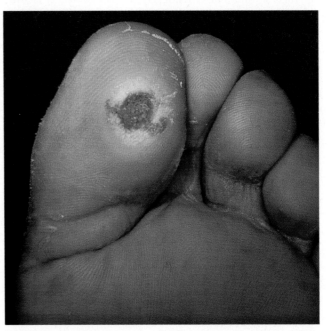

Figure 7–18 An intense local necrosis with adjacent tissue maceration and blister occurred after a single application of 1.0% cantharidin to a plantar wart.

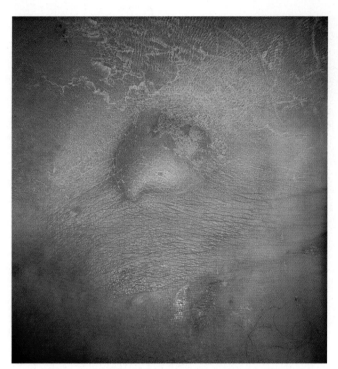

Figure 7-19   An extreme local tissue reaction occurred after a small amount of topical podophyllin was used for the treatment of a plantar wart. The patient suffered severe local pain and allergic-like symptoms after the treatment.

this compound is not recommended for the treatment of lower extremity warts.

Formalin is very rarely used today for the treatment of warts but may be considered in those resistant lesions where other more conventional treatments have failed. The technique involves trimming the overlying tissue and painting the wart frequently with concentrated formalin solution and covering the area. Alternatively, the entire foot may be soaked for 20 to 30 minutes daily in a 4% formalin solution. Sensitization to formalin may occur with this technique.

Phenol has also been used in a similar method to monochloroacetic acid with similar results. Phenol causes more allergic reactions and is less predictive than many other topicals and is generally not favored for the primary treatment of warts. It is, however, frequently used to paint the area of a wart after other acids or treatments have removed the majority of abnormal tissue.

Cryosurgery with carbon dioxide snow (Fig. 7-20) or liquid nitrogen destroys the epithelium through single or multiple freeze-thaw cycles. Necrosis occurs with ice formation, cellular dehydration, and, ultimately, vascular stasis. Cryotherapy on the plantar aspect of the foot may cause a deep and painful blister that is very slow to heal. Multiple light applications of freezing are less likely to cause problems than are single aggressive applications. The wart or warts are treated with or without anesthesia with the cryoprobe, applicator wand, or

cotton swab until the entire lesion is frosted white (Fig. 7-21). Immediately after the cryotherapy the wart blanches. The tissue is then allowed to slowly thaw, which produces an inflammatory response, and additional light freezing is performed again. The depth of freeze is about one and one-half times the lateral spread. This process is repeated two or three times on each visit. Several days later the tissue will blister, and in 1 to 2 weeks sloughing usually occurs. During the treatment process the patient may complain of intense burning, but most adults can tolerate the therapy. Children do not fare well with this approach, and it is not therefore generally recommended in the treatment of pediatric warts.

Intralesional bleomycin sulfate is an effective method of treatment for periungual warts and an alternative method for resistant plantar and mosaic warts of the lower extremities. Bleomycin is injected in a concentration of 1 unit/ml, and no more than 2 units should be injected as a total cumulative dose. A volume of 0.1 ml is injected into warts measuring less than 5 mm in diameter, and 0.2 ml is injected into warts greater than 5 mm in diameter. This treatment may be very painful but is generally well tolerated by adults. The wart that is responding usually shows hemorrhagic eschars and blackens and sloughs during the week after treatment. A second injection may be necessary after a 1-month interval. One or two injections are usually all that is necessary to resolve a wart with this technique. One of the problems with this technique is the cost of the product. It is not provided in a multidose vial and is considered to be unstable after approximately 12 hours. Therefore, each treatment requires the use of an additional new vial, which is expensive and inefficient.

5-Fluorouracil is a fluorinated pyrimidine that causes necrosis of proliferative tissue. Excessive sloughing and erosion may occur if too large an area is treated or too much 5-fluorouracil is applied. Systemic toxicity is also possible. Regimens of topical application of small amounts of 5-fluorouracil 1% applied daily for 1 week is effective (>50%) for the treatment of single warts. Intradermal injections of 0.1 to 0.4 mL of 5-fluorouracil, depending on the size of the wart, have shown greater than 90% cure rate. This is an effective procedure; however, several of my patients showed excessive hyperpigmentary changes in the area immediately surrounding the infiltrative injection sites. These changes all resolved with time, but the patient should be forewarned of this possibility for cosmetic reasons.

Electodesiccation with curettage is an effective method for removing small warts (Fig. 7-22). The electrodesiccation technique involves the use of a Hyfrecator unit with a needle-tip applicator on a hand-held instrument. The wart area is anesthetized with a local anesthetic agent, and the surrounding area is prepped. The current is advanced until a visible spark occurs between the instrument tip and the wart tissue. The wart

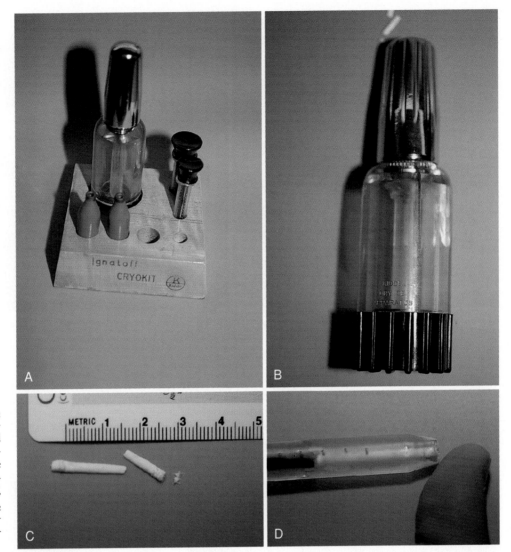

Figure 7–20 *A,* CO_2 cryokit with chamber, CO_2 cartridges, applicator syringes, and holder. *B,* Close-up of CO_2 chamber, which houses the cartridge in the metal part and the applicator syringe in the glass part. *C,* Compressed CO_2 snow. *D,* CO_2 application with applicator syringe. (Courtesy of Kidde. Ignatoff Cryokit.)

area is lightly charred, and the residue is curetted away. The wart will become firm, and it is possible to completely remove the wart base intact. Additional Hyfrecator treatment is applied to the underlying base to reduce any residual verrucal tissues that might be present.

Blunt dissection along with curettage is one of the most consistent and effective methods of removing lower extremity warts. This simple surgical technique is fast and usually nonscarring as long as the underlying dermal skin layers are not penetrated.

The technique begins with local anesthesia with epinephrine delivered around and under the involved wart. One technique uses a jet injector to administer a small amount of lidocaine at the four corners surrounding the wart. Additional infiltration may then be performed from these anesthetized skin areas. A plane of dissection is established with tissue nippers, dissection scissors, or small surgical blade (Fig. 7–23). This outer cut should extend through the epidermal layer only and

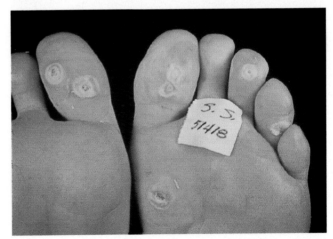

Figure 7–21 Multiple small plantar warts have been frosted with liquid nitrogen with several applications, allowing thawing to occur between each freeze. (Courtesy of Dr. Robert Wendel.)

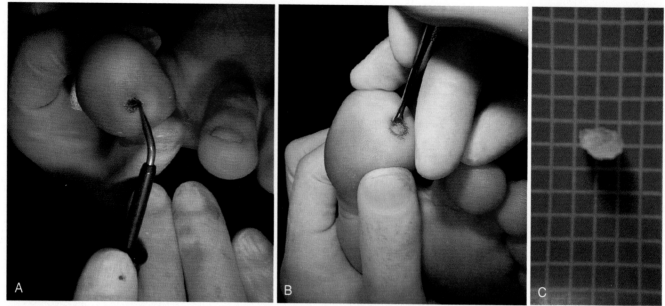

Figure 7–22   *A,* A small plantar wart is lightly desiccated with a Hyfrecator. *B,* The wart is curetted from its base, and the base is again lightly electrocauterized. *C,* The wart is removed as a single unit with its capsule intact.

should not involve the dermis if possible. Once the plane of the wart has been established by cutting the skin circumferentially outside the wart capsule or lining, the blunt dissector (or end of a small curette) is inserted in the plane of cleavage and the wart is gently separated from the underlying normal dermal layer (Fig. 7–24). The technique involves short, firm, and even strokes that will "push" the wart tissue off in a single unit. Once the wart has been removed from the area, the curette is then applied lightly to

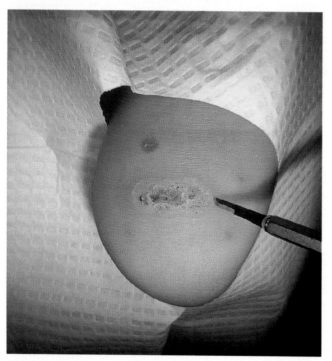

Figure 7–23   A small surgical blade is used to establish a dissection plane by very shallow scoring of the tissue outside the visible wart capsule.

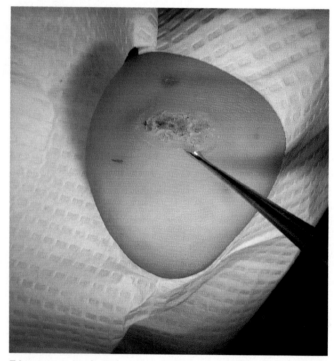

Figure 7–24   The blunt dissector or end of the curette is used to bluntly elevate the wart and its capsule away from the underlying dermal skin layer.

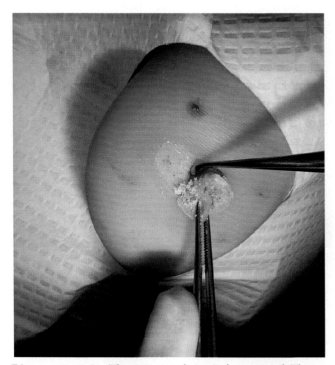

Figure 7–25 The entire wart lesion is then removed. The underlying dermal base is lightly curetted to remove any residual wart tissue.

the base to smooth any rough spots and to remove any residual wart tissue that may remain on the dermal layer (Fig. 7–25). The outer edge of the crater resulting from the wart removal is smoothed using a scalpel technique. This creates a very shallow crater, which seems to greatly enhance the speed of healing. Bleeding is controlled by lightly coagulating the bleeding areas or applying topical Monsel's solution. The exposed area is then painted with a fluorinated corticosteroid cream and covered with a nonadherent gauze pad (Fig. 7–26). A bandage is placed on the wound, and the patient is seen in 3 to 4 days for follow-up. At this visit the dressing is changed and the corticosteroid cream is applied once again. The patient is then seen 1 week after surgery, and all dressings are removed. Thereafter, the wound is left exposed, unless weight bearing, and warm water Epsom salts soaks are started until healing is complete in 2 or 3 weeks. This combination of blunt dissection (excochleation), curettage, and topical steroid under mild compression (Fig. 7–27) has provided the highest long-term success for the resistant plantar verrucae in my practice.

Many other treatments for warts are available with variable results. Topical and injectable corticosteroids, CO_2 and argon laser therapy, dinitrochlorobenzene immunotherapy, alpha interferon treatment, and x-irradiation have all been proposed as treatment options for warts. I have no experience with these modalities.

MOLLUSCUM CONTAGIOSUM

Molluscum contagiosum is a communicable viral disease confined to the skin and mucous membranes and is caused by a large DNA virus that is a member of the Poxviridae. It is more common in children and adolescents but may occur in adults. Molluscum contagiosum is commonly found on the face, upper body, and lower extremities and occasionally on the feet.

The early lesions are dome-shaped papules that are pearly, flesh-colored, or pink (Fig. 7–28). Older and more mature lesions and those on the plantar aspect of the foot may appear white (Fig. 7–29). On the plantar foot, molluscum contagiosum has been misdiagnosed as plantar warts, tylomas, and keratoacanthomas. The lesions frequently have a central umbilication with a mildly erythematous base. The umbilicated center may be filled with a white curd-like core that may be expressed with lateral compression. These discrete lesions may range from 3 to 6 mm in diameter, and several papules are usually present. Rarely, giant molluscum contagiosum may be identified on the lower extremities measuring as large as 3 cm in diameter (Fig. 7–30).

Most lesions are self-limiting and spontaneously resolve in 2 to 9 months; however, they may last as long as 3 years. Unless they become secondarily infected the lesions heal without scarring. Spread of the lesions is by contact, autoinoculation, or scratching. Genital lesions are spread by sexual contact. Diagnosis is by the distinctive clinical presentation of the lesion, by light microscopy of the stained smears of the expressed core,

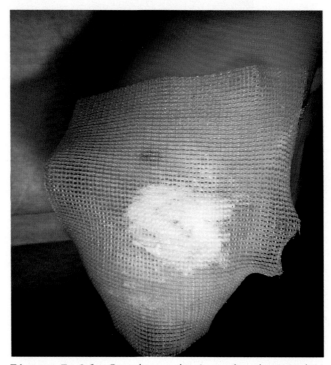

Figure 7–26 Once the procedure is complete, the exposed tissue is painted with topical corticosteroid cream and a nonadherent gauze dressing is applied. Mild compression is then recommended.

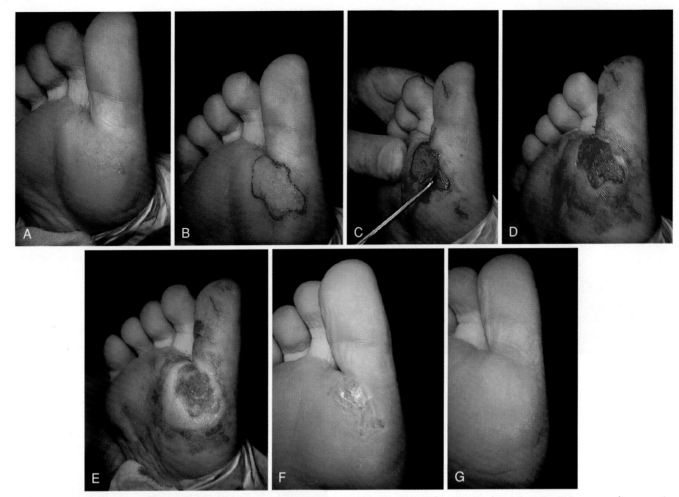

Figure 7–27   Blunt dissection, curettage, and topical corticosteroid treatment of resistant plantar warts. *A,* Long-standing mosaic plantar wart resistant to other treatments. *B,* Circumferential scoring of the epidermis outside the visible wart capsule. *C,* Blunt dissection of the wart in one piece. Note the underlying intact skin lines of the dermis. *D,* Light curettage of the base was done to remove rough areas and any residual wart tissue. *E,* Scalpel removal of the crater edge made it more shallow. *F,* Twelve days after surgery there is complete removal of visible wart tissue. *G,* Final appearance of the treated area with no wart and no scarring.

and by biopsy. Treatment is not always mandatory, but, once the condition is diagnosed, most patients want to be rid of the lesions quickly. The most accepted form of therapy is removal of the lesions with sharp curette and cautery, liquid nitrogen, or topical acid therapy. More than one treatment may be necessary to completely resolve the condition.

HAND-FOOT-AND-MOUTH DISEASE

Hand-foot-and-mouth disease is a very distinctive complex caused by coxsackievirus, usually of the A16 strain. This is an enterovirus of the Picornaviridae. Infections are common in late summer and in the early fall and are usually seen in children younger than 15 years of age. Most cases reported have been in children younger than 10 years of age. Clinically, the patients may have mild prodromal symptoms of malaise, fever, sore throat,

or abdominal pain before the lesions appear. There are a limited number of round or oval, slightly yellow vesicles surrounded by erythema on the hands (Fig. 7–31) and feet (Fig. 7–32). Close-up evaluation of the lesions show 2- to 10-mm gray, oval to round vesicles. The lesions often run in or parallel to the skin lines and are surrounded by a red areola (Fig. 7–33). The vesicles occur primarily on the palms, soles, and oral mucosa. There may be lesions on the dorsal aspect of the toes and fingers and occasionally on the face, buttocks, or legs. The lesions may be tender or totally asymptomatic and heal in 2 to 7 days. Oral vesicular lesions are frequently discernible for only a short period of time and, unless they are painful, may be missed during the examination. The diagnosis is usually based on clinical presentation. Histopathological findings include reticular and ballooning degeneration within the epidermis. This degenerative process leads to multilocular intraepidermal vesicles without giant cells or inclusion bodies.

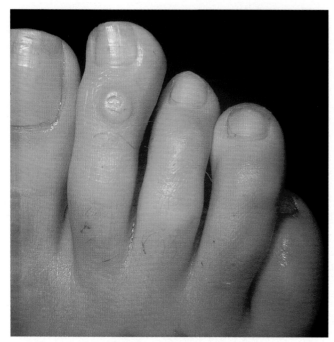

Figure 7–28   Molluscum contagiosum. Single lesion on the dorsal aspect of the second toe is a typical flesh-colored, dome-shaped papule with an umbilicated central core and slightly erythematous base.

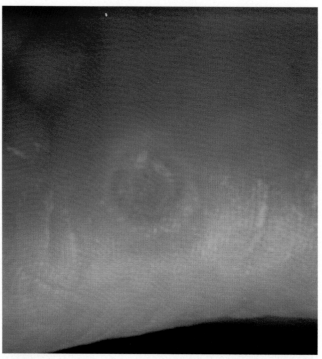

Figure 7–30   Molluscum contagiosum. Giant molluscum contagiosum measuring 2 cm in diameter on weight-bearing surface of the foot was confirmed by clinical appearance, stained smears of central core material, and histopathology.

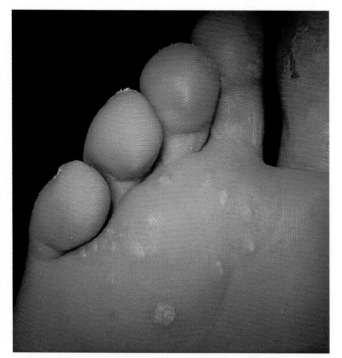

Figure 7–29   Molluscum contagiosum. A swimmer presented with multiple plantar foot lesions. Plantar foot lesions may appear white and flat and may be confused with plantar warts until the diagnosis is confirmed.

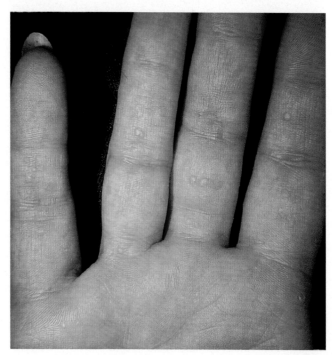

Figure 7–31   Hand-foot-and-mouth disease. Hand lesions are frequently small, oval, slightly yellow vesicles with a fine erythematous rim.

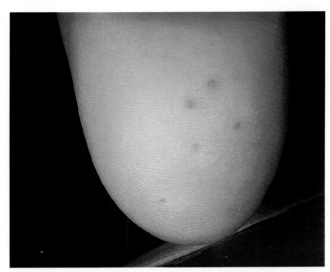

Figure 7–32 Hand-foot-and-mouth disease. On the soles, the lesions may occur primarily as red papules, especially on the heel area.

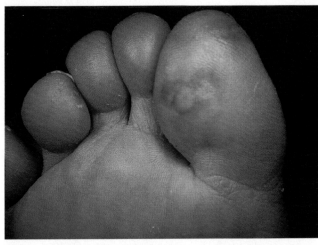

Figure 7–33 Hand-foot-and-mouth disease. On the fingers or toes the lesions may be composed of round to football-shaped vesicles that may coalesce.

In most cases, symptomatic and supportive treatment is all that is required. Dehydration and fluid imbalance should be avoided, and fever and pain should be controlled with non–aspirin-containing products.

BIBLIOGRAPHY

Bartolomei FJ, McCarthy DJ: Cutaneous manifestations of viral diseases, In McCarthy DJ, Montgomery R (eds): Podiatric Dermatology, pp 146–164. Baltimore, Williams & Wilkins, 1986.

Curry SS: Cutaneous herpes simplex infections and their treatment. Cutis 26:41–58, 1980.

Daniel CR: Nonfungal infections. In Scher RK, Daniel CR (eds): Nails: Therapy, Diagnosis, Surgery, pp 120–126. Philadelphia, WB Saunders, 1990.

Davidson MR, Schuler BS: Skin curette and the treatment of plantar verrucae. J Am Podiatr Med Assoc 66:331–335, 1976.

Dockery GL, Nilson RZ: Intralesional injections. Clin Podiatr Med Surg 3:473–485, 1986.

Dockery GL: Podiatric dermatologic therapeutics. In McCarthy DJ, Montgomery R (eds): Podiatric Dermatology, pp 311–335. Baltimore, Williams & Wilkins, 1986.

Ferson MJ, Bell SM: Outbreak of Coxsackie virus A16 hand, foot, and mouth disease in a child day-care center. Am J Public Health 81:1675–1676, 1991.

Fisher AA: Severe systemic and local reactions to topical podophyllin application. Cutis 28:233–235, 1981.

Goette DK: Topical chemotherapy with 5-fluorouracil. J Am Acad Dermatol 6:663, 1981.

Habif TP, Graf FA: Extirpation of subungual and periungual warts by blunt dissection. J Dermatol Surg Oncol 7:553–555, 1981.

Heaton CL: Herpes simplex. In Moschella SL, Hurley HJ (eds): Dermatology, 3rd ed, pp 791–796. Philadelphia, WB Saunders, Philadelphia, 1992.

Johnson RE, Johnson JC, Kloberdanz SJ, Morrill MJ: Recombinant α-interferon and verruca plantaris: A review of the literature. J Am Podiatr Med Assoc 81:253–257, 1991.

Kirby PK: Human papillomavirus infection. In Moschella SL, Hurley HJ (eds): Dermatology, 3rd ed, pp 818–830. Philadelphia, WB Saunders, 1992.

Laskin OL: Acyclovir and suppression of frequently recurring herpetic whitlow. Ann Intern Med 102:494–495, 1985.

Litt JZ: Don't excise—exorcize: Treatment for subungual and periungual warts. Cutis 22:673–676, 1978.

Mancuso JR, Abramow SP, Dimichino BR, Landsman MJ: Carbon dioxide laser management of plantar verruca: A 6-year follow-up survey. J Foot Surg 30:238–243, 1991.

Markus T, Krell B, Reinherz R: CO_2 laser techniques in destruction of verrucae plantaris: Discussion of the blister technique, a more complete method of wart ablation. J Foot Surg 27:217–221, 1988.

McCarthy DJ, Tate R, Rusin J: Intradermal use of 5-fluorouracil in human pedal verrucae. J Am Podiatr Assoc 69:587–597, 1979.

McCarthy DJ, Berlin SJ: The ultrastructural effects of 5-fluorouracil in the management of pedal verrucae. J Am Podiatr Assoc 72:402–411, 1982.

McCarthy DJ: Therapeutic considerations in the treatment of pedal verrucae. Clin Podiatr Med Surg 3:433–448, 1986.

McGregor RR, Wehr GV: Blunt dissection of plantar verrucae using a new instrument. J Am Podiatr Assoc 64:92–96, 1974.

McKendrick M, McGill J, White J: Oral acyclovir in acute herpes zoster. BMJ 293:1529–1532, 1986.

Oranje AF, Folkers E: The Tzanck smear: Old, but still of inestimable value. Pediatr Dermatol 5:127–129, 1988.

Pringle WM, Helms BC: Treatment of plantar warts by blunt dissection. Arch Dermatol 108:79–82, 1973.

Samitz MH, Dana AS: Cutaneous Lesions of the Lower Extremities, pp 54–55. Philadelphia, JB Lippincott, 1971.

Shumer SM, O'Keefe EJ: Bleomycin in the treatment of recalcitrant warts. J Am Acad Dermatol 9:91–95, 1983.

Thiers BH: Herpes zoster and postherpetic neuralgia. In Newcomer V, Young E (eds): Geriatric Dermatology, pp 355–361. New York, Igaku-Shoin, 1989.

Thiers BH, Sahn EE: Varicella-zoster virus infections. In Moschella SL, Hurleys HJ (eds): Dermatology, 3rd ed, pp 797–806. Philadelphia, WB Saunders, 1992.

Thomas I, Janniger CK: Hand, foot, and mouth disease. Pediatr Dermatol 52:265–266, 1993.

Tomczak RL, Hake DH: Near fatal systemic toxicity from local injection of podophyllin for pedal verrucae treatment. J Foot Surg 31:36–42, 1992.

Torre D: Understanding the relationship between lateral spread of freeze and depth of freeze. J Dermatol Surg Oncol 5:51–53, 1979.

Valinsky MS, Hettinger DF, Gennett PM: Treatment of verrucae via radio wave surgery. J Am Podiatr Med Assoc 80:482–487, 1990.

Vardy DA, Baadsgaard O, Hansen ER, Lisby S, Vejsgaard GL: The cellular immune response to human papillomavirus infection. Int J Dermatol 29:603–610, 1990.

Warszawer-Schvarcz L: Treatment of plantar warts with banana skin. Plast Reconstr Surg 68:975–978, 1981.

8

INFESTATIONS, STINGS, AND BITES

INTRODUCTION

There are thousands of mites, bugs, crawling and flying insects, and other creatures that infest, bite, and sting humans. Some of these encounters are to the lower extremities, particularly to the feet and region around the ankles. Wearing shoes and socks can help protect these areas from some potentially harmful insects, which may account for the lower incidence of bites on the lower extremity than on other areas of the body. The conditions described in this chapter vary from infestations of mites, such as scabies, to stings from insects and injury from marine life, such as the jellyfish or sea urchin. Other injuries and infestations include spider bites, ant bites, tick and flea bites, and creeping eruptions.

MITES

Human scabies is a contagious disease caused by the itch mite, *Sarcoptes scabiei* var. *hominis,* which produces highly characteristic lesions when it involves the skin. It may evoke a variety of cutaneous lesions, such as macules, papules, vesicles, pustules, bullae, nodules, and scaling plaques, which may be confused with the lesions of many other skin diseases. The mite is capable of completing its life cycle in humans, and it may remain indefinitely unless an effective topical treatment is employed. The female mite does most of the damage; the male mite is smaller and does not burrow. The female mite is oval and ventrally flat and measures 300 to 450 μm long. The pregnant female mite burrows into the stratum corneum and deposits her eggs and fecal material (scybala). Scybala are dark, oval masses that are easily seen with the eggs when burrow scrapings are examined under a microscope. They may act as an irritant and be responsible for some of the itching. Dur-

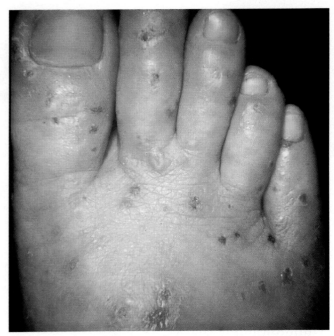

F i g u r e 8 – 2   Scabies. Close-up of infestation on the feet showing vesicles, papules, and excoriations, and the characteristic "burrow" located at the base of the second digit.

ing its 30-day life cycle, the female mite continues to burrow and lay eggs each day. After the completion of egg laying the female dies. The eggs hatch into larvae in 2 or 3 days and promptly emerge on the surface. The larvae reach maturity in 14 to 17 days, and copulation occurs in the adult mites. After impregnation the females then burrow into the skin to start a new life cycle.

Scabies is characterized by small papular pruritic lesions with burrows that contain the female mite and the larvae and eggs. The burrows are slightly elevated, and a vesicle or pustule may be found at the distal end proximal to which the organism itself may be found. These lesions are most commonly seen on the fingers, palms, wrist, axillae, genitalia, buttocks, lower legs, and feet (Fig. 8–1). Infants and young children tend to have more vesicles on the palms and soles. The primary lesions (vesicles) and the elementary lesions (burrows) contain the female mite and eggs. The vesicles are isolated, pinpoint, and filled with serous fluid. Small papules usually represent a hypersensitive reaction or area that has been scratched and rarely contain mites. The burrow is linear, curved, or irregular. The lesions are usually elevated and are the active portion of the infestation (Fig. 8–2). Secondary lesions may confuse the clinical presentation. These lesions result from infection or damage caused by scratching the skin lesions. A hypersensitivity reaction rather than a foreign-body response may be responsible for the lesions, which may delay recognition of the condition. This sensitization begins about 1 month after onset of the infestation. During this 30-day period the mites may be burrowing on the skin without causing pruritus or discomfort. The severe itching develops owing to the sensitization of the

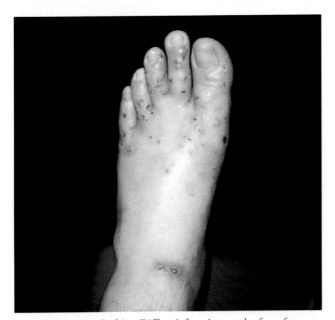

F i g u r e 8 – 1   Scabies. Diffuse infestation on the feet of a young patient. The hands and groin were also involved.

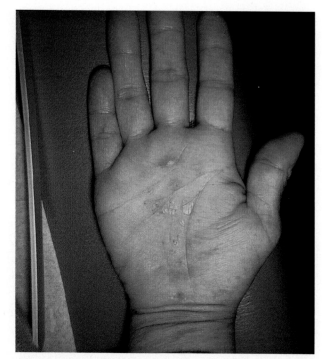

Figure 8 – 3 **Scabies.** Typical appearance on the hand. This is a very common location in men.

host. Small erosions or excoriations may be common. Scaling and eczematous inflammation may result from self-treatment. The main symptom of scabies is intense pruritus. The itching is more pronounced in the evening or at night and after warm baths when the mites appear to be more active. Scratching the lesions causes difficulty in isolating the mite owing to excessive excoriations and the development of secondary bacterial infection. When the condition has been present for a long period of time, eczematization, lichenification, impetigo, and furunculosis may also be present.

Scabies is usually contracted by close personal contact such as sleeping together. It is not transmitted by casual contact, such as shaking hands. If one member of the family becomes infested, the other members may become infested quickly unless treatment intervenes. Infestations may be sexually transmitted between partners. The more parasites the individual carries, the more likely is transmission of the condition to other persons. The average number of mites per patient is 11 and usually less than 20. Transmission is less frequent by the common use of contaminated towels, bed linens, and clothing. The female mite can survive only a few days away from the warm skin of a human.

The distribution of the lesions is characteristic in humans. The most prominent sites are the interdigital spaces of the hands and feet, the flexor surface of the wrists, the elbows, the anterior axillary folds, the breast region in females, the abdominal region of the belt line, the external genitalia in males, and the palms and soles (Fig. 8–3). There is a lack of infestation of the head and neck in most adults. Infants, however, sometimes have

lesions in this area. The lesions may be sparse and less characteristic in persons of excellent hygiene who are daily bathers. One or two of the aforementioned sites almost always are affected. In neglected cases, the lesions may be very extensive and cover large areas of the body.

In extremely severe cases, there may be heavy crusting of the skin on the hands and feet (Fig. 8–4) and there may be excessive nail involvement (Fig. 8–5). This form of scabies is termed *crusted (Norwegian) scabies*, and it is usually seen in elderly patients or in patients with alcoholism, neurological disease, mental disorders, nutritional disorders, or infectious disease, and in immunosuppressed patients. Itching or nocturnal pruritus is usually absent, but in some patients it may be severe. Examination of the crusts shows a large number of mites in all stages of development.

Another clinical variation is termed *nodular scabies*. In this disorder, there are several reddish brown pruritic nodules occurring as the only manifestation of scabies (Fig. 8–6). These nodular infestations usually involve covered areas such as the buttocks, groin, scrotum, axillae, and occasionally the elbows and lower extremi-

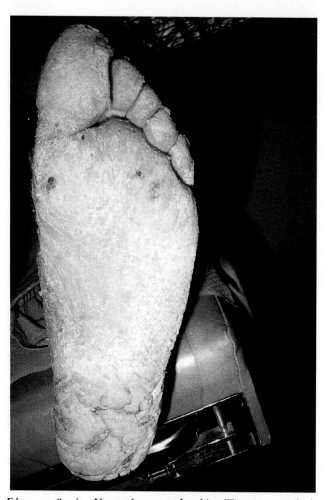

Figure 8 – 4 **Norwegian crusted scabies.** There is severe thickening of the tissues. The crusts are filled with hundreds of mites.

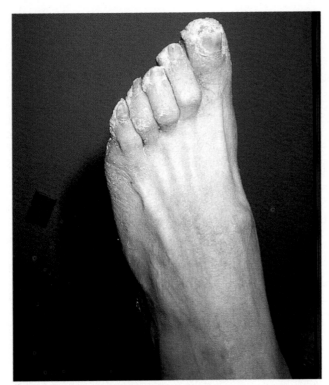

Figure 8–5   Norwegian crusted scabies. The toenails are involved.

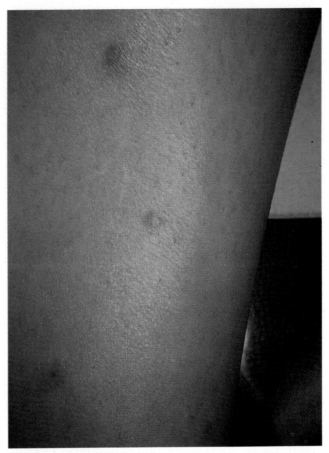

Figure 8–6   Nodular scabies. Diagnosis may be difficult without biopsy.

ties. Because of its clinical presentation this condition may be misdiagnosed as insect bites. The mites are often very difficult to identify in the nodules and are usually found in biopsy specimens. The nodules may still be evident for many weeks or months after the mites are eliminated. If there is persistent itching in the nodules, they may respond to intralesional injections of corticosteroid and a local anesthetic agent.

The definitive diagnosis of scabies is made only by the demonstration of *Sarcoptes scabiei* in a fresh preparation under the light microscope with a low-power objective (Fig. 8–7). This is done by shaving off the burrow with a No. 15 surgical scalpel blade. The blade is held perpendicular to the skin surface of the burrow, and the top is scraped vigorously. The adult female mite is readily seen with a good light microscope or may be identified with a bright light and hand-held magnification lens. The tunnel of an inhabited burrow can be slit open gently by the surgical blade and the mite transferred to a dry glass slide for direct microscopic examination. Some physicians prefer to use mineral oil or saline so that the mite can move and be identified by its activity. Potassium hydroxide may be applied in an attempt to remove the associated stratum corneum. This preparation is not heated as is done in a slide mount of fungal elements.

Treatment must be done thoroughly and conscientiously with good patient compliance and understanding. There are several recognized treatment programs that are very effective and safe, if used as directed. No matter which therapeutic agent is utilized a number of

principles apply. One is to establish the correct diagnosis by finding the organism. Second, the amount of drug should be limited to only what is needed and the concentration should be reduced in children to prevent overusing the local medication. Finally, patients must

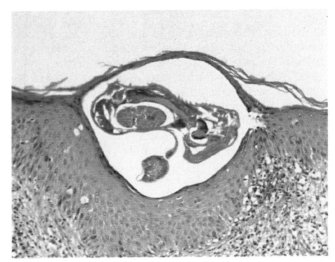

Figure 8–7   Scabies. Microscopic presentation of burrow with female scabies mite.

understand the treatment program and what they are supposed to do. They need to understand that overtreatment can lead to toxic reactions, especially in the debilitated, elderly, or very young.

The three major forms of medications for the treatment of scabies are (1) lindane (1% gamma benzene hexachloride), (2) crotamiton (10% *N*-ethyl-o-crotonotoluide [Eurax]), and (3) sulfur ointment (5% precipitated sulfur).

Lindane 1% (available in cream, shampoo, and lotion) is an extensively used and relatively effective scabicide. One application is usually sufficient to kill the organisms. It should be emphasized to the patient to treat all areas, especially between the fingers and toes, the groin, and the axillae. If there are scabetic lesions on the head and neck (usually seen only in children), they are also treated, but great care is used to avoid the eyes, nose, and mouth. The physician dispenses about 30 g (1 oz) for adults with instructions for the patients to apply the medication to the entire body from the neck down after bathing and to leave it on for 8 to 12 hours (overnight). After the overnight period the patient should bathe or shower to thoroughly remove the medication. The entire family should be treated at the same time. The dosage for children should be diluted by half and applied only for 2 hours or as directed by the physician. If there are any obvious new lesions after 1 week the treatment may be repeated.

Crotamiton is also a very effective and popular scabicide. It is applied in the same fashion as lindane but reapplied in 24 hours, and the patient is instructed to wash 24 hours after the second application of the medication. Therefore, the drug is in contact with the skin for 48 hours before it is washed off. Although it has not been confirmed, crotamiton may have antipruritic properties.

Sulfur ointment, 5%, is not as popular because it is messy, is odoriferous, and stains clothing easily. An acceptable alternative is the water-soluble base in place of the ointment base. The medication is applied for three consecutive nights, and the patient bathes 24 hours after the last application. Because it is considered less toxic it is still frequently recommended for infants and pregnant women; however, the safety of sulfur has never been accurately established.

Alternative medications for the treatment of scabies infestations include permethrin, thiabendazole, and coal tar. Permethrin (pyrethrins 0.33%, A-200 Pyrinate) is a synthetic pyrethrin that is derived from the chrysanthemum. Permethrin 5% cream is a rapid-acting pediculicidal agent that is also very effective against scabies. It is applied to the skin at night and left on for 8 to 12 hours and washed off during a shower or bath the next morning. One application is highly effective and, if necessary, a second application may be repeated a week later if symptoms are not improved. Thiabendazole is an anthelmintic primarily used in the treatment of cutaneous larva migrans. For the treatment of scabies, thiabendazole 10% (Mintezol) suspension is applied twice daily for 5 days and then washed off completely or a 10-day course of oral thiabendazole (25 mg/kg/day) is given.

Several complicating factors of scabies infestations include contact dermatitis, intense pruritus, long-term nodule formation, and secondary infection. Supportive measures may be given in the form of topical corticosteroids, antihistamines, or antibiotics. Patients should be told early in the treatment program that they should not expect itching to stop immediately even though the scabicide may be totally effective. Patients should be seen 2 weeks after scabicidal therapy to determine compliance or possible reinfestation. Special types of scabies such as nodular scabies, persistent scabies, or crusted Norwegian scabies may be very difficult to treat, and these cases might best be managed by a dermatologist.

SPIDERS

Two species of spiders in the United States, class Arachnida, have venom strong enough to produce significant toxic and cutaneous effects in humans. Other spiders may produce cutaneous lesions to a lesser degree. The two main genera are *Loxosceles* and *Latrodectus*. Five different species of *Loxosceles* have been associated with cutaneous loxoscelism (a morbid condition following the spider bite beginning with a painful erythematous vesicle and progressing to a gangrenous slough of the affected area). The most frequent offender appears to be *Loxosceles reclusa*, the brown recluse spider. This spider has six eyes in three pairs and is sometimes referred to as the violin or fiddleback spider because of the violin-shaped design on its dorsal cephalothorax. The brown recluse spider hibernates during the winter months, and most bites occur during the spring and summer and occasionally during the early fall. The web is small and haphazard and sometimes placed in very small areas. The habitat of this spider includes old buildings, storage sheds, garages, and wood piles, and it will move into occupied homes to nest in closets, behind hanging pictures, in stored clothing areas, under beds, and in basements. This makes the spider relatively more accessible to human encounters than other spiders.

The brown recluse spider is 5- to 25-mm long and yellow-tan to dark brown, with a characteristic, dark violin-shaped design, as mentioned previously, located on its back (Fig. 8–8). The broad base of the violin shape is near the head with the stem pointing toward the abdomen. The bites of the brown recluse spider are usually reported to have occurred when a person was working around storage areas or cleaning out the garage. Other scenarios include putting on boots, coveralls, or jackets that have been hanging in storage closets or basements for some time and in which the spider is residing. Bites typically occur on the hands, arms, feet, legs, and buttocks. The actual bite may not be noticed, or there may be minor stinging or burning after an instantaneous sharp pain similar to a bee sting. The variability of the bite may be due to the amount of venom injected or the age or overall medical status of

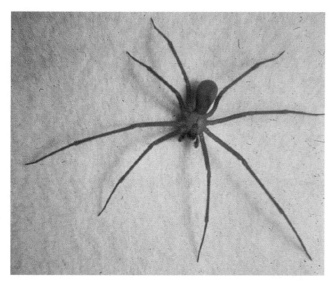

Figure 8–8   Brown recluse spider, *Loxosceles reclusa*, with characteristic fiddle-shaped markings on the cephalothorax.

the victim. The venom contains sphingomyelinase, which acts on the cell membranes and is probably responsible for the dermonecrotic activity, and a lipase that induces disseminated intravascular coagulopathy.

Two general types of reactions occur after the brown recluse spider bite: (1) the localized cutaneous injury (loxoscelism) and (2) the systemic reaction with intravascular hemolysis, acute vasculitis, platelet thrombi, and leukocyte infiltrates. Severe nausea, vomiting, fever, malaise, arthralgia, and generalized weakness may all occur. This severe reaction is rarely fatal and most frequently occurs in children and debilitated patients. Most bites result in local cutaneous reactions that have a benign course.

The local cutaneous reaction to the bite may be minor, with mild to moderate pruritus and an urticarial plaque or very small area of necrosis (Fig. 8–9). In many of these cases the patient will rub or excoriate the area owing to the itching and burning. This effect may make

the clinical diagnosis more difficult. In more involved cases there is increased swelling and erythema with an increase in the pain (Fig. 8–10). With a greater amount of venom the tissue reaction is more intense and cutaneous loxoscelism occurs. The process starts with the development and expansion of a blue-gray, macular halo around the bite site. A cyanotic vesicle or bulla may appear, and the superficial skin may be rapidly infarcted. Pain may be severe at this point. The violaceous macule with a blue center may widen, show extensions into adjacent tissue, and start to indent in the center (Fig. 8–11). The necrotic tissue may extend deeply into muscle. The dead tissue sloughs, leaving a very deep, indolent ulcer (Fig. 8–12). A closer evaluation of the ulcer shows that it has a necrotic, thick, black eschar with ragged edges (Fig. 8–13). There is usually a surrounding zone of erythema that becomes violaceous, and lymphangitis or lymphadenopathy may be present. In a few cases, usually involving children, the tissue reaction is much more severe, with extensive tissue necrosis and subsequent generalized systemic symptoms (Fig. 8–14). Rarely, the systemic reaction progresses with peripheral edema, significant discoloration, and

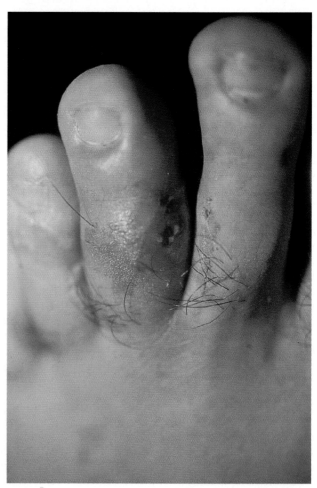

Figure 8–10   Brown recluse spider bite. Local tissue reaction on the toe with swelling, erythema, and pain that occurred 3 days after the envenomation.

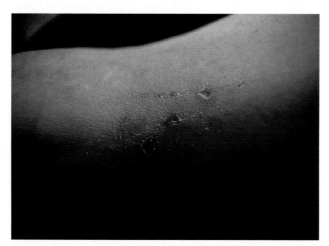

Figure 8–9   Spider bite. Early cutaneous changes with secondary excoriations due to pruritus.

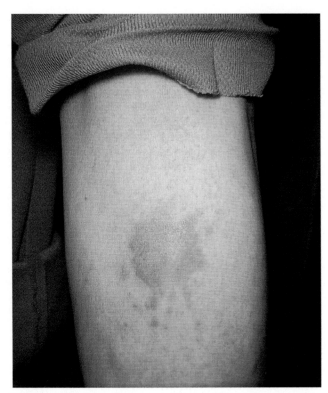

Figure 8-11 Brown recluse spider bite. Cutaneous loxoscelism with a small plaque of necrotic tissue occurring at the anterior calf.

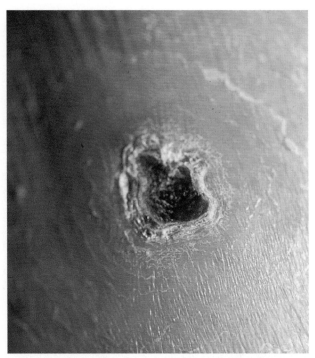

Figure 8-13 Brown recluse spider bite. Close-up shows that the center of the necrotic plaque is sunken below the normal skin ("sinking infarct"). The ulcerated lesion has a firmly attached, thick, black eschar with a ragged edge. (Courtesy of Dr. E. Mollahan.)

generalized ecchymosis (Fig. 8–15). Within 12 to 24 hours after the bite, the patients frequently complain of fever, chills, nausea, vomiting, muscle cramps, joint pain, generalized weakness, and, in some cases, urticaria or hives. The specific diagnosis is made by visual identification of the spider. In many cases, no spider is actually seen or captured but the patient's description

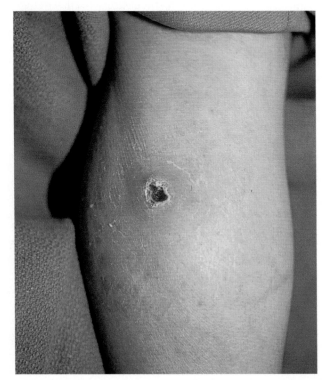

Figure 8-12 Brown recluse spider bite. A deep indolent ulcer occurs on the posterior calf as the tissue necrosis proceeds, in this case, at 10 days after the bite. (Courtesy of Dr. E. Mollahan.)

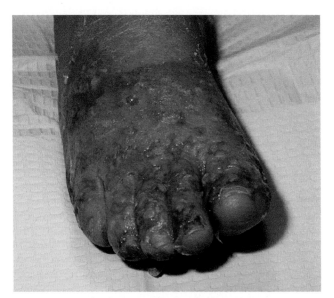

Figure 8-14 Brown recluse spider bite. Extensive tissue necrosis is evident on the forefoot area in this child. Subsequently, very slow healing took place. (Courtesy of Dr. Bradley Whitaker.)

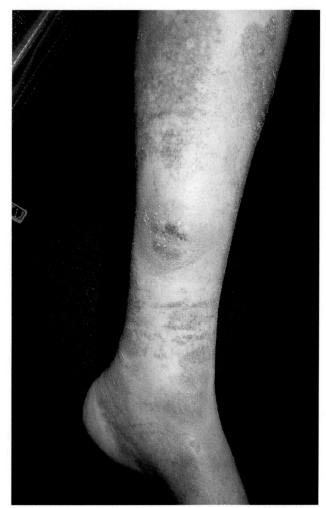

Figure 8–15   Brown recluse spider bite. The bite occurred on the medial lower leg in this girl. There were severe tense edema, ecchymosis, and discoloration of the entire leg, and the characteristic area of the original bite. The bite area ulcerated and required an extended period of time to heal completely.

of activities immediately before the incident combined with the clinical presentation is used to make a presumptive diagnosis.

Treatment of the brown recluse spider bite is symptomatic in lesser involved cases with rest, cold packs, pain control, and antibiotics to prevent infection. In more severe cases, the addition of elevation of the limb, antihistamines for the pruritus, tetanus toxoid (if necessary), and dapsone may be required. Dapsone, a leukocyte inhibitor, is given at 50 to 100 mg/day and may be helpful in preventing severe necrosis. Dapsone may also prevent severe perivasculitis with polymorphonuclear leukocyte infiltration in viscerocutaneous loxoscelism. Treatments and activities that should *not* be instituted include hot compresses, strenuous exercise, early incision or excision of the lesion, and localized compression. Hot packs and exercise will make the lesion much worse. Early incision or excision of the le-

sion will induce more complications and spreading of necrosis. However, once the lesion has passed through all phases of conversion to a dry, necrotic lesion and all of the secondary and systemic symptoms have resolved, surgical excision of the area with skin grafting is the treatment of choice for larger (>1 cm) lesions.

The black widow spider, *Latrodectus mactans*, is one of the most feared of the spider family; however, the fatality rate of those bitten is less than 1%. The black widow spider has eight eyes and is shiny black, usually with a red or orange double triangle or hourglass design on the ventral surface of the abdomen (Fig. 8–16). The female is larger (up to 4 cm total length) than the male, and the venom of the black widow is a neurotoxin that produces symptoms of general toxemia 10 to 15 minutes after the bite. The actual bite may not be felt or may produce an immediate sharp or burning pain that disappears promptly. The black widow injects venom into its victim through its fangs, and if the bite area is examined immediately the two small red fang marks may still be seen. In most cases reported, no local puncture sites are noticed. Local tissue reaction is minimum but may include mild erythema or edema. After the latency period of about 15 minutes to 1 hour the characteristic symptoms appear. Symptoms include muscle spasms and cramps, especially of the legs and abdomen, numbness gradually spreading from the inoculation site to involve the entire torso, marked abdominal rigidity, headache, sweating, increased salivation, eyelid edema, diffuse macular rash, increased deep tendon reflexes, nausea, and vomiting. This series of symptoms is collectively termed *latrodectism*. The acute symptoms last for up to 48 hours and gradually decrease in 2 or 3 days. In some cases there are residual symptoms of generalized weakness, numbness, pruritus, and transient muscle spasms that last for several weeks or months after the acute stage.

Treatment of the black widow spider bite includes cool compresses, ice packs, analgesics (aspirin for mild pain; morphine for severe pain), muscle relaxants (me-

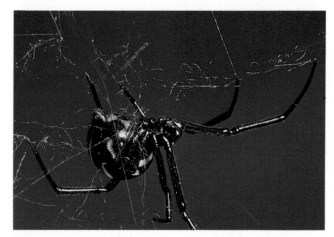

Figure 8–16   Black widow spider, *Latrodectus mactans*, with characteristic "hourglass" marking on the underside of the abdomen.

thocarbamol or diazepam), intravenous calcium gluconate (10 mL of 10% solution), and in very severe cases or in the young or debilitated patient, antivenin *(Lactrodectus mactans)* (available from Merck, Sharp and Dohme, West Point, PA), 2.5 mL intramuscularly. The antivenin is prepared from horse serum, and therefore a 1-mL vial of normal horse serum for eye sensitivity testing is supplied. [Some patients may be allergic to the serum, and this quick test is supplied to check.] Treatments that are *not* recommended include the application of hot packs to the bite site, lancing or suction of the injection area, tourniquet application proximal to the site, or surgical incision or excision of tissue.

ANTS

Ants belong to the order Hymenoptera, which also includes bees, wasps, and hornets. The three main stinging and biting ants are the fire ants, harvester ants, and pharaoh ants. The fire ant, *Solenopsis* species, is prominent in the southeastern Unitied States and its method of stinging produces a typical cluster of cutaneous lesions (Fig. 8–17). The fire ant grasps the skin with its jaws while it pivots and stings repeatedly with its abdominal stinger in a circular fashion. Two red puncta may be seen at the center of the stings. Immediate pain results, which usually quickly resolves. Small red wheals form and convert to vesicles within 3 to 4 hours. After 24 hours the lesions typically are pustules with an erythematous rim that will resolve in about 10 days. Multiple ant stings may cause a more serious systemic allergic reaction similar to those caused by other Hymenoptera species (Fig. 8–18). The bite area is treated

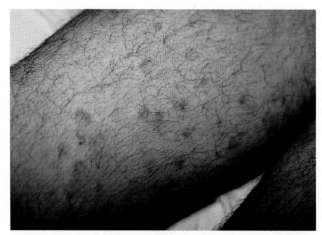

Figure 8 – 1 8   Fire ant stings. Multiple stings may cause generalized edema and systemic symptoms.

with cool compresses, antipruritic lotions, oral antihistamines, and scrupulous cleansing of the area to prevent secondary bacterial infection.

Harvester ants (*Pogonomyrmex* species) are large (up to 1 cm long), red-brown, and sometimes winged ants found in the southern portion of the United States. Like the fire ants, the harvester ants may attack in large numbers and inflict vicious stings. The stings are usually several in number and tend to form a linear pattern (Fig. 8–19). Unlike the fire ant bites the lesions of the harvester ant do not form pustules and they usually clear within a few days. Treatment is of symptoms only.

The pharaoh ant (*Monomorium* species) is found in the warm southern states. This small brown ant may inflict a small but painful sting that is considered milder than the stings of the fire ant and the harvester ant. The sting area generally stays red for several days and then resolves. No treatment is usually necessary.

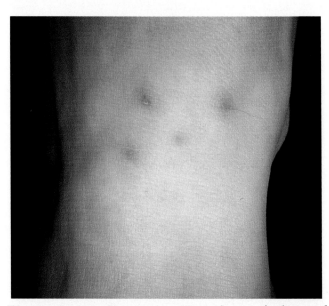

Figure 8 – 1 7   Fire ant stings. Fire ant bites on the dorsum of the foot are diagnosed by evidence of typical circle of stings with two tiny red dots in the center where the jaws were attached.

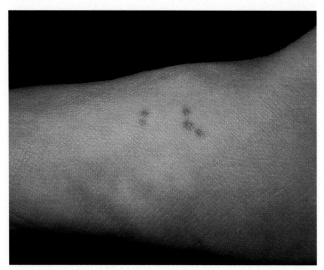

Figure 8 – 1 9   Harvester ant stings. These stings are typically very red and may form a linear pattern.

STINGING INSECTS

The bumblebee, honeybee, wasp, hornet, and yellow jacket are the more prominent stinging members of the order Hymenoptera. The combined stinger unit and venom sac is a modified ovipositor apparatus, and only the honeybee leaves its barbed stinger and venom sac in the wound. The stingers of the others in this group are not barbed and may be used multiple times. Hymenoptera venoms contain histamines and other vasoactive agents, which are both hemolytic and neurotoxic. Lower extremity stings usually occur in the spring and summer, and patients are frequently in shorts and shoeless while mowing the grass or working in the garden. The clinical picture after a sting in a nonallergic individual includes moderate to severe pain, a localized wheal, erythema, pruritus, and edema (Fig. 8–20).

Because the honeybee leaves its barbed stinger, venom gland, and viscera imbedded in the skin, it should all be scraped away with a knife or fingernail. Forceps and tweezers should not be used. If the apparatus is grasped or handled, the venom sac will compress and inject additional venom into the skin, causing a more severe sting (Fig. 8–21). In some patients a more extensive local reaction may occur marked by severe pain, prolonged edema, and intense erythema (Fig. 8–22). These symptoms usually last for more than 2 days and may extend for as long as a week. Infection and cellulitis may also be seen in these patients. Systemic allergic reactions range from mild to moderate to severe. The moderate reactions include malaise, nausea, vomiting, dizziness, and wheezing. The most severe hy-

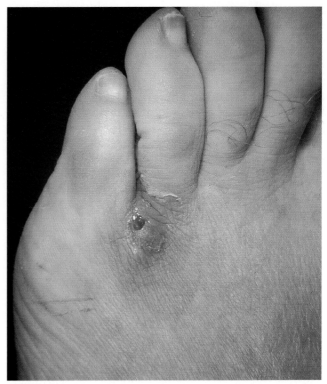

Figure 8–21   Honeybee sting. The stinger apparatus was grasped with the fingers, injecting the area again and causing an intense local reaction. The stinger was then removed along with a piece of the skin.

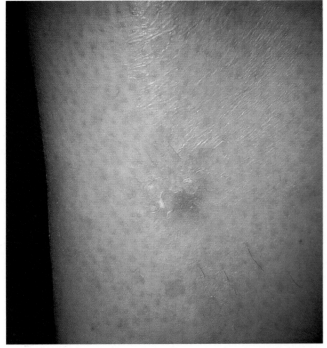

Figure 8–20   Bumblebee sting. Local reaction on the lower leg with blister formation and surrounding wheal in a nonallergic individual.

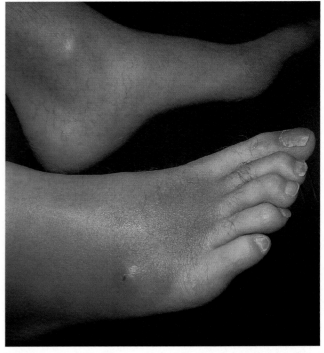

Figure 8–22   Hornet sting. Note intense erythema, edema, and pain in a patient with hypersensitivity to bee stings.

persensitivity reactions are anaphylactic and involve hypotension, bronchospasm, and laryngeal edema.

Localized stings in nonallergic individuals are treated with cool compresses or ice, elevation of the part, and a topical lotion composed of equal parts of water and meat tenderizer. Localized reactions in allergic patients are treated in the same manner but these patients are given antihistamines to reduce the inflammatory component of the reaction. In delayed local reactions that appear after 24 hours, a short course of systemic corticosteroids may be very effective. In more severe allergic manifestations in adults, subcutaneous injections of aqueous epinephrine 1:1000 in a dosage of 0.3 to 0.5 mL are given. This injection may be repeated in 20-minute intervals for a total of three injections. Prepackaged bee-sting kits with epinephrine (1:1000)–loaded syringes, tourniquets, and antihistamine tablets are available. Persons with known sensitivity should be advised to keep one of these kits available at home and during travel to prevent serious anaphylactic episodes.

TICKS

The tick bite is usually inconsequential by itself, but the tick may act as a carrier of several organisms that cause rickettsial, spirochetal, bacterial, and parasitic infections. Some of the more important conditions and diseases include Rocky Mountain spotted fever, relapsing fever, Colorado tick fever, Lyme disease, erythema chronicum migrans, tularemia, tick bite paralysis, and Western equine encephalitis. Ticks are blood-sucking ectoparasites that typically live in grass, brush, and wooded areas. Adults are usually infested on the legs and feet while walking through heavy grass or in the woods.

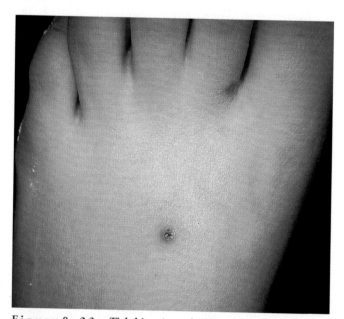

Figure 8–23   Tick bite. An embedded tick on the dorsal surface of the foot was noticed after a hunting trip. There was no pain, but mild pruritus was present.

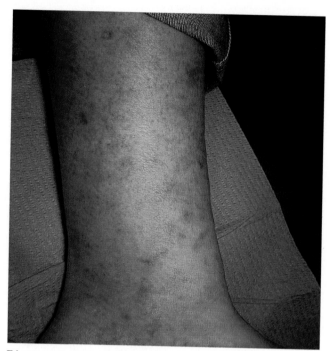

Figure 8–24   Rocky Mountain spotted fever. A generalized macular petechial eruption of the entire cutaneous area includes the palms and soles.

The adult tick can reach 1 cm in length and has eight legs and a large teardrop- or oval-shaped body. The two main families of ticks are soft-bodied and hard-bodied ticks. Hard ticks are vectors for most of the tick-borne diseases. Ticks are dark, grayish brown to black with a leather-like shell. Hard ticks may remain attached to the victim for up to 10 days, whereas the soft tick will usually release in a few hours after filling with blood. The tick bite itself is usually painless and may go unnoticed until a lump is found or a local reaction of an urticarial wheal or a pruritic area forms around the tick (Fig. 8–23).

Rocky Mountain spotted fever occurs in many parts of the United States but is prevalent in Oklahoma, Texas, and the South Atlantic states. This condition is caused by *Rickettsia rickettsii* transmitted in the tick bite. The infection is seasonal, with most cases reported between April 1 and September 30, which corresponds to the increased activity of ticks. The principal vector in the western states is the wood tick, *Dermacentor andersoni*; in the eastern states it is the dog tick, *Dermacentor variabilis*; in the south central states it is the Lone Star tick, *Amblyomma americanum*. The tick will transmit the disease after it has been attached for at least 6 hours. The incubation period ranges from 3 to 12 days, and the onset of early symptoms is abrupt with fever, chills, headache, myalgia, arthralgia, and generalized rash. The rash usually appears first on the wrists and ankles. The forearms, palms, and soles become involved within hours, and then symptoms become generalized (Fig. 8–24). In the beginning of the rash presentation the macules will blanch with pressure, but this phenomenon ceases when the lesions become petechial in 3 or 4 days. In blacks the rash may be very hard to see; in about 15% of all cases the rash does not appear (spotless fever), making the diagnosis even more difficult. Symptoms and signs include fever, headache, myalgia, arthralgia, cough, nausea, vomiting, abdominal cramps, rash, and generalized illness.

Prevention of tick bites is best performed by wearing protective socks and boots with pant cuffs tucked into the socks while outdoors in tick country, inspection of all skin areas regularly for ticks, and treating socks and other outer clothing with repellents, such as permethrin. Treatment involves the immediate removal of the tick once it has been identified.

Tick removal requires care and should not be performed with the fingers because of the danger of contracting a rickettsial infection. The soft-bodied ticks are much easier to remove than the hard-bodied ticks that cement their mouth parts into the skin. The proper technique for tick removal is to use forceps, tweezers, or thread attached as close to the skin surface as possible and pull upward with steady even pressure for several minutes until the tick is removed. Care should be taken not to squeeze the tick's body, which will cause infectious fluids to enter the skin. The tweezers should not be rotated or twisted during the removal process because this may allow the forepart to break off within the skin. If the mouth parts do not come away or portions are left in the skin, they may be removed with a small punch biopsy. If the mouth parts are left below the skin surface, they may produce a nodule known as a tick-bite granuloma.

Once the tick has been removed the area should be cleansed well with warm water and soap and disinfected with isopropyl alcohol. Additional treatment should include tetracycline for all patients older than 8 years of age (except pregnant women) or chloramphenicol for children younger than 8 years and pregnant women. Both drugs are given at 50 to 100 mg/kg/day with a maximum of 2 g/day for children and 4 g/day for adults. Treatment is continued for up to 1 week after the patient becomes afebrile. Treatments that should *not* be performed include applying hot packs, handling ticks with the bare hands, twisting the tick off, cutting or puncturing the tick's body, applying hot items to the tick's body (hot items tend to induce the tick to regurgitate infected fluids into the skin), or giving the patient sulfonamides, because they appear to enhance rickettsial infections.

Colorado tick fever is a nonexanthematous febrile disease occurring in the Rocky Mountain regions of the United States where the tick vector (*Dermacentor andersoni*) of the causative virus is prevalent.

Tick-borne relapsing fever occurs worldwide with increasing incidence in the Rocky Mountain regions of the United States. Many different species of ticks serve as vectors for transmission of the condition of this acute septicemic process caused by one of several species of spirochete of the genus *Borrelia*. As the name implies, this condition is characterized by recurrent paroxysms of fever with or without a body rash. The onset of the fever is abrupt and may reach a very high temperature (>104°F) with chills, headache, abdominal cramps, nausea, vomiting, myalgia, and dry cough. Treatment is with erythromycin or tetracycline, either of which is more effective in the clearing of spirochetemia than the penicillins. Pretreatment with corticosteroids and acetaminophen reduces most toxicity.

Lyme disease is a multisystemic condition that involves the skin, nervous system, joints, and heart. It is caused by a tick-borne spirochete, *Borrelia burgdorferi*. This malady is named for Lyme, Connecticut, where the first cases were reported in children. Lyme disease is now recognized on six continents and in at least 20 countries; persons of all ages and both sexes are equally affected. Most of the reported cases in the United States are from Massachusetts to Maryland in the northeast and in Wisconsin and Minnesota in the upper midwest. Many other states have reported cases of Lyme disease as well. The clinical picture is one of headache, stiff neck, myalgia, arthralgia, fatigue, and fever (with a temperature of up to 105°F). Lyme disease has three primary stages. Stage 1 (sometimes called the flu-like stage) is the early infection phase with erythema chronicum migrans (85% of cases) at the site of the tick bite with other early symptoms of minor constitutional complaints and regional lymphadenopathy. Stage 2 (the cardiac and neurological stage) is the disseminated infection phase with the characteristic signs and symptoms in the cutaneous system, nervous system, and musculoskeletal sites. Stage 3 (chronic arthritis and neurological syndrome stage) is the late persistent infection phase with severe progressive arthritis, chronic encephalomyelitis, chronic fatigue syndrome, ataxic gait, spastic paresis, and polyradiculopathy.

Routine laboratory testing is not helpful in diagnosing Lyme disease. There may be nonspecific findings, including mild anemia, elevated erythrocyte sedimentation rate, and elevated liver function studies. An IgM-specific response to the spirochetemia is seen 3 weeks after infection. Approximately 6 weeks later there is a slow rise in IgG-specific antibody level, which remains elevated. The early treatment with antibiotics may abolish the antibody response. There may even be no diagnostic levels of antibodies developed in cases of chronic Lyme disease.

Diagnosis is frequently made solely on the knowledge that the individual was bitten by a tick and subsequently developed a skin lesion in the general area. The skin lesion, erythema chronicum migrans, is therefore the most characteristic finding in Lyme disease. Unfortunately, erythema chronicum migrans does not occur in all cases of Lyme disease and may even appear as an isolated case in patients who do not recall any tick bite. The skin lesion begins as a small vesicle or papule at the tick bite site. The bite site may clear, become indurated, or ulcerate. The lesion then slowly enlarges, forming an erythematous ring or oval with a gradually clearing central area. The central clear zone may return to normal skin color or may be slightly blue. The erythematous ring blanches on pressure and may be slightly elevated but does not scale or vesiculate. Over the next few days the erythematous lesion expands rapidly away from the bite area to form a single or double, broad, round-to-oval area of erythema. After about 1 week the lesion starts to clear centrally and the advancing ring may continue for several days or weeks (Fig. 8–25). Many cases involve reports of multiple concentric rings with minimal pruritus and tenderness, although burning has been noted. During the early stage with the skin lesion present, patients may develop fever and minor constitutional symptoms. The lesions usually disappear within 4 weeks of the infection.

Treatment of Lyme disease and erythema chronicum migrans is early administration of oral tetracycline, 250 to 500 mg four times a day, or doxycycline, 100 mg twice a day for 3 weeks. Amoxicillin, 250–500 mg three times a day (20–40 mg/kg/day) for 3 weeks, is recommended for children younger than 8 years of age and in pregnant or lactating women. In patients allergic to the penicillins, erythromycin, 250 mg four times a day (30 mg/kg/day for children) for 30 days is recommended.

FLEAS

The flea is a blood-sucking parasite from the order Siphonaptera, which contains two important groups or families: Pulicidae (human, dog, cat, bird fleas) and Tungidae (sand fleas). Fleas found on the beaches on the eastern coast of the United States and Mexico are frequently called sand fleas, but they are almost always of the Pulicidae family rather than the Tungidae fam-

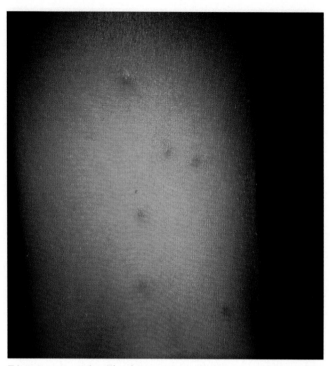

Figure 8–26   Flea bites. Note typical cluster pattern on the lower leg.

ily, which are distributed in South America, Africa, and the West Indies. The human flea, *Pulex irritans*; the dog flea, *Ctenocephalides canis*; the cat flea, *Ctenocephalides felis*; and the bird fleas, *Ceratophyllus gallinae* and *C. columbae,* all feed on humans. Fleas are small, reddish brown to black, hard-bodied, flat-sided, wingless insects that have the ability to jump about 2 feet. The adult flea can survive for several months without eating. They live in rugs, furniture, sand, grass, and pet sleeping areas. Human attacks from fleas are more often from those in the furniture or carpet region than from a pet. Most fleas found on pets prefer their host animal but will occasionally bite humans in the same house. An increase in flea bites is sometimes noticed when the pet is lost or gone from the living area. Flea bites frequently occur on the lower extremities in irregular clusters because the flea likes to sample several adjacent areas while feeding (Fig. 8–26). Individuals at the beach will sometimes get multiple flea bites about the feet and ankles while sitting in the sand (Fig. 8–27). These bites are not from the burrowing sand flea but usually from fleas from an animal. Fleas will also feed in a characteristic linear pattern of three or four bites in a row, sometimes called, "breakfast, lunch, dinner, and bedtime snack" (Fig. 8–28). These papules with a hemorrhagic punctum may be intensely pruritic. In some highly sensitive individuals the papules will evolve into blisters and ulcerate with an intense erythematous border (Fig. 8–29). Impetiginization or secondary bacterial infections may result from scratching these pruritic lesions.

Treatment begins with local skin treatment for the pruritus with topical corticosteroids. Administration of

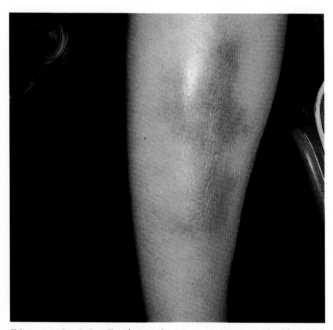

Figure 8–25   Erythema chronicum migrans. A double broad oval of violaceous erythema has slowly migrated from the central area adjacent to the tick bite on the lower leg.

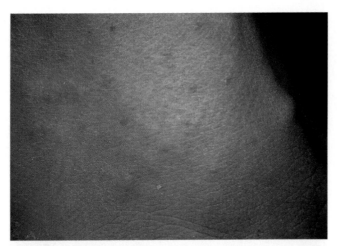

Figure 8–27   Flea bites. Multiple small bites on the ankle were acquired at the beach and are frequently called sand flea attacks.

vitamin B_1 (thiamine), 25 to 50 mg/day in two doses, may be helpful. Oral antihistamines may be necessary in the sensitized individual. If impetiginization or secondary infection has occurred, treatment consists of appropriate oral antibiotics. Elimination of the fleas and larvae from the living environment may be done with insecticide sprays and powders for all suspected flea breeding and living grounds. All sources must be treated, including the pets and their bedding areas. Commercial house foggers are sometimes necessary with a large infestation problem. New products available from veterinarians may be given to dogs to kill the female flea's eggs before they hatch.

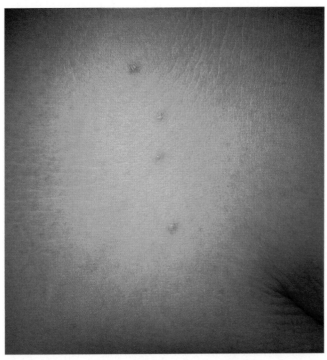

Figure 8–28   Flea bites. These bites occurred in a characteristic pattern of "breakfast, lunch, dinner, and bedtime snack."

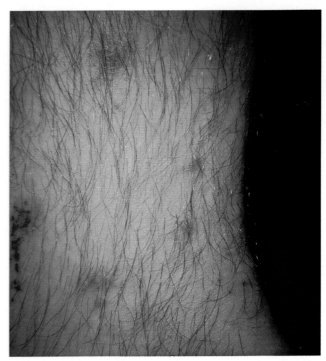

Figure 8–29   Flea bites. These bites occurred on the lower legs in a sensitive individual, resulting in blisters that ulcerated with intense erythematous borders. This lesion was extremely pruritic and caused increased excoriations.

HOOKWORMS

Cutaneous larva migrans is caused by hookworm larvae of various nematode parasites. The cat or dog hookworm, *Ancylostoma braziliense,* is the most common species in the southeastern United States, South America, and many tropical countries. *Ancylostoma canium* is also implicated in the formation of creeping eruptions. The adult nematodes are found in the intestines of dogs and cats, where they deposit ova that are secreted in the feces. The ova hatch into larvae in the sand or soil where they were deposited. The larvae then penetrate human skin that comes into contact with them. This usually occurs as the person is sitting, standing, or lying on the soil or sandy beach. The condition is extremely common on the hands, feet, legs, and buttocks region. As the name implies, the larvae then begin to creep or migrate under the skin, causing an inflammatory reaction in a bizarre pattern (Fig. 8–30). Several larvae may be present in the epidermis, creating many different lines of involvement. Most patients complain of moderate to intense pruritus. In a few sensitive individuals, the larva migrans eruption is accompanied by an intense urticarial reaction and eosinophilia (Fig. 8–31). The larva stays deep in the epidermis directly ahead of the advancing tip of the serpiginous tract. The parasite migrates between the stratum corneum and the stratum germinativum. Because the larva is not in the actual lesion but is ahead of it, biopsy specimens infrequently show the organism. Specimens that are collected approximately 1 cm ahead of the advancing tip may show

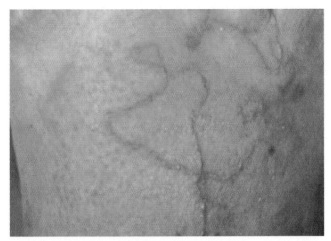

Figure 8–30 Cutaneous larva migrans. Note the characteristic wandering-type pattern of the larva beneath the skin.

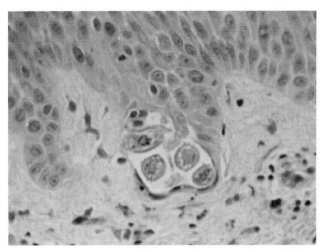

Figure 8–32 Cutaneous larva migrans. In this photomicrograph the larva is seen in cross section deep within the epidermis.

the parasite in cross section (Fig. 8–32). As a rule, punch biopsies are not necessary to make the diagnosis because the clinical picture is so distinct.

Treatment of cutaneous larva migrans begins with light freezing of the advancing border tip of the larva tract and the area of predicted travel of the larva with ethyl chloride spray. Even if this does not kill the larva, it will usually stop its forward progression. Topical thiabendazole 10% aqueous solution is recommended for the treatment of mild infections during the early stages of the infestation. It is applied four times a day for 7 days to the affected area and 2 cm in front of the advancing border. Oral thiabendazole (Mintezol) is supplied in chewable 500-mg tablets or as a suspension, containing 500 mg/5 mL. A dosage of 25 mg/kg of body weight taken twice daily after meals for 2 days is usually effective in resolving the pruritus in less than 12

hours and the migration of larvae in less than 1 week. If necessary, an additional 2 days of treatment may be warranted. Side effects from the oral dosage include dizziness, nausea, and vomiting. Topical corticosteroids are prescribed if there has been an urticarial or eczematous inflammatory response.

MARINE LIFE

Hard coral injuries to the feet and legs usually occur when swimmers or waders step on or brush against the razor-sharp external skeletons of calcium carbonate (Fig. 8–33). Fragments of the calcareous material and animal protein may be left behind in the cuts or puncture wounds. Itchy red wheals (coral poisoning) occur around the wound (Fig. 8–34). These relatively minor wounds are very painful, pruritic, and slow to heal and often become infected. A large part of the condition is probably a result of a foreign-body reaction and secondary infection. These injuries should be scrubbed vigor-

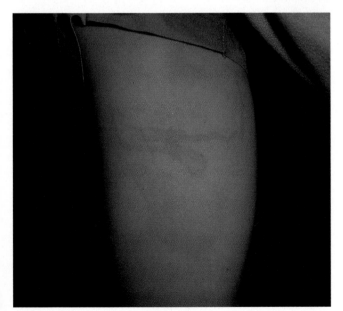

Figure 8–31 Cutaneous larva migrans. In this young patient a hypersensitivity reaction produced an intense urticarial response.

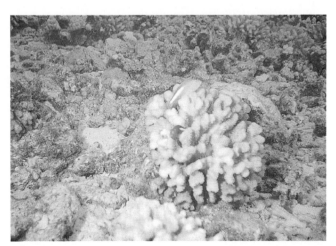

Figure 8–33 A small coral head on the sea floor is easy for ocean bathers to brush bare skin against or step on.

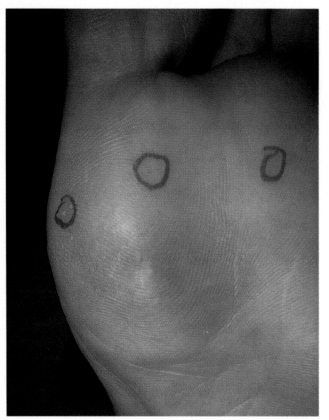

Figure 8–34   Coral cuts. These wounds on the plantar aspect of the foot with pruritic erythematous wheals are typically difficult to heal and often become infected.

ously with soap and water, irrigated with hydrogen peroxide and alcohol, and painted with povidone-iodine solution. Repeated aggressive wound care is recommended until the lesions clear. Small superficial pieces of the coral or other debris may be removed; however, this process may cause a delayed, foreign-body reaction. If chronic coral granulomas occur, they may be treated with intralesional injections of short-acting corticosteroids.

Fire coral, *Millepora alcincornis,* of the phylum Cnidaria (formerly, Coelenterata) and from the class Hydrozoa, is not considered a true coral, but it has the same general appearance. Almost all coelenterates possess nematocysts, which are stinging cells that contain a toxic venom that can inject the skin on the slightest contact. A common misconception regarding fire coral is that it must be red or bright orange. In most cases, fire coral is dull brown or yellow-green. It also appears very soft and fuzzy, and inexperienced divers have a tendency to want to touch it. The stinging coral has many small nematocysts on its external exoskeleton of lime carbonate and when they discharge into the skin of a diver there is immediate burning or stinging, followed by erythema and vesicle formation (Fig. 8–35). The first two actions that most individuals take after a fire coral injury are the two that should be avoided: rubbing the area with the hand or a towel and washing

the injury with fresh water. Both of these activities will spread the venom and activate any unfired nematocysts on the skin. Any remaining nematocysts may be inactivated by alcohol (rubbing alcohol, liquor, after-shave, cologne), vinegar, or acetic acid. Hot sea water as a rinse has been advocated by many divers. Other applications that may be helpful include meat tenderizer, formalin solution, baking soda, flour, talcum, or boric acid and sea water made into a paste to cover the affected area. Topical corticosteroids may be necessary later to reduce some of the inflammation. Appropriate systemic or topical antibiotics are recommended if secondary infection is present.

Jellyfish stings are very common marine injuries experienced by swimmers, ocean bathers, snorkelers, and scuba divers. The long beautiful tentacles, containing stinging nematocysts, trail out underneath or several feet behind the body of the jellyfish. If the tentacles are broken away from the body, they may float free in the water and remain venomous for weeks. Stings are characterized by an instant burning sensation, followed quickly by the formation of linear erythematous streaks (Fig. 8–36). In allergic individuals, these intense reactions are more severe with pustule formation and desquamation of the skin. These patients may suffer additional systemic effects of muscular pain, cramps, fever, chills, nausea, and dyspnea. Fortunately, most

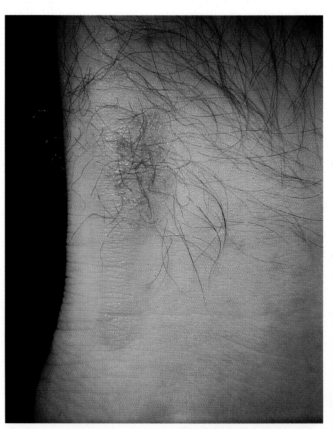

Figure 8–35   Fire coral injury. Dermatitis occurred on the posterior ankle of this diver and resulted in an intense burning sensation that resolved in several days.

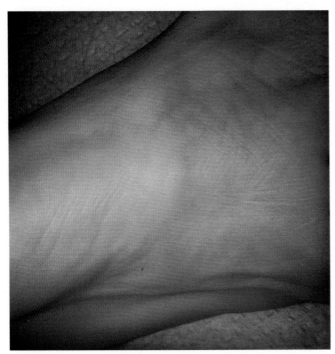

Figure 8–36 Jellyfish sting. Linear erythematous vesicles were produced by nematocysts on tentacles that brushed against the skin of the foot.

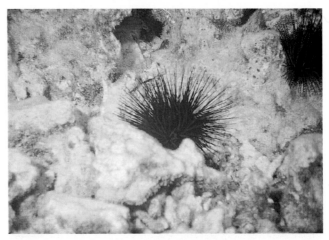

Figure 8–37 Sea urchin with numerous sharp protruding spines. These creatures are usually attached to the rocks on the ocean floor.

stings are not serious. Treatment begins with removing any attached tentacles with gloves and not bare hands. Tentacles and toxin are washed off with sea water that has not been heated because that may cause additional firing of the remaining nematocysts. The area should then be flushed with alcohol or vinegar, followed by the application of a paste made with sea water and baking soda or meat tenderizer. Topical corticosteroids and oral antihistamines may be indicated in severe stings. Treatments that should *not* be done include rubbing the area with bare hands, applying fresh water or hot sea water, rubbing the area with sand or towels, or placing saliva on the wound.

Sea urchins are round-bodied organisms with a calcareous skeleton called a cast that houses the soft body. The cast is studded with numerous brittle, sharp spines made of calcium carbonate covered with pigmented epithelium (Fig. 8–37). The sea urchin is usually found attached to rocks on the ocean floor. Most sea urchin injuries are due to inadvertent contact with the spines, leading to puncture of the skin where the spine tips break off. Reactions to sea urchin injuries are of two types: immediate and delayed. Unlike injuries from stinging organisms, most initial sea urchin injuries do not produce pain out of proportion to a puncture wound. However, in some injuries, severe burning pain with edema may be noticed. This would suggest that some species of sea urchins have a toxin within the spines or the spinal epithelium. Profuse bleeding from the puncture site may also occur. When small tips of the spines have punctured the skin or have broken off within the skin the wound may be pink or violet-black

because of the pigments located on the spine epithelium (Fig. 8–38). This pigmented puncture may give the impression that sea urchin spines are present, but it may just be the pigmented epithelium. Radiographs are important in the early stages to locate spines of calcium carbonate. In the delayed reaction, which may occur several months after the original injury, there is a granulomatous foreign-body–type reaction. Hypersensitivity reactions with granulomatous nodules may not contain foreign bodies. Treatment includes removal of visible spines, but deep probing should be discouraged because this activity may break the friable spines into

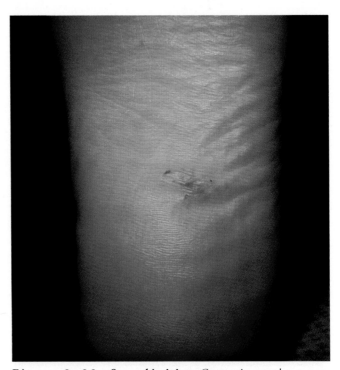

Figure 8–38 Sea urchin injury. Group pigmented puncture wounds on the planar foot with pigmented retained spines.

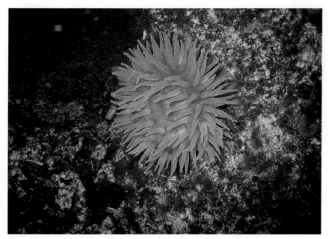

Figure 8–39 Sea anemone with beautiful flower appearance attached to rocks.

many smaller segments. Direct visualization using x-rays or fluoroscopy may allow accurate surgical removal of embedded spines. Intralesional injections of corticosteroid (triamcinolone, 10 mg/mL) may be useful in the treatment of delayed reactions and granulomatous nodules. If there is secondary infection the patient should be treated with appropriate antibiotics.

Sea anemones are sessile coelenterates with finger-like tentacles (Fig. 8–39). These beautiful flower-like creatures are considered true corals and members of the Anthozoa class. Many species of sea anemones have stinging cells on their numerous soft tentacles. The sea anemone attaches itself to the base of sponges and rocks

on the ocean floor, and when divers come in contact with the tentacles there is a burning sensation followed immediately by erythema, vesicles, and localized edema (Fig. 8–40). In highly sensitized individuals there may be additional systemic reactions of fever, nausea, vomiting, and muscle spasms. This reaction is rarely reported. Therapy for sea anemone dermatitis is immediate topical treatment with alcohol, vinegar, or meat tenderizer paste.

BIBLIOGRAPHY

Berger BW: Erythema chronicum migrans of Lyme disease. Arch Dermatol 120:1017–1021, 1984.

Black JR, Fenske NA: Cutaneous infestations. In McCarthy DJ, Montgomery R (eds): Podiatric Dermatology, pp 165–177. Baltimore, Williams & Wilkins, 1986.

Burnett JW, Calton GJ, Morgan RJ: Venomous sea urchins. Cutis 38:151–155, 1986.

Cangialosi CP, Schnall SJ: Pedal spider bite (arachnidism): Report of two similar cases. J Am Podiatr Assoc 71:385–388, 1981.

Dockery GL: Human scabies: A review of diagnosis and current therapy. J Am Podiatr Assoc 70:177–181, 1980.

Enander MW, Adam RC: Cutaneous larvae migrans: A literature review and case report. J Am Podiatr Med Assoc 79:83–85, 1989.

Felman Y, Nikitas JA: Scabies. Cutis 25:32–42, 1980.

Goldenberg E: Soft Tissue Injuries of the Lower Extremities. In Levy LA, Hetherington VJ (eds): Principles and Practice of Podiatric Medicine, pp 967–977. New York, Churchill Livingstone, 1990.

Gutowicz M, Fritz RA, Sonoga AL: Brown recluse spider bite: A literature review and case report. J Am Podiatr Med Assoc 79:142–146, 1989.

Istell R, Bodmer EJ, Bodmer E: Black widow spider (*Latrodectus mactans*) bite of the foot. J Am Podiatr Assoc 69:562–563, 1979.

Kleger SJ, Feldman B: Larva migrans. J Am Podiatr Assoc 56:324–326, 1966.

Marcinko DE, Rappaport MJ: Cutaneous necrotic arachnidism: A case report. J Am Podiatr Med Assoc 76:105–108, 1986.

Needham GR: Evaluation of five popular methods for tick removal. Pediatrics 75:997–1002, 1985.

Pardo RJ, Kerdel FA: Parasites, arthropods, and hazardous animals of dermatologic significance. In Moschella SL, Hurley HJ (eds): Dermatology, pp 1923–2003. Philadelphia, WB Saunders, 1992.

Smith L: Pediatrics. In Zier BD (ed): Essentials of Internal Medicine in Clinical Podiatry, pp 464–529. Philadelphia, WB Saunders, 1990.

Steere AC, Malawista SE, Snydman DR: Lyme arthritis: An epidemic of oligoarticular arthritis in children and adults in three Connecticut communities. Arthritis Rheum 20:7–17, 1977.

Walter JH Jr, Burton M: Marine-related foot injuries. In Scurran BL (ed): Foot and Ankle Trauma, pp 261–269. New York, Churchill Livingstone, 1989.

Woodward TE: Rocky Mountain spotted fever: Epidemiology and early clinical signs are key to treatment and reduced mortality. J Infect Dis 150:465–468, 1984.

Wongs RC, Hughes SE, Voorhess JJ: Spider bites: Review in depth. Arch Dermatol 123:98–105, 1987.

Zebrack SD: Creeping eruptions (larva migrans): A case report. J Am Podiatr Assoc 64:105–107, 1974.

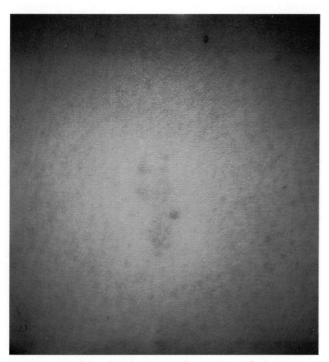

Figure 8–40 Sea anemone dermatitis. Inflammation occurred on the lower leg of a diver.

9

PERIPHERAL VASCULAR DISEASE AND RELATED DISORDERS

INTRODUCTION

A number of lower extremity cutaneous lesions and dermatoses are related to, or are part of, vascular disease. The physician may see the cutaneous effects of small vessel disease, peripheral arterial problems, venous incompetency, or other pathological entities involving the peripheral vasculature long before the condition has been properly diagnosed. A wide range of conditions is discussed in this chapter, and the emphasis is on recognition and treatment of the cutaneous disorder. There is a firm understanding that the underlying pathological process must also be managed.

ARTERIOSCLEROSIS OBLITERANS

Arteriosclerosis is the condition of arteries characterized by a thickening of the intima, loss of elasticity, and increased calcium content in the artery wall. *Atherosclerosis* is the condition of the intimal lining of arteries characterized by focal accumulation of lipids, complex carbohydrates, blood, fibrous tissue, and calcium. There are often changes within the median layer of the artery. Atherosclerosis rarely occurs in the absence of arteriosclerosis. In general, arteriosclerosis refers to hardening of the arteries, whereas atherosclerosis refers to hardened arteries with intimal lining lesions containing lipid.

Arteriosclerosis is also an occlusive arterial disease of the major arteries of the lower extremities. This condition is the most common peripheral arterial problem involving the medium-sized and large vessels and accounts for more than three fourths of all the cases of occlusive vascular disease of the extremities. Chronic and progressive obstruction is produced by the narrowing of the lumen of the medium or large-sized vessels due to atheroma (focal plaque-like lesion of the intima)

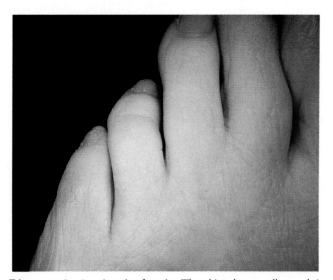

Figure 9–1   Arteriosclerosis. The skin shows pallor and is thin, atrophic, dry, and shiny. There is no hair growth.

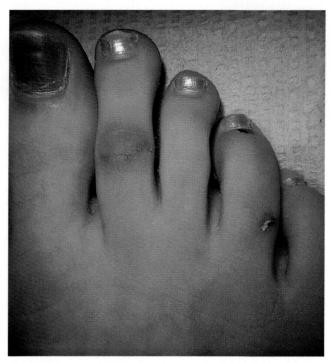

Figure 9–2   Arteriosclerosis. Note distal thickening of the toenails, diffuse color change, and distal gangrene as well as decreased hair growth in a cool extremity.

formation or due to median arteriosclerosis (median coat vessel changes) in the medium-sized vessels or both. The great majority of the occlusive lesions of arteriosclerosis obliterans are atherosclerotic. The condition may be worsened by sudden thrombus of the involved segment. The major symptoms of arteriosclerosis obliterans are those of ischemia, producing complaints of mild intermittent claudication (pain or fatigue in the muscle with activity) to severe, constant pain at rest. The signs of arteriosclerosis obliterans include decreased palpable peripheral pulses, systolic bruits, positional and postural color changes of the lower extremities, temperature changes, edema, trophic skin changes, atrophy of the muscles, thinning or atrophy of the soft tissues and skin, xanthoma formation, and frank gangrene (tissue necrosis due to blood flow obstruction).

Intermittent claudication results when there is moderate to severe chronic ischemia. When the limb is at rest there is usually adequate blood supply. When there is activity, however, the leg muscles reveal the decreased blood flow by fatigue or cramping. Typically, the patient states that he or she can walk for only 10 to 15 minutes, or for only a few blocks, when the calf muscle cramps or starts to burn. After a few minutes of rest the patient can continue for an additional period before having to stop again. In more advanced cases there may be muscle atrophy of the calf or foot. In a few cases, tibial arterial disease produces the claudication symptoms localized to the foot. The thermal changes noted in arteriosclerosis obliterans are usually represented by

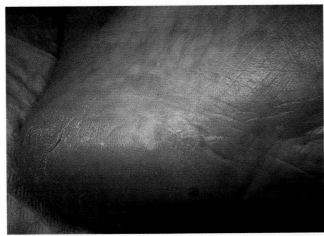

Figure 9–3 **Arteriosclerosis.** Painful heel fissure occurred in patient with one block claudication.

coldness of the distal extremity. Venous thrombosis may also occur in this stage. The color changes may range from pallor, to cyanotic, to erythematous owing to decreased oxygenated blood flow and pooling or congestion of the blood. Patients may complain of pain with rest, especially at night, and they may state that they have to hang the foot and leg over the side of the bed or get up and walk around to obtain temporary relief of the discomfort. Besides being very cold to the touch, the skin may appear to be thin, shiny, and atrophic and show a significant decrease in normal hair growth (Fig. 9–1). The trophic changes include deformed nails, shrinkage of the toes, ulceration, and gangrene (Fig. 9–2). Atrophy of the fat pad of the heel may be noted, and the heel may show a characteristic "fissure," which is painful, except when neuropathy coexists, as in diabetes (Fig. 9–3). In more advanced stages, the fissure is over a small area of cyanosis with one or more necrotic zones (Fig. 9–4). Edema of the foot and leg may also occur in advanced stages, and this condition is attributed to capillary atony (Fig. 9–5).

Ulcerations of the lower extremity secondary to arte-

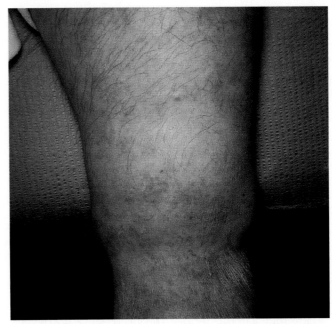

Figure 9–5 **Arteriosclerosis.** Edema of the foot and leg occurred in a patient with an advanced state of vascular disease.

riosclerosis frequently start on the distal toes (Fig. 9–6). The ulcers are usually very shallow, with a dark, dry base and with an atrophic border. Spontaneous ulcerations may start as a dark pustule with a surrounding erythematous zone. This ulcerates and then slowly forms a thin eschar with an underlying necrotic base (Fig. 9–7). This ulcer may be located over necrotic tissue that is undergoing purulent softening. As the ulceration deepens, the area is frequently contaminated with bacteria and becomes secondarily infected (Fig. 9–8). An atherosclerotic ulcer may be very painful, es-

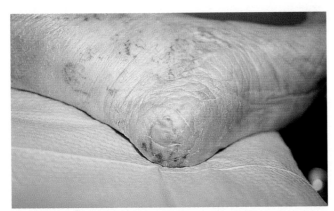

Figure 9–4 **Arteriosclerosis.** Fissures occurred over area of cyanosis accompanied by necrotic skin changes of the inferior heel.

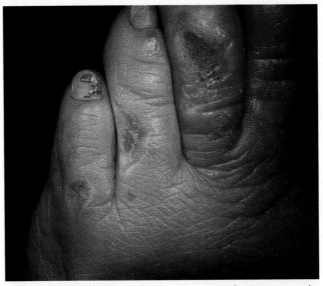

Figure 9–6 **Arteriosclerosis.** Ulcers may first appear on the dorsal or distal toes.

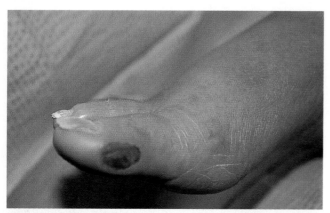

Figure 9–7   Arteriosclerosis. Ischemic ulceration occurred on the medial hallux. This is a characteristic site for arteriosclerotic ulcers but not for venous ulcers.

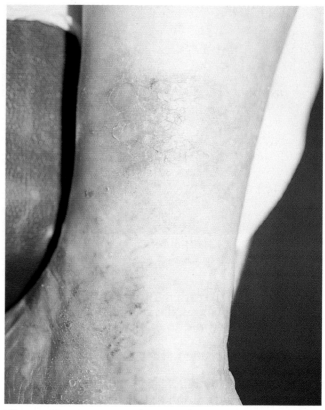

Figure 9–9   Arteriosclerosis. Atherosclerotic ulcer is evident on the lower leg.

pecially at night. These ulcers are found primarily on the lower leg (Fig. 9–9), ankle (Fig. 9–10), heel (Fig. 9–11), and dorsum of the foot.

Another variant, termed the *hypertensive ischemic ulcer,* is due to arteriosclerosis and ischemia occurring in the presence of hypertensive disease (Fig. 9–12). The disease is seen predominately in women older than 50. These ulcers are extremely painful and may be deep, with sharp borders, and are difficult to treat. Hypertensive or ischemic ulcers may be single or multiple, are usually seen around the lateral leg and ankle, and may have black areas of necrosis. Cutaneous "infarction" resulting in gangrenous lesions on the lower extremity is the final stage of severe ischemia (Fig. 9–13). Acute arterial occlusion and severe ischemia may be secondary

to embolism or thrombosis. Acute arterial embolism is occlusion of the lumen by a plaque, clot, or other tissue that has traveled to the site of obstruction from a more proximal site. The most common source of emboli is the heart, but microemboli frequently arise from plaques in the terminal portion of the aorta or large proximal branches. Of the two major forms of atheromatous emboli (atheroembolism and cholesterol microembolism), cholesterol showers affect the smaller terminal or digital vessels (Fig. 9–14). The clinical pre-

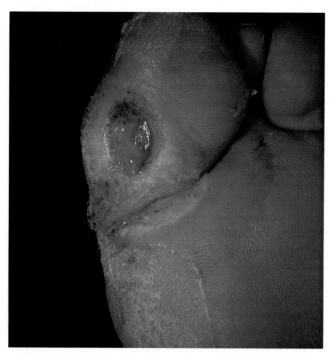

Figure 9–8   Arteriosclerosis. Ischemic ulceration on the medial hallux has become secondarily infected.

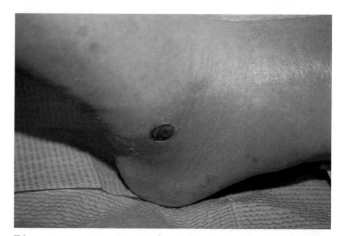

Figure 9–10   Arteriosclerosis. Lateral ankle ulceration that was very painful.

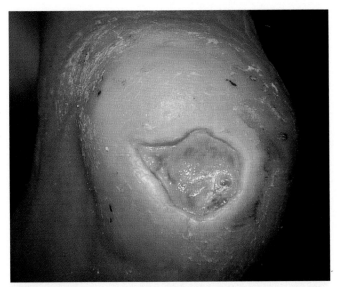

Figure 9–11 Arteriosclerosis. Plantar ischemic heel ulcer. The heel is a very characteristic location for arteriosclerotic disease but not for venous disease.

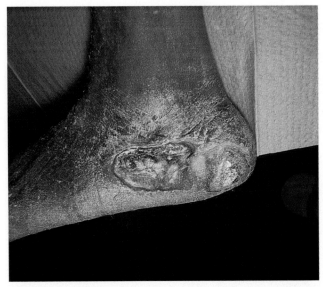

Figure 9–13 Arteriosclerosis. Infarction has occurred, and a black eschar is present in the ulceration on the lateral heel.

sentation varies from digital lesions with ischemic pallor, erythema, or cyanosis to ulceration and necrosis. Complete small vessel occlusion resulting in progressive ischemia leading to cyanosis or "blue toe syndrome" may be seen (Fig. 9–15). Gangrene may follow in a single digit (Fig. 9–16) or in several digits at the same time (Fig. 9–17).

Treatment of arteriosclerosis obliterans is largely conservative. The primary considerations include meticulous foot care and regular foot inspections to detect early problems, weight reduction to decrease lower extremity stresses, decreased consumption of substances

(especially nicotine and caffeine) causing vasoconstriction, and improvement of exercise tolerance. It is also imperative to control diabetes mellitus and hypertension. When resting or sleeping, the patient should keep the extremity horizontal or slightly below horizontal. Lesions that become secondarily infected must be attended to with debridement and appropriate antibiotic therapy. Treatments and conditions that should be avoided include the application of heat or cold, the wearing of elastic compression stockings or of tight stockings or shoes, and elevation of the part. Referral

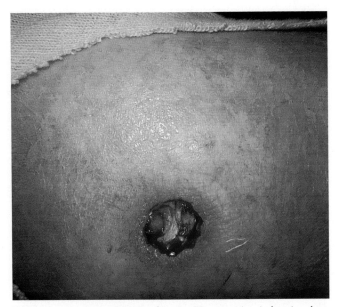

Figure 9–12 Arteriosclerosis. Hypertensive ischemic ulceration of the lower leg. These ulcers are extremely painful, deep, and well demarcated.

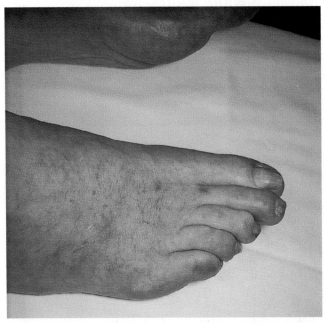

Figure 9–14 Cholesterol microemboli. Ischemic pallor, distal necrosis, and ulcerations and discoloration of the toes were noted.

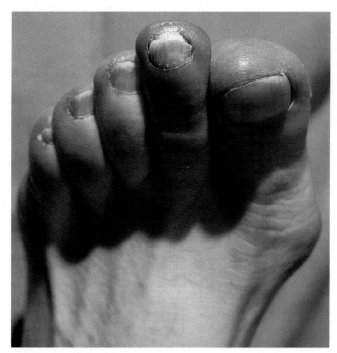

Figure 9–15   Blue toe syndrome. Second toe was cold, cyanotic, and painful.

to a vascular specialist for consideration of surgical procedures including balloon angioplasty and bypass grafting is recommended. In selected cases of digital gangrene, amputation of the affected part may be necessary. Before this procedure is undertaken a complete vascular examination and consultation are required.

THROMBOANGIITIS OBLITERANS

Thromboangiitis obliterans (Buerger's disease) is a progressive vascular disorder that affects the distal extremities in men between 25 and 40 years of age. The condition is relatively rare in women, but the incidence

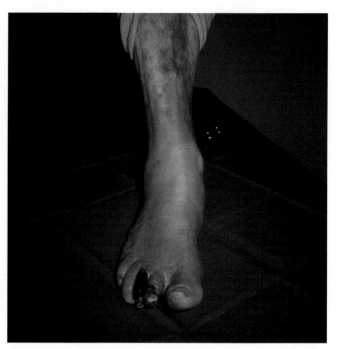

Figure 9–17   Distal ischemia. Digital gangrene of the entire third toe and a portion of the second toe occurred in a patient with blue toe syndrome.

may be increasing. The condition involves the small and medium-sized arteries and may include the veins. It predominantly affects the lower extremities with the possibility of involvement of the small arteries of the hands. Smoking is implicated as the cause of Buerger's disease in most cases reported, and no other cause has been substantiated. The onset of the disease may follow a traumatic event, cold exposure with frostbite, or

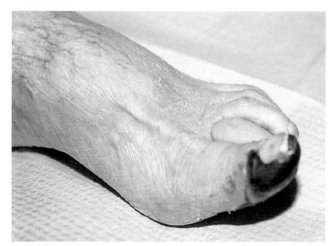

Figure 9–16   Distal ischemia. Digital gangrene of the hallux was secondary to peripheral arterial embolism.

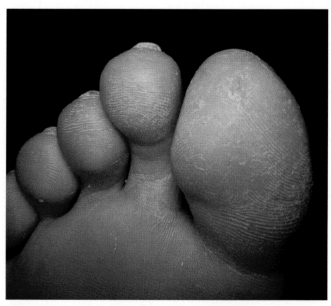

Figure 9–18   Thromboangiitis obliterans. A young male smoker presented with complaints of early distal digital ischemia, coldness, pain, trophic changes, and small ulceration.

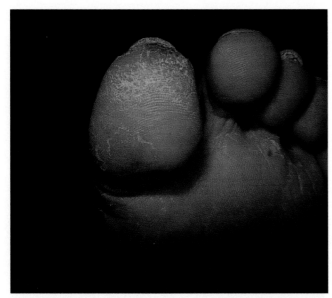

Figure 9–19   Thromboangiitis obliterans. Distal hallux subungual ulceration and trophic changes of the hallux are common findings.

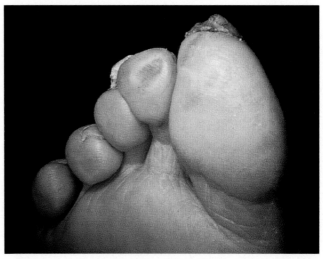

Figure 9–21   Thromboangiitis obliterans. Distal digital ulcerations with ischemia, nail changes, and pallor in a patient with Buerger's disease.

chronic repetitive trauma to the digits. The clinical presentation is one of excruciatingly painful toes with trophic changes and coldness (Fig. 9–18). Additional findings include periungual or subungual ulcerations

(Fig. 9–19), distal digital rubor and nail changes (Fig. 9–20), and distal digital ulcerations (Fig. 9–21). It is common for patients with Buerger's disease who continue to smoke to lose one or more toes secondary to the ischemic ulcerations and subsequent gangrenous changes that occur (Fig. 9–22).

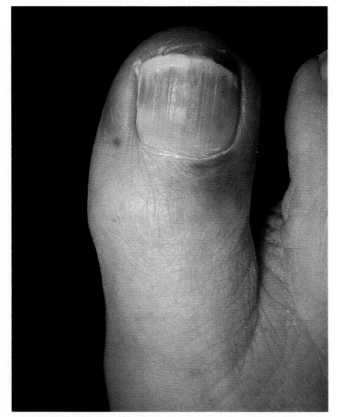

Figure 9–20   Thromboangiitis obliterans. Distal digital rubor and trophic nail changes with ischemic pain.

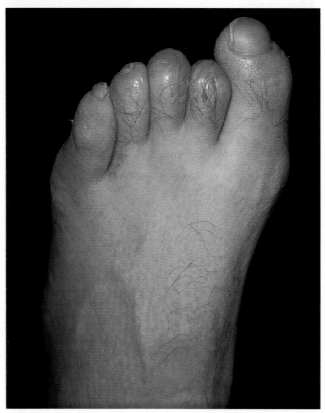

Figure 9–22   Thromboangiitis obliterans. Loss of multiple digits due to ischemia and gangrene in a young male patient who continued to smoke throughout treatment.

Treatment of thromboangiitis obliterans is predominantly the withdrawal of tobacco and provision of analgesics for pain, sympathetic nerve blocks, sympathectomy, and digital amputation. Amputation is reserved for those cases in which the conservative care is not successful, such as severe unremitting pain and gangrene.

THROMBOPHLEBITIS

Thrombophlebitis is the inflammation of a vein associated with thrombus formation. The causes of thrombophlebitis include prolonged recumbency (including sitting for long periods of time), preexisting varicosity, trauma to the leg muscles or veins, infection, carcinoma, and oral contraceptives. Three basic factors of thrombus formation include changes in the vessel wall, changes in the blood itself, or slowing of the blood flow. Thrombophlebitis may be either superficial or deep. The vein occlusion by thrombus causes a block in venous return, and the increased venous pressure produces cyanosis and

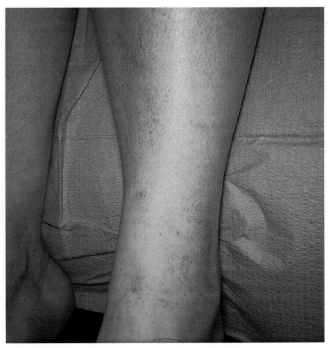

Figure 9–24   Deep venous thrombophlebitis. The limb was swollen with areas of petechiae.

edema. Deep venous obstruction may block circulation to the point of causing gangrene. Deep vein thrombophlebitis of the deep veins of the calf due to prolonged recumbency, especially postoperatively, is the most common variety of thrombophlebitis, and it is the primary cause of pulmonary embolism. Thrombophlebitis occurring within the saphenous vein and its tributaries is the next most common variety. This form is capable of extending into the deep veins of the calf or into the femoral vein and precipitating an embolism. An idiopathic thrombophlebitis is known to occur in young women taking oral estrogenic contraceptive medications.

Clinically, the manifestations of thrombophlebitis include swelling of the limb, mild to severe pitting edema (Fig. 9–23), fullness of the veins, cyanosis of the limb, tenderness or pain in the deep calf, and petechiae in the area if the thrombosis is diffuse and the capillaries are fragile (Fig. 9–24). When the superficial veins are involved, the obstruction is evidenced by painful, warm, erythematous induration of the overlying skin, and the involved vein may be felt as a tender cord and usually leaves no clinical sequelae.

Treatment of acute events involves anticoagulant therapy with heparin, thrombolytic therapy with streptokinase or tissue plasminogen activator, and, in severe cases, balloon catheter thrombectomy. Treatment is directed toward removing the underlying cause, relieving edema, and preventing pulmonary embolism. Oral anti-inflammatory drugs will reduce some of the pain and swelling. Additional therapies with local moist heat, limb elevation, and hydration are also important. Compression support stockings are recommended after the acute episode.

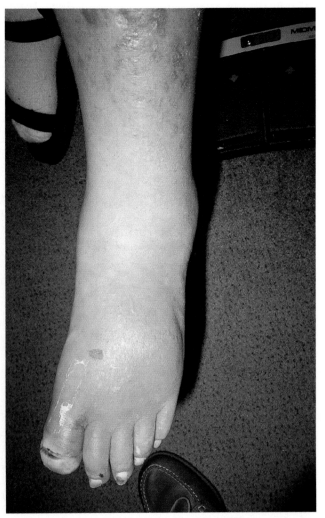

Figure 9–23   Deep venous thrombophlebitis. Note severe swelling and pitting edema of lower leg and foot. There is generalized cyanosis of the limb and tenderness in the deep calf.

POSTPHLEBITIC SYNDROME

Postphlebitic (post-thrombotic) syndrome may occur after deep vein thrombophlebitis secondary to the greatly increased venous pressure in the deep veins. This condition results in chronic venous insufficiency and varicose veins. The clinical presentation of postphlebitic syndrome includes chronic edema, significant increase in pigment formation, scaly stasis dermatitis, and painful, indurated cellulitis (Fig. 9–25). The purpura and pigmentation usually begin at midcalf and extend onto the foot. A chronic eczematous dermatitis with ulceration may occur in the areas of increased congestion. Indurated cellulitis secondary to chronic low-grade inflammation may occur that produces a hard, brawny induration of the subcutaneous tissue. When this involves the entire lower leg it creates a disabling and painful condition referred to as "piano leg" or "champagne bottle leg" (Fig. 9–26). Chronic ulcers may appear at the medial malleolus area that heal very slowly with scar formation (Fig. 9–27). Other conditions that may complicate postphlebitic syndrome include subcutaneous calcification, periostitis of the underlying bone below ulcers, and development of basal cell or squamous cell carcinomas (Fig. 9–28).

Treatment of postphlebitic syndrome is centered on reduction of the swelling and edema of the limb with bed rest, elevation of the leg, and continuous application of pressure-gradient compression stockings. The chronic dermatitis and ulcers are treated with local skin care, debridement, and proper ulcer management with occlusive wound dressings. The superficial infections are treated with topical or systemic antibiotics. Resistant ulcers or malignant lesions may be excised and closed primarily or skin grafted as needed.

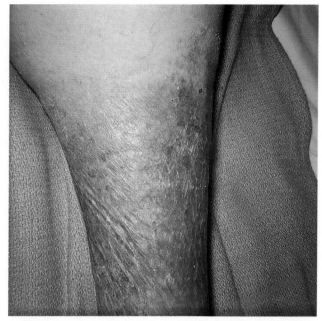

Figure 9–26 Postphlebitic syndrome. Chronic indurated cellulitis has produced the "piano leg" or "champagne bottle leg" appearance.

STASIS DERMATITIS

Stasis dermatitis is an eczematous dermatitis seen primarily on the lower legs and feet in patients with

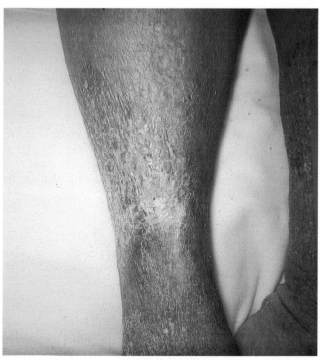

Figure 9–25 Postphlebitic syndrome. Stasis dermatitis is present with pigmented purpura and chronic eczematous dermatitis.

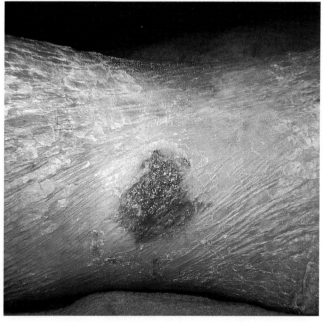

Figure 9–27 Postphlebitic syndrome. Chronic stasis dermatitis with a slow-healing medial ankle ulcer. These ulcers may become secondarily infected and may heal with a very atrophic scar.

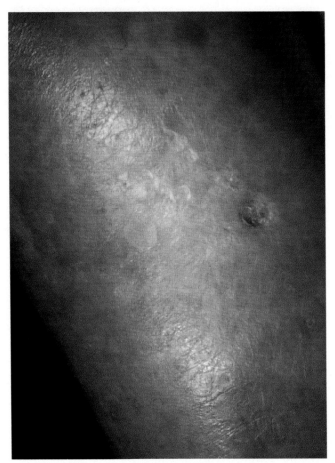

Figure 9-28   Postphlebitic syndrome. Chronic nonhealing ulcer on lower leg was diagnosed as squamous cell carcinoma.

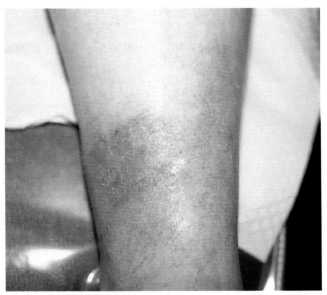

Figure 9-29   Stasis dermatitis. Acute inflammation in the early stages shows an area of weeping vesicles and crusts and adjacent cellulitis.

The secondary pruritus that occurs induces scratching, which will increase the eczematous dermatitis. Attempts to reduce the dryness and itching with topical lanolin, drying lotions (e.g., calamine), or topical antibiotics (e.g., Neosporin) exacerbate the inflammation and increase the dermatitis.

Chronic stasis dermatitis is usually due to recurrent attacks of inflammation causing increasing damage to the skin. This recurrent dermatitis leads to thickening

venous insufficiency syndrome. The term *stasis dermatitis* is a misnomer because the condition is secondary to high blood flow in the capillary bed (venous hypertension) rather than true stasis or pooling of blood. Still, the term is in common use today. This condition may be acute, subacute, or chronic. It may be accompanied by significant pigmentary changes or ulceration, usually involving the medial aspect of the ankle or lower leg. Not all patients with venous insufficiency, deep venous thrombophlebitis, or varicose veins develop stasis dermatitis.

Acute stasis dermatitis begins as an erythematous, superficial, pruritic area that suddenly appears on the lower leg (Fig. 9–29). The lesion may be eczematous and show adjacent cellulitis. There may be a vesicular eruption that is very pruritic, and the involved area may be warm to the touch. This acute inflammatory condition is easily misdiagnosed as contact dermatitis, nummular eczema, or infection.

Subacute stasis dermatitis usually shows an increase in brown pigmentary changes (hemosiderin deposits) that form slowly over several months (Fig. 9–30). The hemosiderin deposits are iron pigment left in the skin after breakdown of the red blood cells that have leaked out of veins because of the increased venous pressure.

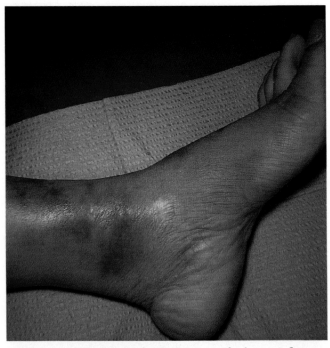

Figure 9-30   Stasis dermatitis. Area of subacute inflammation shows increased hemosiderin deposition in the skin and pruritic erythema around the medial malleolus.

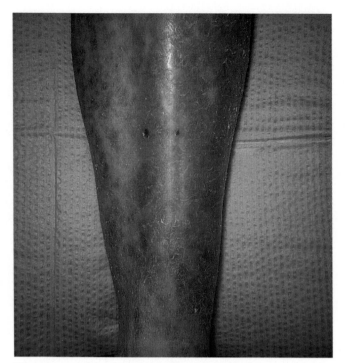

Figure 9-31 Stasis dermatitis. Chronic inflammation was accompanied by increased postinflammatory hyperpigmentation of the lower limb with slow-healing ulcers on the anterior shin.

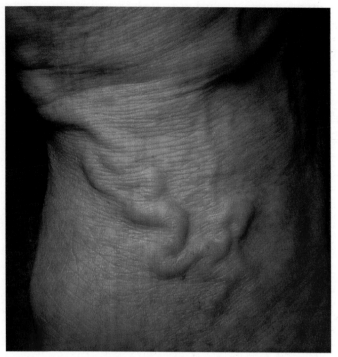

Figure 9-33 Stasis dermatitis. Large tortuous dilated veins were evident on the dorsal surface of the foot, indicating venous hypertension.

of the skin with increasingly darker pigmentary changes (postinflammatory hyperpigmentation) and chronic slow-healing ulcerations of the skin, usually about the anterior shin or medial ankle area (Fig. 9–31).

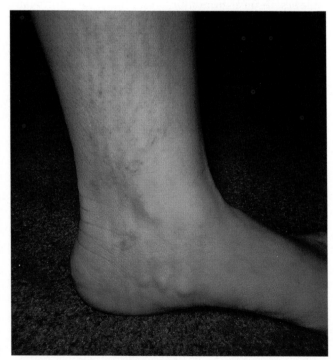

Figure 9-32 Stasis dermatitis. Venous hypertension was associated with dilated veins on the medial side of the foot and heel.

Additional findings that may be seen in cases of stasis dermatitis include small bulging veins secondary to venous hypertension (Fig. 9–32) and large tortuous varicose veins on the foot (Fig. 9–33). *Atrophie blanche* is a condition that results from atrophy and necrosis of the skin and is a small white plaque of sclerosis with a typical hyperpigmented rim (Fig. 9–34). The condition usually occurs on the legs and ankles, may be extremely painful, and is more common in young and middle-aged women. This finding may suggest that thrombosis has occurred in the inferior vena cava or the iliac veins, but it usually does not signal an underlying systemic disease. Variants of the typical atrophie blanche are a multiple-patterned atrophie blanche, seen in cases of diffuse chronic stasis dermatitis and in livedoid vasculitis (Fig. 9–35), and a leaf-pattern atrophie blanche usually noted on the posterior calf (Fig. 9–36). Atrophie blanche probably represents the end-stage of vascular damage to the skin, and the term *vasculopathy* probably describes this disorder more appropriately than the term *vasculitis*. There is no evidence that this condition arises without vascular damage, and it is more likely a clinical manifestation of a nonspecific reparative process during subdermal or ulcer healing. Atrophie blanche may be divided into two clinical classifications: primary (idiopathic atrophie blanche) and secondary forms (Table 9–1).

Treatment of atrophie blanche includes bed rest; elastic stockings; silver nitrate cautery; topical, intralesional, and oral corticosteroids; fibrinolytics (phenformin, ethyloestrenol); warfarin and minidose heparin;

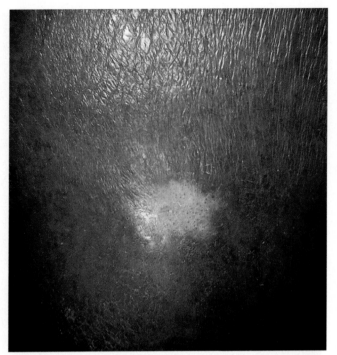

Figure 9–34   Atrophie blanche. A single white plaque of sclerosis occurred as a result of necrosis of the skin in stasis dermatitis. Hyperpigmentation is usually present around the area of hypopigmentation.

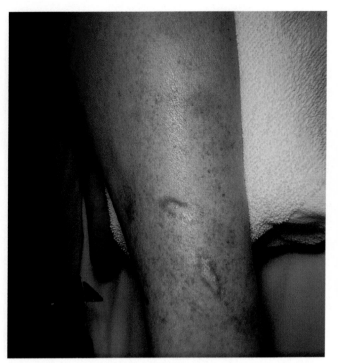

Figure 9–36   Atrophie blanche. A leaf pattern of sclerosis occurred on the posterior calf in stasis dermatitis.

nifedipine; nicotinic acid; anti-inflammatory drugs; sulfapyridine; sulfasalazine; and pentoxifylline.

Treatment of stasis dermatitis is usually of symptoms and is conservative. The acute and subacute inflammatory stasis dermatitis responds to cool, wet compresses, topical group V or VI corticosteroids, and systemic antibiotics. Topical antibiotics (especially Neosporin and Mycolog) should be avoided because there is a very high rate of contact dermatitis, called *dermatitis medicamentosa*, noted with these agents in this condition (Fig. 9–37). Chronic stasis dermatitis is managed with leg elevation while sleeping, prevention of prolonged sitting,

TABLE   9–1 Classification of Atrophie Blanche

Type I: Primary (Idiopathic) Atrophie Blanche
Absence of underlying diseases
Limited to the lower extremities

Primary Lesions
Recurrent, painful, purpuric macules and papules that undergo superficial necrosis and ulceration

Secondary Lesions
White, atrophic scars with peripheral telangiectasia and hyperpigmentary changes

Type II: Secondary Atrophie Blanche
Arteriosclerosis obliterans
Connective tissue diseases
   Systemic lupus erythematosus
   Rheumatoid arthritis
Diabetes mellitus
Dysproteinemia
Hypertension
Stasis dermatitis
Varicose veins

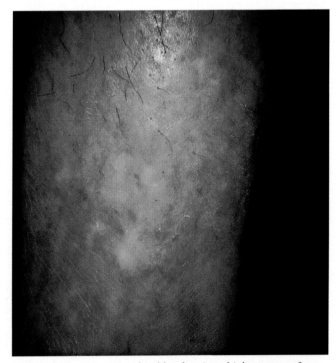

Figure 9–35   Atrophie blanche. A multiple pattern of atrophic white plaques is seen in this patient with stasis dermatitis and livedoid vasculitis.

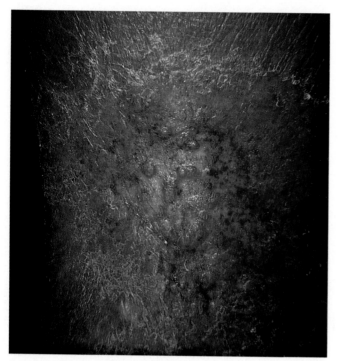

Figure 9–37 Stasis dermatitis. Dermatitis medicamentosa is a contact dermatitis that may result from medicaments such as topical antibiotics. This patient was sensitized to Neosporin that was being used to treat stasis eczema.

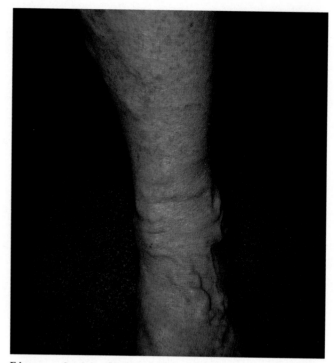

Figure 9–38 Varicose veins. Note large tortuous incompetent dorsal venous arch and great saphenous vein.

avoidance of constrictive hosiery or garments, and wearing of external support gradient-pressure stockings during ambulation.

If ulceration is present, wet to dry compresses are applied with surgical debridement, followed by covering with a biological dressing or occlusive wound dressing. These dressings protect the ulcer base, prevent drying by retarding water loss, and prevent further contamination of the wound. The application of an Unna boot paste dressing (a gauze bandage impregnated with zinc oxide paste) will help to reduce much of the excessive leg edema. An Unna boot is applied by wrapping from the distal toe area, just behind the metatarsophalangeal joint, toward the ankle with even overlapping edges to continue up to just below the knee. This causes a reverse pressure gradient necessary to reduce the edema in the lower leg. This bandage should be replaced on a weekly basis until the ulcer heals. Atrophie blanche has been treated with minidose heparin and with a combination of phenformin and ethylestrenol. Referral to a wound care clinic or a vascular specialist may be required if the ulceration persists after applying these therapeutic measures.

VARICOSE VEINS

Varicose veins refers to a disorder of the lower legs and feet in which the superficial veins are dilated and tortuous (Fig. 9–38). Additionally, varicose veins may show multiple areas of small thromboses and extrava-

sations of hemosiderin into the adjacent tissues (Fig. 9–39). Varicose veins are three times more common in women than in men older than 45. There are two major groups of varicose veins: primary and secondary. Primary varicose veins of the lower extremity result from

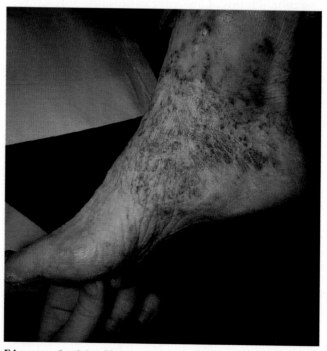

Figure 9–39 Varicose veins. Multiple small varicose veins with thromboses are present with loss of blood pigment into the adjacent skin.

congenital agenesis of the valves or from defective valves of the great and small saphenous veins or the ankle perforating veins. Secondary varicose veins result from venous valves that become incompetent from deep vein thrombosis or arteriovenous fistulae, leading to enlargement and varicosity of the superficial veins.

Varicose veins may develop from increased deep venous pressure, lack of competency, absence of iliofemoral valve, or increased distensibility of the venous wall. Increased deep venous pressure may be caused by pelvic obstruction and venous obstruction due to abdominal masses or pregnancy. Pregnancy may cause or worsen primary varicose veins through vein relaxation, expansion of blood volume, and increased pelvic pressure, which elevates the venous pressure in the iliac and therefore the femoral and saphenous systems.

Venous lakes are blue-purple, soft, compressible papules that are dilated venules and capillaries (Fig. 9–40). Microscopically, these lesions are composed of multiple, tortuous vessels filled with red blood cells and lined by flattened endothelial cells in the upper and middle dermis. Clinically, these lesions are compressible and empty or disappear with external pressure (diascopy). Venous lakes may be found anywhere on the body but are usually noted on the face, lips, and ears in older patients.

Treatment of varicose veins includes rest, elevation of the limbs, leg exercises, functional orthotic foot devices, and graduated compression stockings. Special maternity pantyhose–style pressure gradient compression stockings are available. The combination of injection and compression sclerotherapy has been effective in treating certain forms of lower leg varicosities. Surgical vein stripping or ligation may also be very beneficial. Treatment of venous lakes is usually not necessary on the foot, but when required they may be removed by surgical excision, sclerotherapy, electrodesiccation, and laser ablation.

Sodium tetradecyl sulfate (Sotradecol) is a sterile sclerosing solution containing sodium tetradecyl sulfate, 10

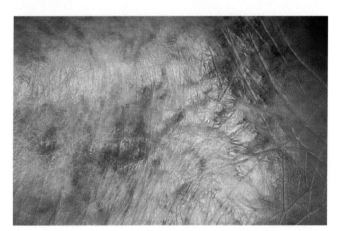

F i g u r e 9 – 4 0   Venous lake. This blue-purple, soft, compressible papule composed of tortuous vessels will empty or disappear with compression, which differentiates it from a thrombotic vessel.

mg (1%) or 30 mg (3%), in water for injection with 0.02 mL of benzyl alcohol and a buffering agent. The combination solution is used for sclerosing small varicose veins and other uncomplicated vascular disorders such as venous lakes of the lower extremities. The dosage should be less than 1 mL for each injection, and the initial injections should be 0.1 to 0.5 mL. This early smaller dosage is important to rule out any possibility of local tissue reaction, allergic reaction, or anaphylactic shock before the injection of larger doses. Once the lesions have been injected it is important to apply firm compression dressings to the area for 24 to 48 hours. This combination of sclerotherapy and compression appears to enhance the final results of eliminating varicose veins and associated vascular lesions.

VENOUS ULCERATION

Ulcerations of the lower extremities are common in patients with varicose veins and stasis dermatitis. In most cases, the patients either have neglected the condition or have been given poor advice on care of their ulcerations. The recognition along with diagnosis of venous ulcerations is the first step in the overall management of this condition.

Treatment of venous leg ulcers begins with treatment of the overlying eczematous inflammation and cellulitis (see accompanying flow chart[74]). Cool wet compresses with saline or 0.5% silver nitrate will rapidly control inflammation and superficial infection. Saline solutions may be prepared by adding 2 teaspoons of salt to 1 quart of water. Burow's solution is made with one packet or tablet of aluminum subacetate dissolved in 1 pint of water. Wet dressings must be replaced hourly for the first 24 to 48 hours. Group V or VI topical corticosteroids are applied lightly two or three times daily and may be covered with the wet dressings. As mentioned earlier, Mycolog, Neosporin, and lanolin products should be avoided because many patients with venous ulcers will develop a topical allergic reaction to these products.

Cellulitis and superficial infections may be treated with appropriate systemic antibiotics and topical application of erythromycin, silver sulfadiazine, or mupirocin ointment to the ulcer bed. Regular debridement of the ulcer exudate and crust should continue until the eczematous inflammation and cellulitis are under control. If the ulcer base is filled with exudate, additional debridement may be performed with the use of absorbing granule beads, which absorb low-molecular-weight substances but not plasma proteins or fibrin. This procedure helps to remove exudate quickly and reduces local tissue inflammation. The dry beads are poured into the ulcer base and covered with a dry dressing. When the beads have become saturated there is a color change. At this point the material is cleansed from the wound and new dry beads are applied. This process is repeated until the ulcer base is dry. Hyperkeratotic tissue (callus) must be removed from the rim of the ulcer

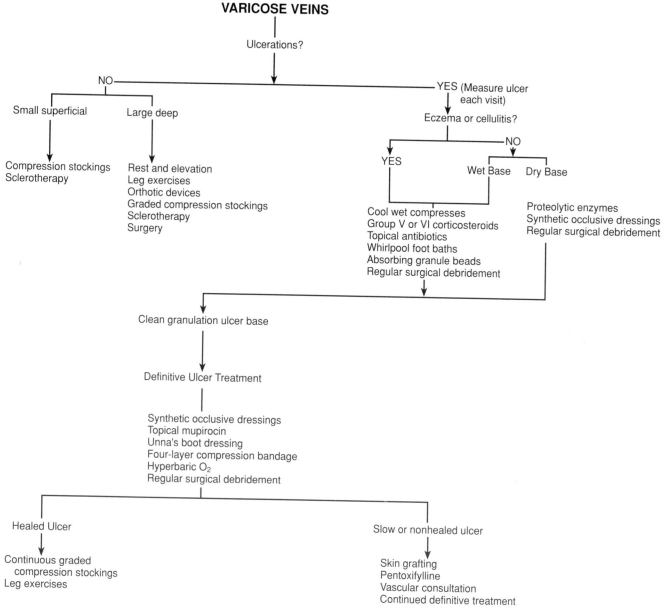

Flow chart for treatment of varicose veins and venous ulcerations

at this time. If the ulcer base is dry with an adherent crust, the treatment involves using synthetic occlusive dressings, proteolytic enzyme ointments, and regular surgical debridement. Either one of these treatment programs should leave the ulcer with a clean granulation base that will allow better healing.

Once no inflammation or cellulitis is present, and the ulcer base has a pink or red granulation layer, the application of external compression is started. Unna's boot dressing may be applied directly over the ulcer next to the skin. The dressing should be applied in the early morning when swelling and edema are minimal. The dressing is applied in layers with even overlapping of each turn, starting at the metatarsals and ending just below the knee. It is very important to prevent creases and wrinkles in the gauze while it is being applied because these will be irritating to the skin when the bandage dries. The moist bandage will dry in 1 to 2 hours to create a firm splint dressing. The paste bandage is covered in a layer wrap of dry gauze, stockinette, and an Ace-type elastic bandage. This combination generates approximately 30 mm Hg of mean pressure below the malleolus that gradually reduces to less than 6 mm Hg below the knee. The pressure decreases rapidly after the first 48 hours. For convenience and cost purposes, the boot is changed weekly. It may be changed sooner if there is exudate draining through the bandage. The ulcer is cleansed, measured, and carefully debrided until it is healed.

A much more efficient compression bandage system

than the Unna boot dressing is the four-layer high compression bandage system (Profore; Smith & Nephew United, Inc., Largo, FL). The four-layer bandage system applies four layers of differing properties incorporating elastic bandages to apply 40 mm Hg of mean pressure at the ankle, graduated to 17 mm Hg below the knee. This pressure is maintained until the bandages are removed in 1 week. The technique involves the sequential application of orthopedic wool wrap, cotton crepe, elastic wrap bandage, and cohesive bandage. The orthopedic wool wrap is designed to absorb exudate and moisture and redistribute pressure around the ankle, protecting the bony prominences such as the malleoli, tibial crest, and the dorsum of the foot from excessive pressure.

The 10-cm bandage is applied without tension in a loose spiral, from the base of the toes to the knee. The 10-cm cotton crepe bandage increases absorbency and smooths the orthopedic wool wrap, thereby preserving the elastic energy of the main compression layers. The crepe is also applied in a spiral, from toe to knee. The conformable compression elastic wrap layer is applied at midstretch in a figure-of-eight fashion from toe to knee with a 50% overlap. This gives a mean pressure of 17 mm Hg on ankles measuring 18 to 25 cm. The final layer is a lightweight, elastic, cohesive bandage, which is applied at midstretch with a 50% overlap spiral from the toe to the knee. This adds an ankle pressure of 23 mm Hg. This layer maintains the four layers in place until removal and adds durability to the bandage system.

Different limb circumferences are accommodated within the regimen, ensuring that all patients receive the correct pressure. Small limbs are protected from excessive pressure by adding extra padding, whereas large limbs require a stronger elastic bandage to ensure that adequate compression is applied. Reduction in edema may also necessitate changing the bandage regimen after the initial application, so that all limbs should be remeasured after 1 week. Once healing has occurred, pressure gradient compression stockings are fitted and applied each morning to prevent recurrence.

TELANGIECTASIA

Telangiectasia is a permanent dilatation of the small cutaneous venules, capillaries, or arterioles. The bright-red or purple lesions may appear as fine lines, heavy cords, or spider macules. There are generally four types of telangiectases: sinus or simple (linear), arborizing (tree-like branching), star or spider, and punctiform (hemorrhagic). The five etiological groups in which telangiectases are classified are those that are (1) associated with an acquired internal disease, (2) a component of a primary cutaneous disease, (3) inherited, (4) the result of hormonal imbalances, and (5) secondary to physical damage (Table 9–2).

Sinus or *simple linear telangiectases* are single or grouped, dilated, blue veins of less than 1 mm diameter. They are frequently noted in the skin around the nail bed or subungual areas (Fig. 9–41) in lupus erythematosus, scleroderma, dermatomyositis, alcoholism, and scurvy. They may be dysplastic but are frequently associated with degenerative processes. This type is a very common form of telangiectasia, and most persons have one or more forms of linear telangiectasia at some point in their lives.

Arborizing or *branching telangiectases* are more involved forms than the simple linear type, and they are usually

TABLE 9–2 Etiological Factors of Cutaneous Telangiectasia

I. Acquired Disease (With Secondary Cutaneous Component)
Collagen-vascular diseases
  Discoid lupus erythematosus (DLE)
  Systemic lupus erythematosus (SLE)
  CREST syndrome (calcinosis, Raynaud's phenomenon, esophageal dysmotility, sclerodactyly, telangiectasia)
  Dermatomyositis
  Progressive systemic sclerosis (scleroderma)
Carcinoma telangiectasia (metastatic tumors)
Cirrhosis of the liver

II. Primary Cutaneous Disease
Basal cell carcinoma
Capillaritis
Dego's disease (malignant papulosis)
Necrobiosis lipoidica diabeticorum (diabetes)
Poikiloderma atrophicans vasculare
Pseudoxanthoma elasticum
Rosacea
Varicose veins (stasis dermatitis)

III. Genetic Inheritance
Bloom's syndrome (dwarfism, photosensitivity, telangiectasia)
Cockayne's syndrome
Congenital neuroangiopathies
  Ataxia-telangiectasia
  Klippel-Trenaunay-Weber syndrome
  Maffucci's syndrome
  Sturge-Weber syndrome
Congenital poikiloderma
Diffuse neonatal hemangiomatosis
Essential progressive telangiectasia
Generalized essential telangiectasia
  Acquired (infectious or hormonal stimulation)
  Familial (autosomal dominant)
Hereditary hemorrhagic telangiectasia
  (Rendu-Osler-Weber disease)
Unilateral nevoid telangiectatic syndrome
Vascular nevi
  Nevus araneus (vascular spider)
  Nevus flammeus (capillary hemangioma)

IV. Hormonal Imbalance
Corticosteroid-induced
  Cushing's syndrome
  Estrogen therapy
  Iatrogenic (topical, intralesional, or systemic corticosteroids)
Pregnancy

V. Physical Skin Damage
Actinic (solar) dermatitis
Physical injury (trauma)
Postoperative (especially around or in suture lines)
  Laser surgery
  Cryosurgery
  Electrosurgery
Radiodermatitis

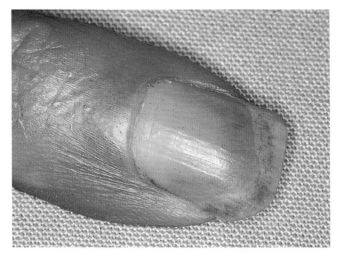

Figure 9–41 Linear telangiectasia. Small fine vessels are noted in the subungual area in this patient with clinical scurvy.

larger in diameter (>1 mm) (Fig. 9–42). In some cases, they are grouped to form a mat of ectatic veins and are frequently associated with varicose veins. Generalized essential telangiectasia is seen primarily in women and

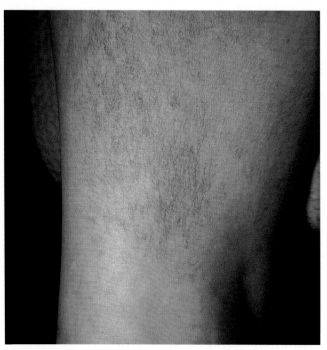

Figure 9–43 Generalized essential telangiectasia. Note the multiple branching telangiectases seen on the inner thigh in a 38-year-old woman with no underlying systemic disease.

is predominately on the legs, especially the inner thighs; it may be unilateral (Fig. 9–43). This lesion may occasionally be symptomatic but is usually of cosmetic concern only.

Star ectasias or *spider telangiectases* are arterial and characterized by a central point that may pulsate. There are radiating and dilated branches from the central punctum that may give the lesion the characteristic starburst or spider-legs appearance (Fig. 9–44). They occur idiopathically in normal persons and frequently are found in women and children. These lesions are permanent and usually do not spontaneously resolve or bleed. Spider telangiectases may be nevoid or acquired

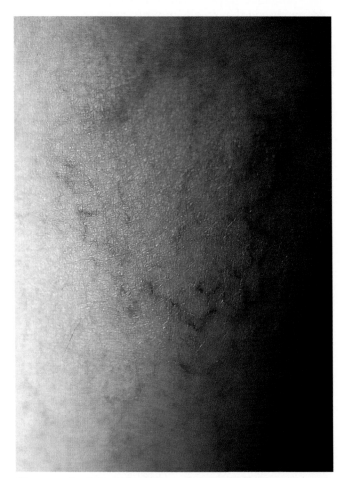

Figure 9–42 Arborizing or branching telangiectasia. This lesion may have the appearance of a lightning bolt, tree branches, or cracked glass and is commonly found adjacent to varicose veins.

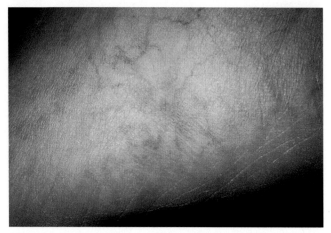

Figure 9–44 Star or spider telangiectasia. Well-defined dilated red vessels radiate from a central point, and the "legs" usually blanch quickly with diascopy.

and tend to be solitary. They increase in numbers in pregnancy, with elevated estrogen intake, in liver diseases (cirrhosis and carcinoma), and with hemorrhagic telangiectasia.

Punctiform or *punctate telangiectasia* is characterized by small, flat, ovoid telangiectases that may bleed easily when engorged (Fig. 9–45). They are considered to be venous. As noted earlier, generalized essential telangiectasia is seen primarily in women and may be familial. The lower extremity lesions slowly progress to other areas of the body and are not associated with systemic problems. The punctiform lesions may form linear, mottled, or net-like patterns. Punctate telangiectasia may be seen in other conditions such as hereditary hemorrhagic telangiectasia (Rendu-Osler-Weber disease), unilateral nevoid telangiectasia syndrome, scleroderma, telangiectasia macularis eruptiva perstans, and ataxia-telangiectasia.

Treatment of telangiectasia is usually not necessary, but in some cases the cosmetic appearance or location of the lesion dictates its removal. Spider telangiectases are the most common lesions to be removed. I commonly use two major forms of therapy to remove spider lesions: electrodesiccation and sclerotherapy.

Electrodesiccation is relatively simple and involves destroying the central arteriole. Before starting, the central puncta should be marked with a skin scribe. Local anesthesia is usually not necessary but, if needed, may be induced peripheral to the lesion. The blood is forced out of the spider telangiectasis and, while pressure is maintained on the lesion, the central arteriole is carefully exposed and gently electrodesiccated. Desicca-

tion is performed by inserting a 0.5-inch 30-gauge needle or an epilating electrosurgical tip into the central punctum and delivering a small current burst into the lesion. Care should be taken not to damage the dermis with vigorous desiccation. Once the central punctum has been destroyed the lesion will blanch and will not refill the radiating capillaries. In a few cases the radiating spokes may need to be destroyed as well. Compression of the treated site for 24 to 48 hours may enhance the results.

Sclerotherapy by injection of sodium chloride (20%) is also an effective treatment for spider telangiectases and other ectasias of the lower extremities (Fig. 9–46). The technique is similar to that of electrodesiccation. Sodium chloride (20%) sterile injectable solution with lidocaine added to give a final strength of 0.4% can be prepared by the local pharmacist and is useful in eradicating small superficial lesions and unsightly vascular lesions, such as spider telangiectases and small varicose veins. This solution must be used carefully because of its sclerosing properties, and because it is injected superficially, pigmentary changes and ulcerations are possible. The solution is slowly injected into the central core of the lesion using a tuberculin syringe with a 0.5-inch, 30-gauge needle, with the bevel turned up. It is recommended that small amounts, ranging from 0.1 to 0.4 mL, be injected during the first visit. After the first session, several lesions may be injected for a total of up to 3 mL as necessary.

When the injection is performed for telangiectasia, there is immediate blanching of the vessel and associated tributaries, followed by a report of a burning sensation from the patient. This discomfort is almost always gone before the patient leaves the office. Care should be taken to prevent extravasation into adjacent tissues. If this occurs, the needle should be withdrawn and pressure placed over the injection site to help diffuse the solution. Treatments should be scheduled for 1- to 4-week intervals until the desired results are obtained. The patient should be told that results are slow and the goal is to improve the appearance by 80% over several months. Once again, compression for the first 24 to 48 hours after injection appears to enhance the end results.

PURPURA

Purpura is discoloration of the skin resulting when blood extravasates into the intracutaneous or subcutaneous areas. Unlike telangiectasia and erythema, purpura is variable in color (from pink to purple and from red to brown) and does not blanch on external pressure. It appears as petechiae or ecchymoses. When the lesions are small (less than 3 mm diameter), red to purple macules they are called *petechiae* (Fig. 9–47); when the lesions are larger and of variable shape and color they are termed *ecchymoses* or common bruises (Fig. 9–48). *Vibices* are linear areas of hemorrhage often due to trauma, toxins, or envenomations (see Fig. 8–15). A contusion usually represents a trauma-

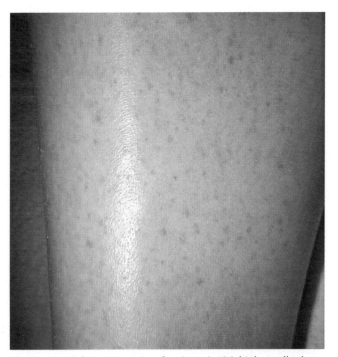

Figure 9–45   Punctate telangiectasia. Multiple small telangiectases were noted on the lower leg in a 40-year-old woman with generalized essential telangiectasia.

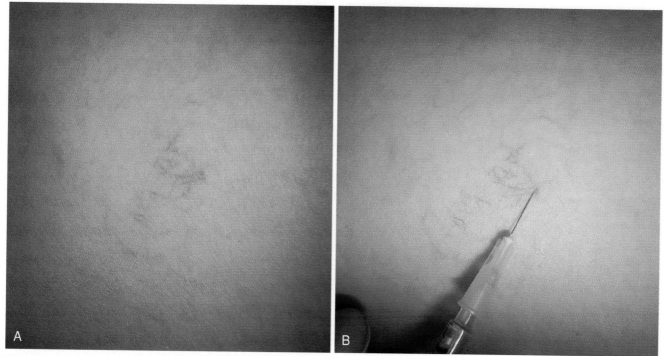

Figure 9–46 Spider-like ectasia. *A,* On the lower extremity, note the darker central punctum with branching spokes. *B,* The central punctum was injected with 0.4% sodium chloride solution.

induced hemorrhage with soft tissue injury. When there is considerable bleeding there may be blistering. Purpura may also occur spontaneously, especially in older persons, without evidence of underlying hemor-

rhagic disorders. This is sometimes referred to as senile purpura (Bateman's purpura), but these ecchymotic lesions seen on the backs of the hands and forearms probably represent changes due to degeneration of the collagen that normally surrounds and protects the vessel

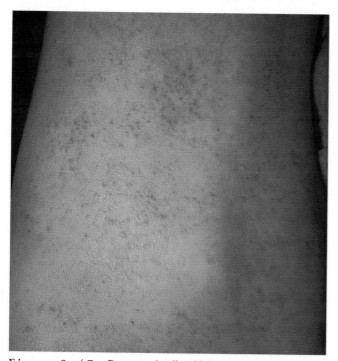

Figure 9–47 Purpura. Small reddish purple macules that do not blanch on pressure are known as petechiae. The lower extremities are the usual sites.

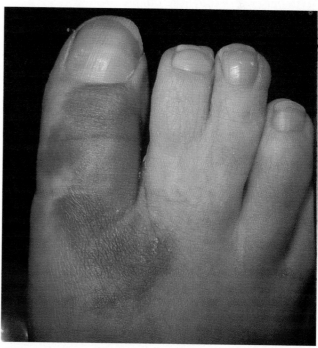

Figure 9–48 Purpura. Large purpuric lesions are known as ecchymoses.

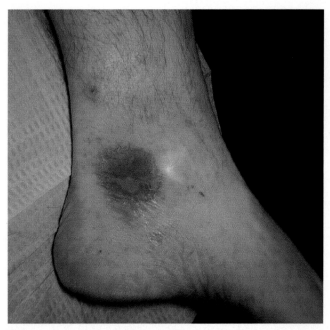

Figure 9-49 Purpura. Chronic use of a fluorinated corticosteroid on the ankle caused a large purpuric lesion.

TABLE 9-3 Simplified Classification of Causes of Purpura

Blood Vessel Defects
Congenital defects of vessel walls
  Ehlers-Danlos syndrome
  Hereditary hemorrhagic telangiectasia
Damage to the vessel walls
  Emboli (tumor, clot, or fat)
  Infections
  Trauma (injury, factitial)
  Vasculitis
Fragility of the vessel walls
  Solar or senile purpura
  Corticosteroid purpura
Increased vascular permeability
  Vitamin C deficiency (scurvy)
  Diabetic purpura
Increased vascular pressure
  Progressive pigmented purpura
  Stasis purpura

Blood Disorders
Coagulation abnormalities
  Hemophilia
Plasma protein abnormalities
  Hypergammaglobulinemic purpura
  Primary macroglobulinemic purpura
Platelet abnormalities
  Idiopathic thrombocytopenic purpura
  Secondary thrombocytopenic purpura
    Carcinoma
    Drug-induced
    Irradiation
    Leukemia

walls. Advanced age is not the cause of this change but rather excess exposure to ultraviolet sunlight. Similar changes are seen in patients who have used potent corticosteroids on their skin for long periods of time (Fig. 9-49). The color of purpura depends on several factors: location, severity, and duration. As blood pigments break down in the skin there are changes in the hue, chroma (color), and intensity of the lesions. Purpura should be distinguished from telangiectasia and erythema by diascopy (see Chapter 3).

The diagnosis may be evident from the clinical presentation and from the patient's history but, in general, if the diagnosis if obscure one should rely on laboratory investigations to reveal the cause of purpura. Purpura results from trauma, vessel wall damage, defective number or function of blood platelets, faulty coagulation, defective quality of perivascular support, or a combination of faulty hemostatic factors. A simplified classification of purpura includes those conditions secondary to blood disorders and those caused by blood vessel defects (Table 9-3).

The most common forms of purpura seen in clinical practice include actinic or senile purpura (Fig. 9-50), purpura of alcoholism or scurvy (Fig. 9-51), stasis purpura (Fig. 9-52), progressive pigmented purpura (Fig. 9-53), traumatic purpura (see Fig. 9-48), diabetic purpura or necrobiosis lipoidica (Fig. 9-54), and drug-induced purpura (Fig. 9-55).

The progressive pigmentary purpura conditions collectively show grouped petechiae on the lower extremities and occasionally elsewhere on the body. These lesions are most often found in men and are usually asymptomatic but may cause mild pruritus. In most cases no associated systemic disease is found. The cuta-

neous manifestations result from increased capillary fragility or from dilatation and increased pressure in vessels in the upper dermis. The primary lesion is a group of purpuric petechiae with pigmentation from hemosiderin. Telangiectasia also occurs secondary to capillary dilatation. When the lesions are pruritic, there may be scaling macules and papules, and lichenification may occur owing to rubbing or scratching.

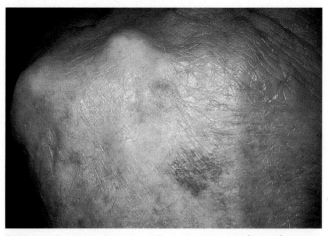

Figure 9-50 Purpura. The most common form of purpura is called senile or solar purpura and is frequently seen on the upper extremities and hands in patients who have had excessive sun exposure for many years.

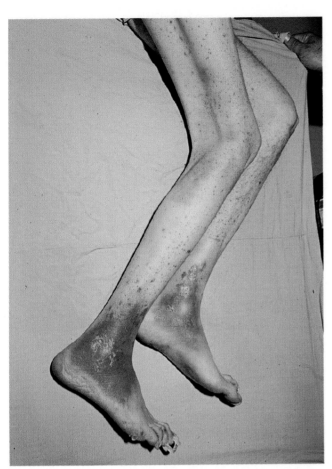

Figure 9–51 Purpura. This patient had chronic alcoholism and vitamin C deficiency (scurvy). The purpura of the skin in scurvy appears in the keratotic follicles and as ecchymoses of the lower extremities.

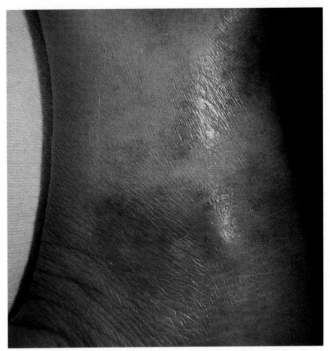

Figure 9–52 Purpura. This stasis purpura is secondary to raised venous pressure and is found in association with varicose veins or stasis dermatitis around the ankle.

The four main classifications of this progressive purpuric condition include (1) progressive pigmented purpuric dermatosis of Schamberg, (2) pigmented purpuric lichenoid dermatosis of Gougerot and Blum, (3) purpuric annularis telangiectodes (Majocchi's disease), and (4) disseminated pruritic purpura of Lowenthal. These idiopathic dermatoses are considered to be variants of the same pathological process and are separated according to their clinically distinctive presentations. These conditions all may persist for months to years, and treatment is symptomatic with systemic corticosteroid and topical corticosteroid therapy in the severely pruritic form. Occlusion with topical corticosteroids may eliminate localized areas of pruritic purpura. Gradient pressure stockings, topical anti-inflammatory or antipruritic medications, and oral antipruritics may be necessary in some cases. Not wearing woolen pants or stockings has also been shown to be beneficial if a sensitivity to wool oil is present.

Progressive pigmented purpuric dermatosis of Schamberg is an asymptomatic disease of males from 15 to 40 years of age (Fig. 9–56). The orange to fawn-colored macular lesions with "cayenne pepper" spots within or on

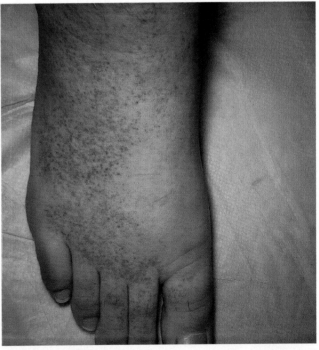

Figure 9–53 Purpura. Schamberg's progressive pigmented purpuric dermatosis is frequently found in young men and is characterized by orange to fawn-colored macules with "cayenne pepper" spots within or on their borders.

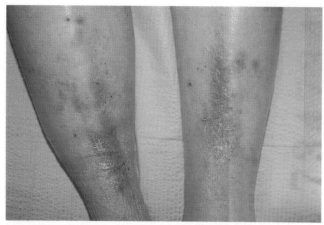

Figure 9–54   Purpura. Diabetic purpura with lesions consistent with necrobiosis lipoidica on the anterior shins of a 60-year-old man. The slightly raised plaques have small telangiectases in the central zone.

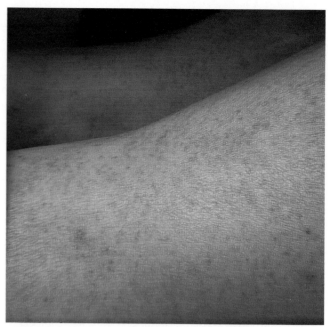

Figure 9–56   Schamberg's progressive pigmented purpuric dermatosis. A 23-year-old man presented with asymptomatic purpura and pigmentation that began on the toes and slowly spread to above the ankles.

their borders are representative of the progressive pigmented purpuras. This condition is most commonly found on the shins, ankles, and tops of the feet and toes. The pinhead lesions are quick to appear initially and then slowly progress with peripheral spread. The purpura gradually darkens after a few months with increasing brown pigmentation due to the presence of heme pigments. The condition may also spontaneously resolve after it has been present for many years. Histologically, an infiltrate is widespread in the subpapillary layer. Small ectatic blood vessels occur with swollen endothelia and hyaline degeneration of the vessel walls.

Pigmented purpuric lichenoid dermatosis of Gougerot and Blum resembles Schamberg's disease with the exception that it is found in older men between 40 and 70 years of age. The characteristic lesions are minute, rust-

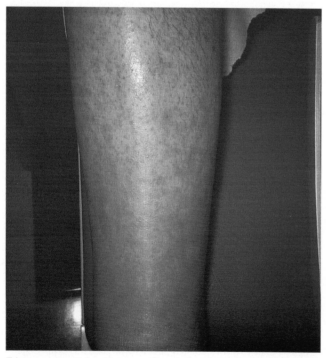

Figure 9–55   Purpura. Drug-induced purpura involving both legs and arms secondary to a reaction to oral generic furosemide.

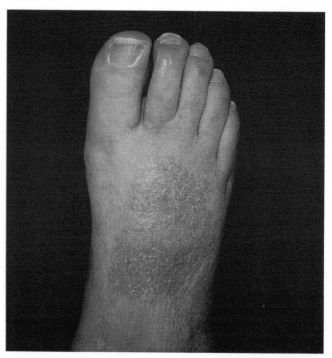

Figure 9–57   Pigmented purpuric lichenoid dermatosis of Gougerot and Blum. A 65-year-old man presented with two consolidating lesions on the top of the foot and similar lesions on the lower legs and thighs.

colored, lichenoid papules that tend to fuse into plaques with indistinct borders. The plaques may contain many papules of different colors on the lower extremities and lower trunk area. This condition may also be seen on the dorsal aspect of the foot (Fig. 9–57). This dermatosis has a more exaggerated histological process with the upper cutis containing a moderate lymphocytic infiltration and hemosiderin. Ectatic vessels with endothelial proliferations are also found. The primary differences between this condition and Schamberg's disease are the age of the patient, the distribution of the lesions, the presence of lichenoid papular elevations that group into plaques, and the fact that it tends to be less chronic.

Majocchi's purpuric annularis telangiectodes is an asymptomatic condition seen primarily in adolescent to young adult males (Fig. 9–58). The lesion is characterized by brownish yellow to dark red annular macules from 1 to 3 cm in diameter. The macule has multiple cayenne-pepper spots and red punctiform lesions with telangiectases. The central part of the lesion may gradually fade with resultant slight atrophy. Few or many lesions may be present with adjacent findings similar to those of Schamberg's disease. The condition may persist for many months to years and spreads centrifugally.

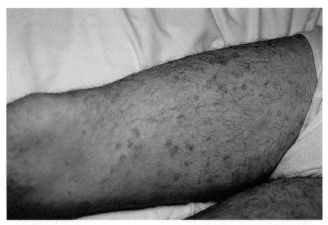

Figure 9–59   Disseminated pruritic purpura of Lowenthal. A 30-year-old man presented with disseminated and intensely pruritic purpura present for several months with no underlying disease or recent drug ingestion. The lesions were located on both lower extremities, buttocks, and lower trunk.

The eruptions usually begin on the lower extremities or ankles and slowly spread up the leg to involve the buttocks, trunk, and, in some cases, the arms. Histologically the condition is the same as Schamberg's disease and is probably secondary to the same process.

Disseminated pruritic purpura of Lowenthal is also termed *itching purpura, eczematoid-like purpura,* and *disseminated pruritic angiodermatitis.* It is an extremely pruritic eruptive hemorrhagic dermatitis that affects young men (Fig. 9–59). The lesions appear as erythematous, fawn-colored macules with punctate purpura. Lichenoid papules with scales may be present owing to rubbing and scratching. Disseminated pruritic purpura is commonly located on the lower legs with dissemination to the thighs, trunk, and finally to the upper extremities. It may persist for many months with periods of remission and exacerbation, especially during the warmer months. The condition may spontaneously clear with or without treatment. Histologically, the eruptions show spongiosis of the malpighian zone in addition to capillaritis. The remaining histopathology is similar to Schamberg's disease. Treatment is usually symptomatic due to the intense itching that occurs. Topical antipruritic agents and corticosteroids may cause improvement in the eruption, but the condition may flare with discontinuation of treatment.

VASOSPASTIC CONDITIONS

Vasospastic disorders differ from the occlusive arterial diseases in that there are no demonstrable intraluminal mechanical obstructions to blood flow. These diseases involve aberrations of the normal vasoconstriction of small arteries in response to chemical, emotional, and cold stimuli. Vasospasm in the peripheral vasculature may be only an incidental finding in the physical examination with no primary subjective complaints from the patient. It may also, in other instances, be persis-

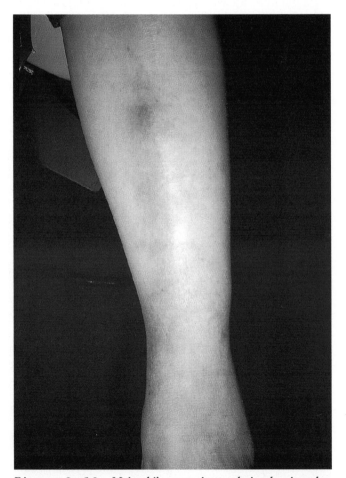

Figure 9–58   Majocchi's purpuric annularis telangiectodes. A 17-year-old boy had characteristic asymptomatic lesions on the anterior shin and thigh.

T A B L E   9 – 4   Comparison of Signs and Symptoms of Major Vasospastic Disorders

Feature	Raynaud's Disease	Acrocyanosis	Livedo Reticularis	Cold Injury
Type of color change	Blue, red, white, mottled, or diffuse	Blue, diffuse	Red, blue, mottled, and reticulated	Variable and exposure
Location of vascular symptoms	Fingers, toes; nose and ears rarely	Hands usually; toes, feet occasionally	Legs usually; arms occasionally	Exposed parts
Duration of symptoms	Intermittent	Permanent	Permanent	Variable; worse in winter
Local symptoms	None or burning pain	Usually none, exept cold digits	None or coldness or pain	Pain, dysesthesia, paresthesia
Effect of cold on symptoms	Increased	Increased	Increased blueness	Increased
Effect of heat on symptoms	May decrease greatly	Little change noted	Less blueness	Usually decreases
Effect of posture on symptoms	Little change	Cyanosis decreased with elevation	Cyanosis decreased by elevation or exercise	Elevation decreases
Ulceration or gangrene	Slight or none, tips of digits	None	Occasionally, feet and legs	Both possible in severe injuries

From Feller SR, Dockery GL: Vasospastic Diseases. Clin Podiatr Med Surg *3:463–471, 1986.*

tent, painful, and a sign of disease with a poor prognosis in which ulceration and gangrene are the end results. Acute digital ischemia not due to thromboembolism may be the result of either a primary vasospastic disorder (Raynaud's disease, acrocyanosis, livedo reticularis) or regional or traumatic disorder (Raynaud's syndrome, cold injury) (Table 9–4).

Raynaud's Phenomenon and Disease

Raynaud's phenomenon describes a clinical picture in which there is pallor or sequential blanching (arteriospasm) (Fig. 9–60), cyanosis (venous stasis) (Fig. 9–61), and rubor (reactive hyperemia) (Fig. 9–62) of the digits induced by cold exposure or emotional stimuli. This is the so-called patriotic or red, white, and blue syndrome. Pain and paresthesia may also be present. This condition is considered to be primary

(*Raynaud's disease*) when associated systemic disease is absent. If other systemic disease is present, this form of vasospasm is secondary and is termed *Raynaud's phenomenon.*

Raynaud's disease typically affects young women. Men, however, may demonstrate Raynaud's phenomenon, especially when secondary causes are present, such as collagen-vascular diseases, systemic sclerosis, or other connective tissue disorders. There are many secondary causes of Raynaud's phenomenon (Table 9–5). Diagnosis of Raynaud's phenomenon is primarily based on the patient's history of a secondary medical condition. These patients may describe episodes of symmetrical attacks of color changes in the hands or feet when exposed to cold or emotional stress (Fig. 9–63). They may also relate disappearance of the symptoms on warming of the part or cessation of the stress.

Physical examination is used primarily to distinguish Raynaud's disease from Raynaud's phenomenon or

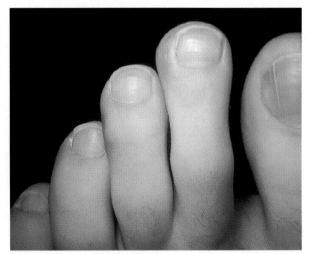

Figure 9–60   Raynaud's disease. Digital pallor is secondary to arteriospasm.

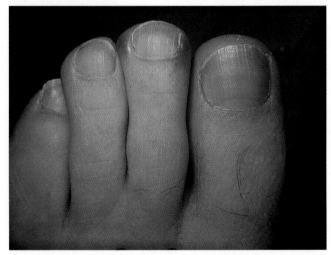

Figure 9–61   Raynaud's disease. Digital cyanosis is secondary to venous stasis.

Chapter 9 ■ PERIPHERAL VASCULAR DISEASE AND RELATED DISORDERS   125

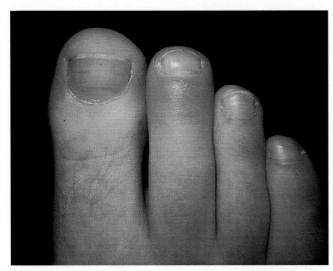

Figure 9–62   Raynaud's disease. Digital rubor is secondary to reactive hyperemia.

syndrome associated with secondary causes. The diagnosis of Raynaud's disease will be correct 95% of the time if (1) the condition is precipitated by cold or emotional stress (Fig. 9–64); (2) the presentation is bilateral; (3) gangrene is absent; (4) no associated secondary causes are noted; and (5) the condition is present for at

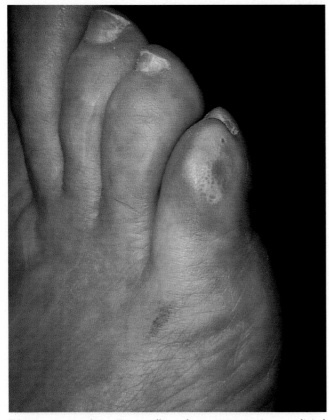

Figure 9–63   Raynaud's phenomenon. Acute digital ischemia is evident in a patient with rheumatoid arthritis after minor cold exposure.

TABLE 9–5 Causes of Raynaud's Phenomenon

Collagen-Vascular Disease
Arteritis (small and large vessel)
Dermatomyositis-polymyositis
Mixed connective tissue disease
Polyarteritis
Rheumatoid arthritis
Sjögren's syndrome
Systemic lupus erythematosus
Systemic sclerosis
Vasculitis

Drugs
Beta-adrenergic blockers
Bleomycin
Cisplatin
Clonidine
Ergotamine
Heavy metal intoxication (lead, arsenic)
Methysergide
Tobacco

Hematologic Disorders
Antiphospholipid syndrome
Cold agglutinins
Cryoproteinemia
Dysproteinemias
Macroglobulinemia
Polycythemia
Thrombocytosis

Neurogenic Disorders
Carpal tunnel syndrome
Hemiplegia
Multiple sclerosis
Poliomyelitis
Reflex sympathetic dystrophy
Syringomyelia
Tarsal tunnel syndrome
Thoracic outlet syndrome

Occupational or Environmental Conditions
Disorders in pianists, typists
Meat cutters
Pneumatic hammer operators
Vibratory tools
Vinyl chloride
Toxic oil syndrome

Vaso-occlusive Disease
Arteriosclerosis obliterans
Arterial embolism
Thromboangiitis obliterans

Miscellaneous Conditions
Hypothyroidism
Occult carcinoma
Pheochromocytoma
Primary pulmonary hypertension
Pseudoxanthoma elasticum

least 2 years. Less than 1% of patients with Raynaud's disease will develop ulcerations or gangrenous changes at the distal tips of digits; however, a much larger percentage of patients with Raynaud's phenomenon will develop small areas of ulcers on the fingers and toes (Fig. 9–65).

Management of this disorder is aimed at protection of the digits from cold and trauma. Wearing loose-fitting, warm, multilayered clothing that covers as much of the body as possible to avoid the cold, includ-

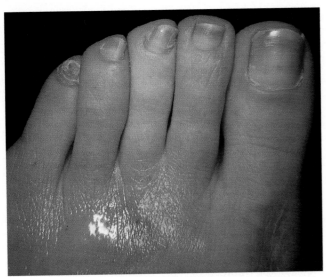

Figure 9–64   Raynaud's disease. Cold challenge with ice cube to top of foot was followed by immediate pallor of the central toe.

ing protection of the feet and hands, is essential when outdoors. Additionally, reassurance of the patient regarding the nature of the disease and its prognosis is equally important. Use of tobacco, as in other arterial diseases, should be discouraged because nicotine induces vasoconstriction. Various nonpharmaceutical modalities such as biofeedback and behavioral modification have been helpful in some patients.

Various medications have been found of use in decreasing the frequency and degree of vasospasm. The calcium-channel blockers nifedipine and verapamil have been chosen to treat Raynaud's disease and phenomenon. Calcium-channel blockers inhibit flux through the slow calcium channel, allowing arteriolar vasodilatation and increased peripheral blood flow. These drugs may be taken with regular daily oral administration or prophylactically with sublingual doses before cold exposure only. I have extensively prescribed phenoxybenzamine, an alpha-adrenergic receptor blocking agent, in doses of 10 mg one to four times daily. This is particularly useful in limiting symptoms during exposure to precipitating factors, such as cold exposure in skiers. Because of possible side effects due to adrenergic blockade, such as postural hypotension, miosis, and nasal congestion, the dosage frequently must be adjusted to achieve efficacy but limit adverse reactions. The adverse reactions also tend to decrease with continuation of therapy. In most of my patients, the optimum dose of phenoxybenzamine has been 10 mg daily taken at bedtime.

Sympathectomy is reserved only for severe, recalcitrant cases of Raynaud's disease and is indicated only when enough time has elapsed for exclusion of associated disease. Lastly, if symptoms persist despite careful management, the possibility of moving to a warmer and drier climate should be discussed with the patient.

Acrocyanosis

Acrocyanosis, like Raynaud's phenomenon, involves coldness and cyanosis of the digits, although the cyanosis in this disorder is much more persistent (Fig. 9–66).

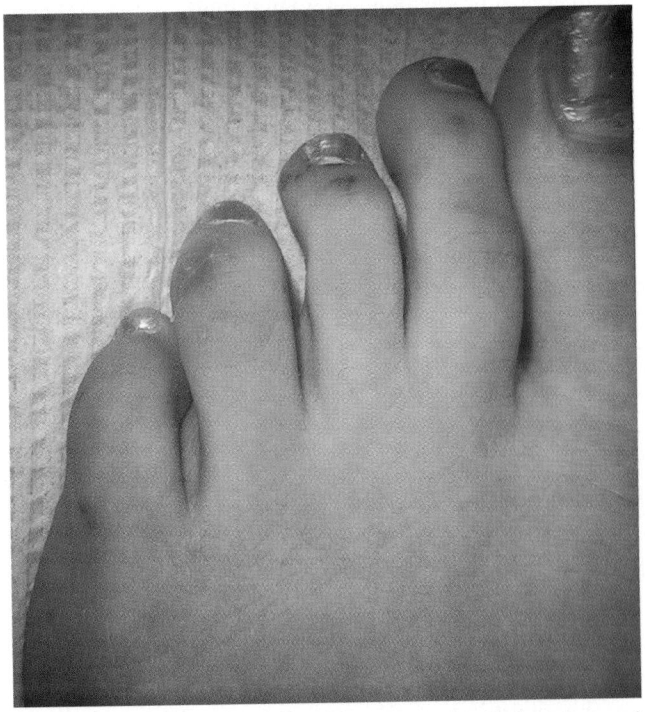

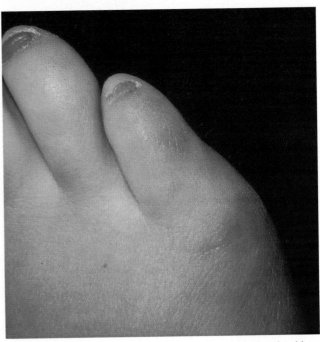

Figure 9–66   Acrocyanosis. Persistent cyanosis and coldness in the digits were evident most of the time in a young woman with no other symptoms.

Figure 9–65   Raynaud's phenomenon. Small ulcerations and gangrene occurred on the toes of a 38-year-old woman with Sjögren's syndrome.

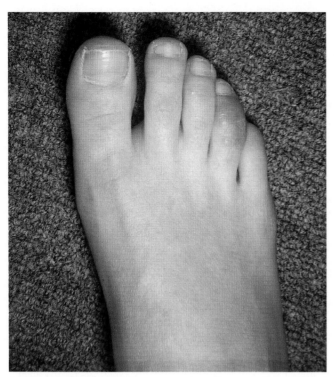

Figure 9–67 **Acrocyanosis.** In the pallor stage after prolonged elevation, the darkest areas of cyanosis will sometimes remain red or purple, but the overall cyanosis returns immediately with dependency.

Acrocyanosis is more prevalent in adolescent females but may be seen at any age and in males. In a study group of 18 patients with acrocyanosis, I found that there were 12 females and 6 males ranging in age from 16 to 34 years. The condition is almost always worse in cold, damp weather but is never completely relieved by warm weather.

The changes are usually symmetrical and are most severe in the hands (fingers) and feet (toes), extending gradually toward the elbows and knees. Pallor, or blanching, being a prominent feature in Raynaud's disease, is much more subtle in the uncomplicated cases of acrocyanosis. Erythema or mottled blue coloration may occur at different times, but generalized cyanosis is present most of the time. Prolonged elevation of the lower extremity will allow mild to moderate pallor to occur, which immediately returns to cyanosis when the extremity is dependent (Fig. 9–67). Unlike in Raynaud's phenomenon, the digital cyanosis may lessen or disappear during sleep and local cooling fails to produce vasoconstriction. Symptoms in most cases are limited to coldness, slight swelling, or numbness of the toes.

The cause of the disorder is unknown, but it is intensified by coldness and emotional upset. The cyanosis results from arteriolar spasm, which is followed by secondary dilation of the subcutaneous venous plexus. The color changes usually persist throughout life, although they may lessen in later years. Usually, the only treatment indicated in acrocyanosis is protection from cold and trauma. I regularly recommend that patients also decrease their intake of caffeine (colas, teas, coffee, chocolate) and nicotine and avoid stressful situations whenever possible. Trophic changes, ulceration and gangrene, do not usually occur, and the prognosis is good in most patients. In cases in which the symptoms of severe coldness in the digits interfere with the patient's job or recreation, I have recommended oral phenoxybenzamine, 10 mg daily, with excellent results. Generally, treatment with primary vasodilators or sympathectomy is not necessary.

Livedo Reticularis

This vasospastic disorder is characterized by reticular or blotchy cyanosis of the skin in a "fish-net" pattern, which gives a reddish blue discoloration of the skin of the extremities, digits, and possibly the trunk (Fig. 9–68). The skin within the webs of the fish-net pattern is normal to pale. The cyanosis is worse in cold weather but frequently persists in warm weather. In true livedo reticularis the pattern is fixed and unresponsive to rewarming. Coldness, numbness, paresthesia, or aching of the extremities may be associated with the disease, al-

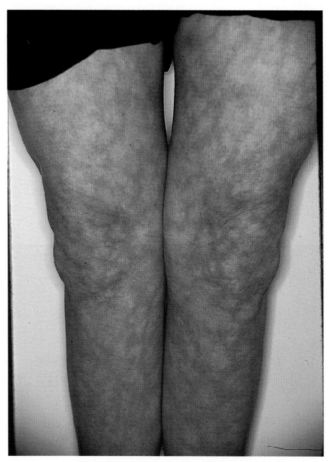

Figure 9–68 **Livedo reticularis.** Classic presentation of reticulated "fish net" pattern on lower extremities. (Courtesy of Dr. Jeffrey C. Page.)

though cosmesis is commonly the patient's main complaint.

The pathophysiology is thought to involve spasm of cutaneous arteries, and cyanosis develops in the area drained by dilated venules. The portions of the extremities displaying the reddish blue discoloration correspond to the arborizations of the peripheral capillaries from arterioles that pierce the cutis from below. Histological study of cutaneous ulcerations in persons with livedo reticularis may show arteriolar occlusion with intimal proliferation, dilatation of capillaries, and nonspecific infiltrate in the skin. Patients usually first notice the physical changes while in the second and third decades of life. It is most common in women younger than age 40 but may occur at any age. In males, this disorder may occur at any age. If the symptoms are of sudden onset and ulcerations are present, a primary disease, such as periarteritis or other collagen disease, immune deficiency, or drug reaction, should be strongly suspected. Treatment is usually aimed at protecting the affected parts from cold exposure. Patients with primary livedo reticularis should be reassured that the disorder is not serious and the prognosis in most cases is good.

Vasodilators offer little help in this disorder. Likewise, sympathectomy offers, at best, limited and temporary relief of symptoms.

Cold Injuries

Vasospasm plays a central role in the development and sequelae of cold injuries. *Cold injury* is a general term used to include pernio (chilblain), immersion foot, and frostbite. Clinical features in these conditions are similar, and differences in the signs and symptoms are probably due to differences in environmental conditions, length of cold exposure, and variations in the reaction of the peripheral vasculature to cold.

Vasospasm begins in the affected part during the actual exposure to cold. Vasoconstriction often persists, even after warming. Constriction occurs primarily in

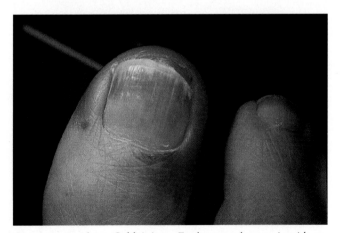

Figure 9–69   **Cold injury.** Erythema and cyanosis with severe discomfort in toes that followed cold injury several months earlier.

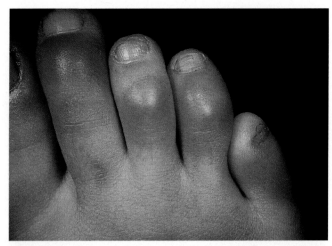

Figure 9–70   **Cold injury.** Painful, swollen, and erythematous toes resulted from cold exposure while hunting.

less-injured areas and extends centrally, while dilatation appears in areas of severe damage, leading to perivascular edema and intravascular stasis with erythrocyte agglutination and fibrin deposition. This often results in thrombosis and tissue loss. Symptoms of cold injury range from sensitivity to cold, with color changes in the extremities suggesting vasospasm (Fig. 9–69), to a persistent causalgia-like syndrome with burning pain. Patients may also complain of dysesthesia, paresthesia, and vague aching of the affected parts. The "hunting reaction" is a paradoxical cold-induced vasodilation that is manifested by an intensely painful erythematous swelling of the toes when exposed to cold (Fig. 9–70). It can result from outdoor exposure in winter (as in hunters and other sports enthusiasts) with inadequate foot protection. This exaggerated reaction may cause disabling pain in some patients. Treatment is usually with rewarming and prevention of reinjury.

Pernio or *chilblain* is characterized by local cyanosis and doughy subcutaneous swelling in digits exposed to cold (Fig. 9–71). Painful red-purple papules, nodules, or plaques may form on the tips of the toes, and mild trauma may produce hemorrhagic bullae. Changes are usually noted within 24 hours of cold exposure. Pain, burning, or pruritus may persist for many weeks. The onset of pernio is usually in late fall with worsening during winter and spontaneous disappearance during the spring and summer months. Treatment of pernio consists of prevention of cold injury, protection of the toes and fingers during outdoor activities, rewarming after cold exposure, and oral medications, such as nicotinic acid, nifedipine, and phenoxybenzamine.

Exposure to cool or cold water for extended periods may result in *immersion foot*. This condition may also be termed *trench foot, seaboot foot, swampfoot,* or *fisherman's foot,* depending on the circumstances of the exposure to wetness (Fig. 9–72). Clinically, there are three stages of immersion foot: the hyperemic stage, the edema and pain stage, and the post-hyperemic stage. The hyperemic stage may last for over 6 weeks. The second stage

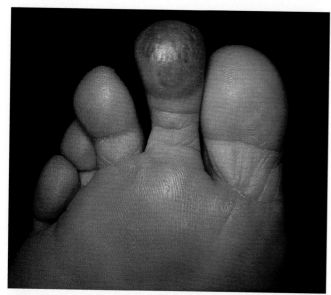

Figure 9–71 Pernio. Digital swelling, cyanosis, and nodule formation followed cold exposure in a 60-year-old woman who shoveled snow in her house slippers.

shows significant erythema, edema, and increased heat of the affected parts with intense burning or throbbing pain. The symptoms may diminish after 1 or 2 weeks, but the patient may report paroxysmal shooting pains for several weeks. There may be blister formation, ulceration, or superficial gangrene during this stage. The third and final stage is the post-hyperemic stage, which is characterized by hyperhidrosis, hyperesthesia, and coldness of the part with joint pain and stiffness. This

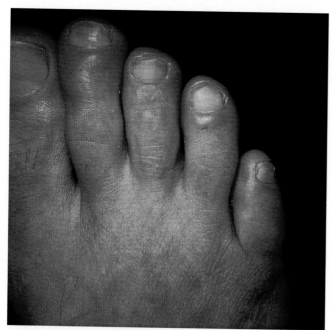

Figure 9–72 Immersion foot, stage 2. A 25-year-old male commercial fisherman with "seaboot foot" had redness, swelling, blister formation, and intense throbbing pain on both feet in a stocking distribution.

condition may continue for many years and may be exacerbated by repeated exposure to cold or damp weather conditions. Treatment is similar to that of frostbite.

Frostbite occurs when ice crystals form in the tissues and involves actual freezing of the skin, which becomes white and anesthetic followed by tissue damage and gangrene. The ears, nose, fingers, and toes are most often affected by this degree of cold injury (Fig. 9–73). Military personnel had long been subjected to the effects of freezing temperatures during war times spent in cold climates. Now, most cases of frostbite are found in outdoorsmen, hunters, skiers, hikers, and snowmobilers who spend extended time in activities in the snow or on frozen ground. *Frostnip* is defined as a superficial, reversible form of frostbite. There is involvement only of the skin, and clinical manifestations include simple erythema, transient anesthesia, and superficial blistering. If exposure to cold is continued, the frostnip will progress to frostbite.

Frostbite is classified into four stages or degrees, based on the depth of tissue damage:

1. First-degree frostbite is characterized by paleness of the part during cold exposure, followed by erythema and edema after thawing. Vesicles or blisters do not form.

2. Second-degree frostbite is confined to the upper dermis, and, along with erythema and edema after thawing, there is vesicle and blister formation within 48 hours. The fluid is slowly reabsorbed leaving an eschar.

3. Third-degree frostbite extends into the subcutaneous layers. After thawing, there is slow-developing, but severe, edema that may last for more than a month. Hemorrhagic vesicles and blisters may form that are smaller than those seen in second-degree frostbite.

4. Fourth-degree frostbite is characterized by full-thickness injury that proceeds to dry gangrene and am-

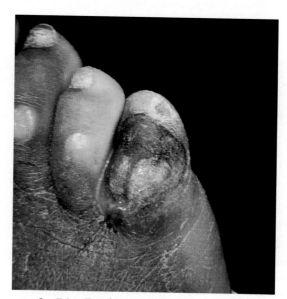

Figure 9–73 Frostbite. Superficial tissue gangrene is evident on small toe after extended cold exposure.

putation. Bone involvement is common. If secondary bacterial infection occurs, a wet gangrene may be seen.

In most cases of frostbite, the classification of superficial or deep frostbite is used because clinically it may be impossible to identify the type of tissue damage by degree.

Treatment of all stages of frostbite centers on rapid rewarming in a warm water bath between 100° F and 110° F. The process should be monitored to prevent thermal injury. During this process there may be considerable pain, and analgesics may be necessary. Rewarming should be delayed, however, if there is any chance of refreezing the part because injury is greatly increased by repeated freeze-thaw cycles. The patient should be hospitalized if at all possible, and the injured part should be elevated and protected. Active range of motion is recommended to prevent additional atrophy, but rubbing and irritation should be avoided. Early debridement and amputation should be discouraged because damage may be much less than predicted. Debridement and amputation may be delayed for many weeks without jeopardizing outcome. Complications include tetanus, gas gangrene, infection, and compartment syndrome. Tetanus prophylaxis, analgesics, and antibiotics all may be administered as needed.

Long-term sequelae of frostbite include cold sensitivity of the injured part, paresthesia and sensory defects, vasospastic color changes, stiffness, loss of toenails and nail dystrophy, atrophy of the toe tips, osteoporosis, coldness, hyperhidrosis, anhidrosis, and dry, cracked skin that is not easily rehydrated (Fig. 9–74).

GLOMUS TUMOR

This small flesh-colored to red nodule may be found on the hands or feet (Fig. 9–75), particularly beneath the nails (Fig. 9–76). The tumor derives from the arteriovenous shunts (subcutaneous neuromyoarterial

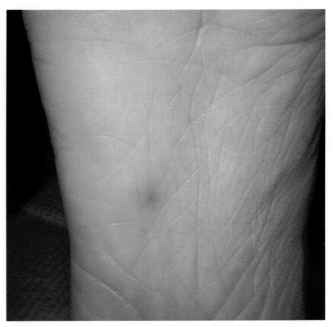

Figure 9–75   Glomus tumor. This plantar foot lesion in an 18-year-old woman is solitary and less than 1 cm in diameter. The diagnosis is usually confirmed by the histopathology report.

glomus) that occur normally in the body. The glomus tumor is a benign, excruciatingly painful neoplasm that may be difficult to identify clinically. The pain is frequently paroxysmal with sudden recurrence or intensification of symptoms, and this is considered the most suggestive clinical feature of the diagnosis. Glomus tumors are hamartomas of glomus bodies and blood vessels; therefore, they are composed of blood vessels

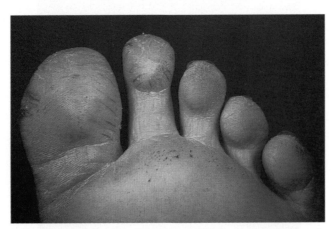

Figure 9–74   Post-frostbite syndrome. A 32-year-old male mountaineer had bilateral skin changes of anhidrosis, dry cracking skin, and persistent rubor after frostbite injury to his feet several years earlier.

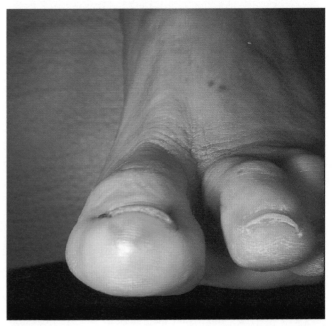

Figure 9–76   Glomus tumor. A 45-year-old woman presented with intense paroxysmal pain at the distal hallux and under the toenail.

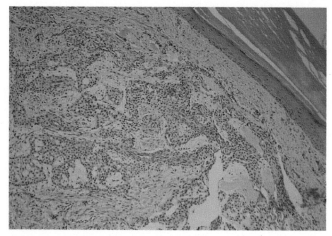

Figure 9–77   Glomus tumor. Photomicrograph shows a collection of vascular spaces surrounded by large numbers of cells with round, basophilic nuclei.

surrounded by uniformly cuboidal cells with round basophilic nuclei (Fig. 9–77). Histologically, the lesion arises from the cells of the Sucquet-Hoyer canal (an arteriovenous coiled shunt composed of an arterial and a venous segment united by a vascular channel). Glomus tumors are richly innervated, and this may account for the painful symptoms. Treatment is complete surgical excision of the lesion. If the lesion is not completely removed, it tends to recur.

BIBLIOGRAPHY

Adlerman DB: Therapy for essential cutaneous telangiectasia. Postgrad Med 61:91–95, 1977.

Au YF: Intralesional electrodesiccation with a 30-gauge needle. J Dermatol Surg Oncol 7:190–191, 1981.

Bauman ML, Steiner I: Schamberg's disease. J Am Podiatr Assoc 70:508–510, 1980.

Bentivegna S, Green R: Blue toe syndrome. J Am Podiatr Assoc 72:467–468, 1982.

Blair ST, Wright DD, Backhouse CM, Riddle E, McCollum CN: Sustained compression and healing of chronic venous ulcers. BMJ 297:1159–1161, 1988.

Borovoy M, Beresh A: Transient vasospasm: The blue toe. J Am Podiatr Assoc 75:656–658, 1985.

Bouché RT, Medawar SJ, Dockery GL: Oral contraceptives and deep venous thrombosis with pulmonary embolism. J Foot Surg 21:297–301, 1982.

Brenner MA, Kalish SR: Glomus tumors with special reference to children's feet. J Am Podiatr Assoc 68:715–720, 1978.

Brown AL Jr, Juergens JL: Arteriosclerosis and atherosclerosis. In Fairbain JF, Juergens JL, Spittell JA Jr (eds): Peripheral Vascular Diseases, 4th ed, pp 159–171. Philadelphia, WB Saunders, 1972.

Brown F, Klein S, Berlin D: Local manifestations of cold injury. J Am Podiatr Assoc 71:595–598, 1981.

Burton CS: Management of chronic and problem lower extremity wounds. Dermatol Clin 11:767–773, 1993.

Dana AS, Rex IH, Samitz MH: The hunting reaction. Arch Dermatol 99:441–450, 1969.

Dockery GL, Nilson RZ: Intralesional injections. Clin Podiatr Med Surg 3:473–485, 1986.

Edwards EA, Coffman JD: Cutaneous changes in peripheral vascular disease. In Fitzpatrick TB, Eisen AZ, Wolff K, Freedberg IM, Austen KF (eds): Dermatology in General Medicine, 3rd ed, pp 1997–2022. New York, McGraw-Hill, 1987.

Faria DT, Fivenson DP, Green H: Peripheral vascular diseases. In Moschella SL, Hurley HJ (eds): Dermatology, 3rd ed, pp 1145–1190. Philadelphia, WB Saunders, 1992.

Feller SR, Dockery GL: Vasospastic diseases: Diagnosis and management. Clin Podiatr Med Surg 3:463–471, 1986.

From L, Assaad D: Vascular neoplasms, pseudoneoplasms, and hyperplasias. In Fitzpatrick TB, Eisen AZ, Wolff K, Freedberg IM, Austen KF (eds): Dermatology in General Medicine, 3rd ed, pp 1059–1077. New York, McGraw-Hill, 1987.

Goldman MP, Bennett RG: Treatment of telangiectasia: A review. J Am Acad Dermatol 17:167–170, 1987.

Gupta AK, Goldfarb MT, Voorhees JJ: The use of sulfasalazine in atrophie blanche. Int J Dermatol 29:663–665, 1990.

Hart ES, Kwasnick R: Blue toe syndrome: A case presentation. J Am Podiatr Assoc 73:635–637, 1983.

Harvery CK: An overview of cold injuries. J Am Podiatr Med Assoc 82:436–438, 1992.

Jetton RL, Lazarus GS: Minidose heparin therapy for vasculitis of atrophie blanche. J Am Acad Dermatol 8:23–26, 1983.

Kidawa AS, Lemont H: Vascular diseases of the lower extremities. Clin Dermatol 1:67–76, 1983.

Kuwada GT, Dockery GL: Contact dermatitis: A review. Clin Podiatr Med Surg 3:551–561, 1986.

Lance BJ, Kirschenbaum SE: Distal ischemia with digital gangrene secondary to Buerger's disease. J Foot Surg 30:534–541, 1991.

McCarthy DJ: Therapeutic considerations in the podiatric care of ulcerations. Clin Podiatr Med Surg 3:487–504, 1986.

Moffatt CJ, Franks PJ, Oldroyd M, Bosanquet N, Brown P, Greenhalgh RM, McCollum CN: Community clinics for leg ulcers and impact on healing. BJM 305:1389–1392, 1992.

Muehleman C, Wise RD: Epidermal culture and grafting: A brief review. J Am Podiatr Med Assoc 83:462–465, 1993.

O'Keefe RG, Pikscher I: Ulcers of the lower extremity. In McCarthy DJ, Montgomery R (eds): Podiatric Dermatology, pp 198–209. Baltimore, Williams & Wilkins, 1986.

Page JC, Dockery GL: The sudden onset of digital ischemia in a diabetic: A case report. J Am Podiatr Assoc 71:443–445, 1981.

Port M, Ottinger ML, Fenske NA: Connective tissue disorders. In McCarthy DJ, Montgomery R (eds): Podiatric Dermatology, pp 264–282. Baltimore, Williams & Wilkins, 1986.

Ratnam KV, Su WP, Peters MS: Purpura simplex (inflammatory purpura without vasculitis): A clinicopathologic study of 174 cases. J Am Acad Dermatol 25:642–650, 1991.

Schamberg JF: A peculiar progressive pigmentary disease of the skin. Br J Dermatol 13:1–4, 1901.

Shornick JK, Nicholes BK, Bergstresser PR, Gilliam JN: Idiopathic atrophie blanche. J Am Acad Dermatol 8:792–789, 1983.

Sperandio CP, McCarthy DJ: Digital arterial embolism: True blue toe syndrome: A histopathologic analysis. J Am Podiatr Med Assoc 78:593–598, 1988.

Stein RS: Purpura: Determining the underlying cause. Diagnosis 9:75–81, 1981.

Turski D, Taylor D, Whittaker D: Unusual ulcerations of the lower extremity. In McCarthy DJ, Montgomery R (eds): Podiatric Dermatology, pp 210–218. Baltimore, Williams & Wilkins, 1986.

Vega M, Rosenfeld S, Rabinowitz AD: Chronic pigmented purpura. J Am Podiatr Assoc 72:412–417, 1982.

10

ECZEMATOUS DERMATITIS

INTRODUCTION

Eczematous dermatitis represents an inflammatory response of the skin to many different external and internal stimulants or agents. The cause of many forms of eczema is unknown, and the diagnosis is often difficult. Eczematous dermatitis is classified by its general appearance, location, and presenting symptoms. It is divided into acute, subacute, and chronic stages, each of which represents a stage in the evolution of the inflammatory process. Spongiosis (intercellular edema) of the epidermis is identified in most cases of eczematous dermatitis, and this condition is extremely helpful in the dermatohistopathological diagnosis.

The eczematous dermatoses may start at any stage and may evolve into another stage. The acute stage involves the formation of vesicles, blisters, or bullae and is usually intensely red with significant pruritus (Fig. 10–1). The subacute stage involves redness, scaling, and fissuring, with a parched or scalded appearance (Fig. 10–2). There is slight to moderate pruritus with stinging or burning pain. The chronic stage involves lichenification with accentuated skin lines, excoriations, and fissurings. Moderate to severe pruritus is present during this stage (Fig. 10–3). Each type of eczema is further divided into subtypes based on distribution or causative agents.

Clinical classifications of eczematous dermatitis are somewhat confusing because of the disputed nomenclature and variations in the classification schemes by different workers. For the purposes of this chapter, all of the conditions are discussed individually without specific classification. Topics described include asteatotic dermatitis, atopic dermatitis, contact dermatitis, drug eruptions, dyshidrotic eczema, exfoliative dermatitis, hand and foot dermatitis, lichen

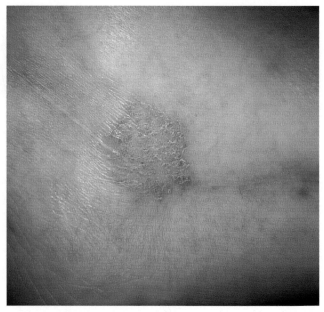

Figure 10–2 Subacute eczematous dermatitis. Erythema, scaling, and mild fissuring in a round pattern are consistent with a nummular pattern.

simplex chronicus, prurigo nodularis, and nummular eczema.

ASTEATOTIC DERMATITIS

Asteatotic dermatitis is also known as chronic winter itch, winter dry skin, eczema craquelé, pruritus hiemalis, and xerotic eczema. This eczematous dermatitis is characterized by dehydration showing redness, dry scaling, and fine superficial cracking of the skin, which is similar in appearance to mild ichthyosis vulgaris (Fig. 10–4). These changes usually occur in patches over several parts of the body but are seen commonly on the anterolateral aspects of the lower extremities, especially in the elderly (Fig. 10–5).

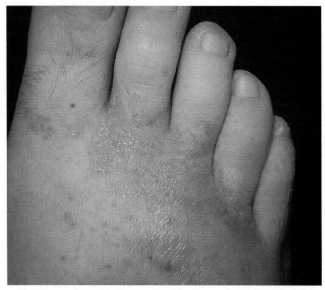

Figure 10–1 Acute eczematous dermatitis. Numerous pruritic vesicles on an erythematous base are secondary to poison ivy dermatitis. The vesicles may become confluent with time.

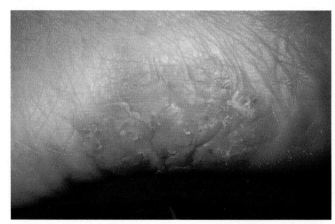

Figure 10–3 Chronic eczematous dermatitis. A plaque of lichenified tissue with accentuated skin lines and eczematous papules represents a case of lichen simplex chronicus.

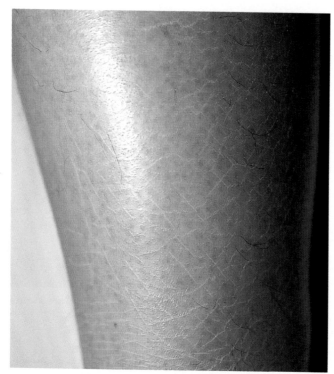

Figure 10–4 Asteatotic eczema. Fine xerosis of the skin shows dry, cracked, and scaly changes in the superficial layers.

This xerotic and pruritic dermatitis is frequently seen during the winter and in areas where the humidity is very low. The skin becomes extremely dry and scaly and starts to show accentuation of the skin lines (xerosis).

As the process proceeds there is redness with thin, long, horizontal superficial cracks appearing with continued drying (Fig. 10–6). Eventually, vertical cracks begin to connect with the horizontal fissures, creating the cracked glass appearance termed *eczema craquelé*. The most severe form of this condition shows an accentuation of the deep fissuring that becomes secondarily infected. Pain is the primary symptom, rather than pruritus, during this stage.

Asteatotic eczematous dermatitis probably develops as a result of decreased skin surface lipids. Cleansers and deodorant soaps defat the stratum corneum, predisposing the patient to water loss and a decrease in the water reservoir within the stratum corneum. This dryness causes generalized pruritus, which in turn leads to rubbing or scratching, which causes disorganization of the surface lipid balance. Frequent bathing in hot water increases water loss from the skin as it dries. Applying lotions or creams aggravates the inflammation and encourages further water loss as evaporation occurs.

Treatment of asteatotic eczematous dermatitis involves educating the patient about skin care, such as using moisturizing soaps in baths but decreasing the number of baths, and encouraging the use of topical emollients containing lanolin, glycerin, urea, lactic acid, or other alpha-hydroxy acids. The use of room humidifiers should also be encouraged. Lowering the heat in living quarters will help reduce skin water loss due to evaporation, and a lesser quantity of moisture is needed to maintain a high relative humidity at the lower temperatures. Group V or VI topical corticosteroids and antipruritics may be necessary in severe cases. Oral corticosteroids should not be used, because the dermatitis will flare within 48 hours of discontinuation of the medication. Antibiotics may be necessary if secondary infection is present. In severe cases that do not respond to avoidance of defatting agents and conservative measures as outlined, diagnostic studies to evaluate thyroid disease, acquired immunodeficiency syndrome, and malignancies should be considered.

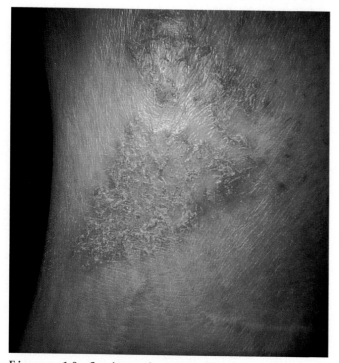

Figure 10–5 Asteatotic eczema. The skin on the anterior ankle is extremely dry, cracked, and scaly.

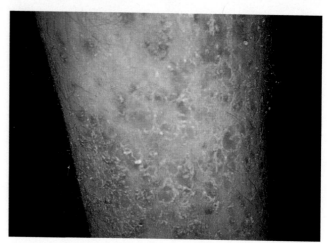

Figure 10–6 Asteatotic eczema. Eczema craquelé occurs over large areas of lower extremities with excessive drying, scaling, and cracking toward the feet.

ATOPIC DERMATITIS

Atopic dermatitis is also known as atopic eczema, allergic eczema, and Besnier's prurigo and is typically referred to as "atopy." *Atopic dermatitis* is the preferred term and represents a chronically relapsing skin eczema that may begin in infancy, childhood, adolescence, or adulthood. There is frequently a family history of atopic dermatitis, associated allergic rhinitis, and asthma. Most cases of atopic dermatitis are present at a very early age. In many of the adolescent and adult cases, eczema was present at an earlier time with remission noted. Atopic dermatitis usually occurs as an erythematous papulovesicular eruption (Fig. 10–7) that evolves into dry, scaly, dermatitis with accentuated skin lines (Fig. 10–8). As the condition progresses over time there is a formation of lichenified plaques (Fig. 10–9). The skin distribution of the rash varies somewhat with age. Infants and children younger than 2 years of age show erythematous papulovesicular lesions on the face, wrists, and extensor surfaces of the arms and legs, usually sparing the diaper area. In older children (2 to 12 years), the flexor surfaces, face, wrists, and ankles show dry maculopapular lesions that are extremely pruritic, leading to chronic rubbing or scratching. In adolescents and adults, flexural surfaces, face, wrists, knees, hands, and feet show xerosis, lichenification, and papulation (Fig. 10–10).

There is no primary lesion in atopic dermatitis, and the diagnosis is made by combining a variety of clinical symptoms, including an extremely pruritic rash, with a typical appearance and distribution and a tendency toward a chronic and recurrent course. The personal or family history of asthma, seasonal allergies, and eczema plays a significant, but not consistent, role in the diagnosis. Sweat retention may be a factor. Secondary superimposed infections, with subsequent sensitization to

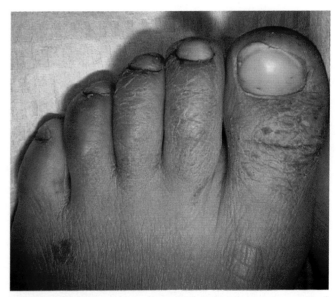

F i g u r e   1 0 – 8   Atopic dermatitis. Lichenification is associated with thickening and exaggeration of skin creases and postinflammatory hyperpigmentation on the feet.

bacterial or fungal elements, may lead to exacerbations. Emotional upsets and increased temperatures may also worsen the pruritus and, subsequently, the dermatitis.

Treatment of atopic dermatitis includes elimination of inflammation and infection, providing hydration, and controlling those factors that cause exacerbations. Topical therapy involves moisturizers with urea or lactic acid after bathing for 20 to 30 minutes in tepid water with bath oils, low-potency group V or VI corticosteroids for mild to moderate rashes and group II to IV corticosteroids for severe lichenified dermatoses applied lightly two or three times a day, and topical tar creams under occlusion. Oral medications include antibiotics if there is secondary infection, antihistamines to control pruritus (hydroxyzine, 10 mg/5 mL three or four times daily), and corticosteroids (prednisone, 5 to 10 mg daily) for a short course in severe resistant cases. The lowest potency of topical corticosteroid that controls a patient's symptoms should be employed, and systemic

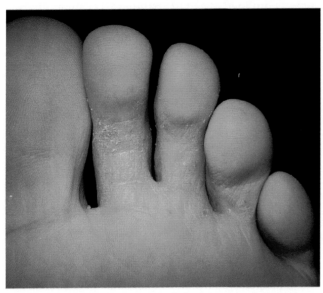

F i g u r e   1 0 – 7   Atopic dermatitis. Symmetrical flexural erythematous papulovesicular rash is evident on the toes.

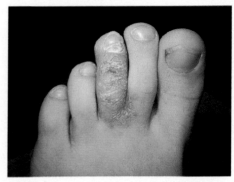

F i g u r e   1 0 – 9   Atopic dermatitis. Lichenified plaques have formed around the pruritic rash on the toes secondary to continued scratching.

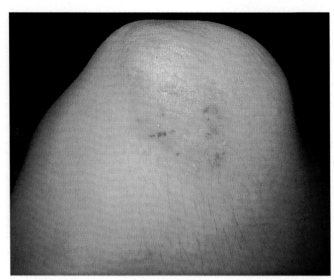

Figure 10–10 Atopic dermatitis. Xerotic and lichenified rash over the knee is present in a 14-year-old patient with atopic dermatitis and asthma.

corticosteroids should be avoided if possible to prevent rebound flares after treatment and to reduce potential side effects. To reduce contact irritant dermatitis and side effects no topical or systemic therapy should be used for prolonged periods. Ultraviolet light therapy and psoralen photochemotherapy (PUVA) has been shown to produce remission in many patients with chronic atopic dermatitis.

CONTACT DERMATITIS

Contact dermatitis can manifest itself in several ways, including primary irritant contact dermatitis, allergic contact dermatitis, and photoallergic contact dermatitis. In primary irritant contact dermatitis, the patient is usually exposed to the sensitizing agent for a brief period of time. Because this is not immunologically mediated, the concentration of an irritant must exceed a threshold before the reaction can take place. This threshold may be very high, according to the irritancy of the compound. It is not necessary for the skin to be previously sensitized; therefore, an irritant reaction may occur immediately after contact with the material. Almost 80% of all cases of contact dermatitis are of the irritant variety.

Allergic contact dermatitis, in contrast, is a delayed or T cell–mediated immune response to the antigen, usually a low-molecular-weight hapten. Unlike irritant contact dermatitis, an induction period of 5 to 7 days is required before the first appearance of hypersensitivity. The peak reaction on the skin occurs 24 to 48 hours after being rechallenged with the same antigen. Allergic contact dermatitis occurs in only 20% of patients suffering from contact dermatitis. In the irritant phase, the skin on the feet responds by localized erythema to

the dorsum of the foot or toes and rarely in the toe web spaces. If the patient is exposed to the sensitizing agent for a sufficient period of time, an allergic phase occurs. This is manifested by inflammation and formation of small pruritic vesicles and papules. If the reaction is severe, the vesicular phase may proceed to bullae formation. If the sensitizing agent is removed, the skin soon heals within a short period of time. However, with repeated exposure to the causative agent, the skin response becomes rapid and severe. The six most common sensitizers of allergic contact dermatitis are the *Rhus* plants, paraphenylenediamine, nickel compounds, rubber compounds, ethylenediamine, and chromates.

One factor that exacerbates allergic contact dermatitis is repeated exposure to heat or constant warmth (as may occur within the shoe), which causes increased perspiration. Many well-recognized sensitizers found within shoe materials can readily be leached out by sweat (Fig. 10–11). This process also promotes spread of the vesicular or pruritic papules by increased vascularity, and the general appearance may lead to a misdiagnosis of tinea pedis. Appropriate treatment of contact dermatitis is frequently delayed because of misdiagnosis and long-term treatment of this condition with topical antifungal agents.

One example of this type of allergic contact dermatitis is a relatively, frequently seen condition secondary to adhesive tape strappings used as a therapeutic arch support (Fig. 10–12). One patient attempted to repeat the same success of tape strapping with a home treatment program using duct tape that resulted in a contact allergic dermatitis (Fig. 10–13). A similar finding can be seen in patients allergic to the adhesive backing of Steri-Strip skin closures (Fig. 10–14). With the advent of transcutaneous electric nerve stimulation and interferential stimulation to control pain there has been

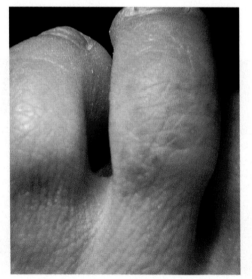

Figure 10–11 Allergic contact dermatitis. An allergy to shoes involved the dorsa of the feet.

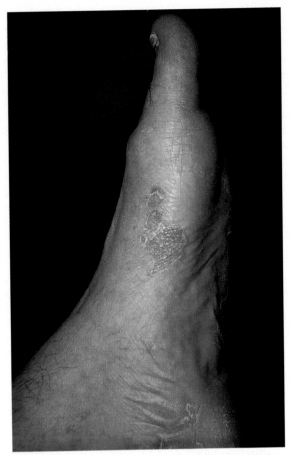

Figure 10–12   **Irritant contact dermatitis.** The cause was adhesive tape strapping of the foot.

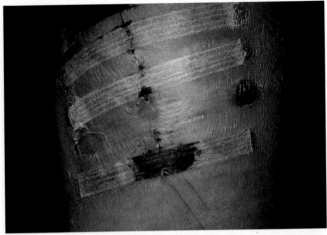

Figure 10–14   **Irritant contact dermatitis.** This was caused by the adhesive in Steri-Strip skin tapes that were used to close an incision.

morphic, with erythema, vesiculation, and edema. Irritant contact dermatitis is generally localized and looks more like a severe burn with large blisters or marked edema and erythema. Microscopically, the acute lesions of irritant contact dermatitis show infiltration of inflammatory cells, vesiculation, spongiosis, and vasodilation.

an increase in cases of irritant contact dermatitis secondary to the adhesive in the electrode pads (Fig. 10–15).

It is difficult to tell the difference between irritant contact dermatitis and allergic contact dermatitis. In general, allergic contact dermatitis appears more poly-

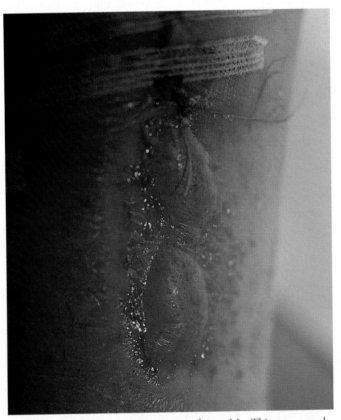

Figure 10–15   **Irritant contact dermatitis.** This was caused by the adhesive in electrode pads used to control pain adjacent to a surgical site. There was no reaction to the Steri-Strip adhesives over the incision.

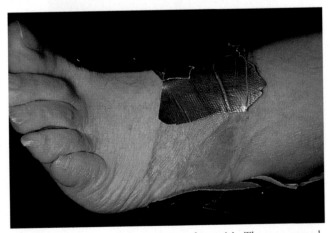

Figure 10–13   **Irritant contact dermatitis.** The cause was adhesive duct tape.

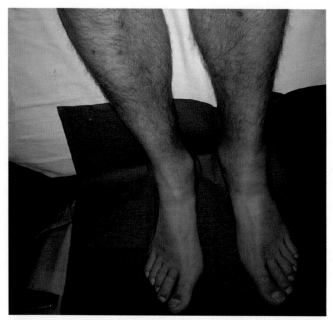

Figure 10–16 Photodermatitis. Patient had sprayed his legs with an insect repellent before sun exposure. The rash appeared quickly and remained for more than 2 weeks.

The more chronic condition of allergic contact dermatitis occurs as hyperkeratosis, parakeratosis, acanthosis, and lymphocytes in the upper dermis.

Photodermatitis (photoallergic contact dermatitis) is less common than the other two forms of contact der-

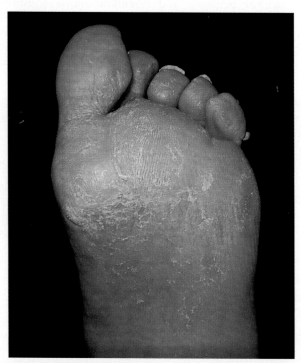

Figure 10–17 Irritant contact dermatitis. A reaction from contact with the insoles of running shoes after their immersion in water is often seen with dyed insoles.

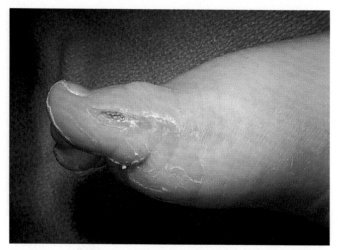

Figure 10–18 Irritant contact dermatitis. Typical pediatric toe-box dermatitis due to rubber lining or rubber cement of the shoe toe-box.

matitis and can occur when certain topical agents are applied to the skin of the lower extremities before sun exposure (Fig. 10–16). Localization on the lower extremities from occupational exposure is uncommon. This type of eruption can be mediated by the T-cell system. If the problem is not immunologically mediated yet sunlight is still required to activate the condition, it is known as a phototoxic reaction.

Shoe chemicals and sensitizing materials found in shoes that can cause contact dermatitis are chromate and potassium dichromate, dye coloring, formalin, formaldehyde, mercaptobenzothiazole (a rubber accelerator), thiuram (a rubber antioxidant), paraphenylenediamine (found in leather), and various materials within the shoes themselves. It has also been reported that the dye found in the insoles of certain running shoes has caused contact dermatitis in runners (Fig. 10–17). In young children there is a condition called toe-box dermatitis that represents a contact dermatitis to the rubber lining of the toe-box of canvas shoes (Fig. 10–18).

Any chemical or material may potentially be a sensitizing agent and some individuals may be allergic to single chemicals or combinations of chemicals reacting together. The external environment harbors many such well-known agents, for example, the pesticides. Plant dermatitis from the *Rhus* plants is the most common contact dermatitis, and this allergen frequently involves the lower extremities (Fig. 10–19). This group includes poison ivy, poison oak, and poison sumac, of which there are over 400 members ubiquitously found through the United States. Between 25% and 60% of Americans are sensitive to the plants. Other plants that are known sensitizers are hops, tobacco, and tulips. Oils found on plant leaves are also known to cause photoallergic contact dermatitis.

Contact dermatitis may be caused by overtreatment with topical medications prescribed for tinea pedis (Fig.

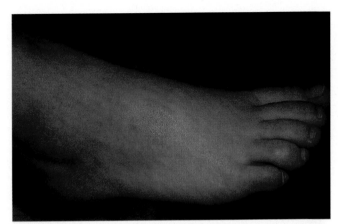

Figure 10–19 *Rhus* **plant dermatitis.** Poison ivy is evident on dorsal aspect of foot and around ankle. Note clear area where shoes were worn.

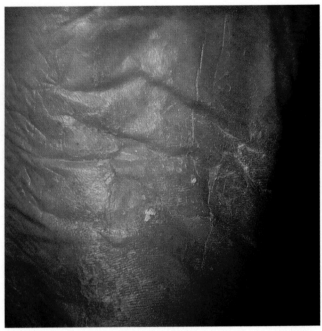

Figure 10–21 Dermatitis medicamentosa. Chemical overtreatment resulted from antiperspirant (aluminum chloride hexahydrate in absolute alcohol) used to treat hyperhidrosis.

10–20) and hyperhidrosis (Fig. 10–21), and by lotions or creams for softening callosities. This condition is usually termed *dermatitis medicamentosa* and may result from ingestion, inhalation, injection, or, more commonly, application of the drug to the surface of the skin. Absorption into the systemic circulation may follow the topical application of medication to the intact skin, superficial lesions (Fig. 10–22), or deep wounds.

I have documented cases in which patients undergoing ultrasound therapy developed a contact dermatitis to the topical gel (Fig. 10–23). When the gel was discontinued, the dermatitis subsided. Benzocaine gel may cause both contact dermatitis (Fig. 10–24) and urticaria. Ethylenediamine and fragrances found in the

perfume of Mycolog cream also cause allergic contact dermatitis (Fig. 10–25). Photoallergies may be seen with substances such as chlorpromazine, promethazine (Phenergan), *p*-aminobenzoic acid, phenothiazines, tincture of benzoin, and povidone-iodine solutions. Povidone-iodine in wound care and surgical scrubs and soaks must be applied cautiously in patients with known sensitivities to iodine or with histories of contact dermatitis, especially if the skin is already damaged

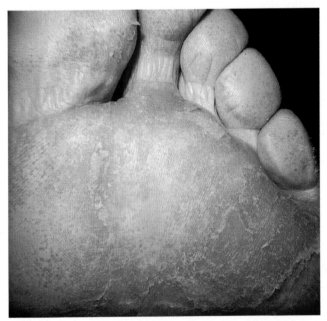

Figure 10–20 Dermatitis medicamentosa. Chemical overtreatment resulted from excessive use of an over-the-counter antifungal medication.

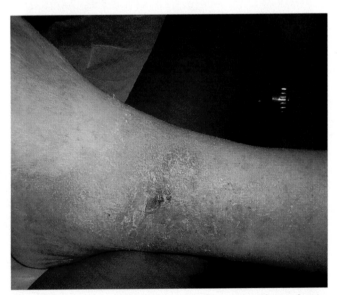

Figure 10–22 Dermatitis medicamentosa. Chemical overtreatment resulted from use of antibiotic ointment (Neosporin) for a superficial ankle lesion.

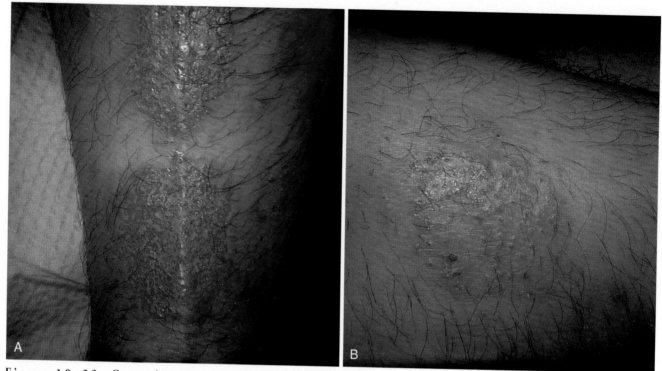

Figure 10-23   Contact dermatitis. *A,* Topical gel used for ultrasound therapy caused a reaction around a surgical site on the posterior lower leg. *B,* Topical gel used for ultrasound therapy resulted in a dermatitis over an area of tendonitis.

(Fig. 10–26). Patients with stasis dermatitis have an excellent chance of developing contact dermatitis to ingredients that are applied to the skin. Certain bath soaps used to moisturize and cleanse dry, scaly skin contain D&C Yellow No. 11 dye, which can cause severe contact dermatitis (Fig. 10–27).

It is not known precisely why some individuals repeatedly exposed to known causative agents do not react. For example, some surgeons scrub their hands daily with povidone-iodine solutions with no long-term problems. Genetic inheritance of certain characteristics affecting the immune system has been theorized as a logical reason why these individuals are not affected.

Darker skins, particularly in blacks, do not allow chemicals to penetrate well. Allergic contact dermatitis based on a true sensitization reaction is rare in infants; however, primary irritant contact dermatitis is very common. In general, children have been found to be less susceptible to the sensitizing agents than adults.

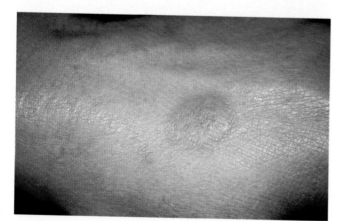

Figure 10-24   Contact dermatitis. The cause was topically applied benzocaine gel.

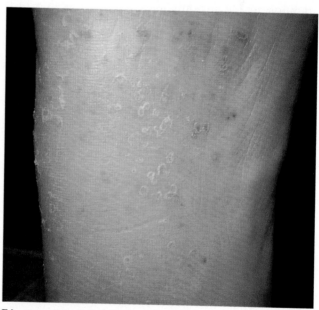

Figure 10-25   Contact dermatitis. The patient was allergic to the perfume base in the Mycolog cream that had been applied to the sole of the foot.

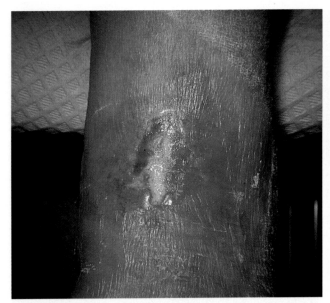

Figure 10–26 Contact dermatitis. Povidone-iodine solution painted regularly on a superficial wound caused a chemical contact dermatitis.

Phytophotodermatitis is due to exposure to plants containing light-sensitive compounds such as furocoumarins (psoralens). This combination may result in intense reactions characterized by distinctive, linear blistering on an erythematous base that is distributed in a bizarre streaky fashion (Fig. 10–28). A history of working in a garden or around plants, lying in a field on a bright day, or having some other similar contact with weeds or plants can be obtained from the patient.

Treatment of contact dermatitis begins with the suspicion of the cause. In many cases the patient already has an idea of the cause of the condition. If not, careful attention to the surrounding circumstances in which the skin problem has occurred and improved in the past may lead to the answer. A thorough history may reveal facts that help in understanding the process. It is helpful to ask questions about whether the eruptions are aggravated by weather changes, employment changes, or vacations away from work or home environments. The history should also include a detailed account of topical cosmetics, creams or ointments, or medications applied, as well as any changes in working environment or clothing, including shoes, hosiery, and socks. Questions regarding any history of skin problems and the family history of similar conditions are also helpful.

A patch test for known and suspected agents should then be employed. Patch tests may be used in two ways. One is to apply a series of the most common sensitizers in the hope that one will show a positive response. The second method is to do a patch test with a specific suspected agent, such as bits of the lining from the shoe, to demonstrate that this particular allergy does indeed exist. Compounds generally provided in patch test kits for shoe dermatitis and common skin sensitizers are listed in Table 10–1. A fairly complete patch and shoe dermatitis test kit may be obtained from Hollister-Stier Laboratories in Spokane, Washington.

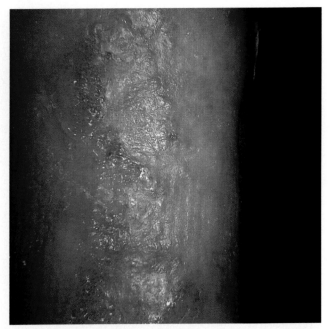

Figure 10–27 Contact dermatitis. Severe contact dermatitis was secondary to D&C Yellow No. 11 dye found in yellow bar soap.

Once the differential diagnosis, including tinea pedis, lichen simplex chronicus, atopic dermatitis, urticaria, and others, is reached and the diagnosis of contact dermatitis is strongly suspected or proved by the patch test, treatment may begin. Exposure to the known causative agents should be avoided throughout the treatment

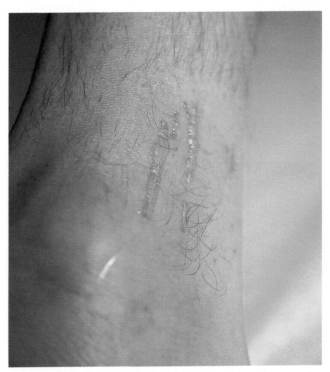

Figure 10–28 Phytophotodermatitis. This is due to an interaction of light-sensitive chemicals in plants and ultraviolet light exposure. Bizarre linear blistering is characteristic.

TABLE 10-1 Compounds Commonly Used for Patch Testing

	Compound	Formulation
Common Sensitizers—Used as Scout Battery When No Particular Contactant Is Suspected	Benzocaine	5% in petrolatum
	Epoxy glue resin	1% in acetone
	Formaldehyde	0.8% aqueous solution
	Lanolin	As is
	Mercaptobenzothiol	1% in petrolatum
	Mercuric bichloride	0.1% aqueous solution
	Neomycin sulfate	20% in petrolatum
	Nickel sulfate	5% aqueous solution
	Paraphenylenediamine	2% in petrolatum
	Potassium dichromate	0.025% aqueous solution
	Tetramethylthiuram disulfide	1% in petrolatum
	Turpentine	25% in olive oil
Battery of Tests for Shoe Dermatitis (in Petrolatum)	Basic chromic sulfate	0.2%
	Bismarck brown	5%
	Formaldehyde	0.8%
	Hydroquinone monomethyl ether	1%
	Mercaptobenzothiazole	1%
	Paraphenylenediamine	2%
	Potassium dichromate	0.5%
	Tetramethylthiuram disulfide	1%

From Lowney ED: Dermatitis and ezema. In Moschella SL, et al (eds): Dermatology. Philadelphia, WB Saunders, 1975.

program and afterward. This is not always as easy as it may seem, because certain components of the allergens may be present in all shoe gear or clothing parts.

Wet dressings and cold compresses help to dry oozing secretions, soften scales and crusts, and cleanse purulent wounds. Cold compresses are also beneficial in relieving burning, itching, and paresthesia caused by irritant contact dermatitis through the cooling and drying effect of the solution. In cases in which the contact dermatitis primarily involves the foot, the area may be completely immersed in a foot bath of plain cold to warm water mixed with aluminum acetate (Burow's solution), diluted 1:10, for 15 to 20 minutes. Epsom salt (magnesium sulfate), diluted 2 tablespoons per pint of water, may also be used; however, it may produce more drying to the skin than desired.

In more inflammatory cases, topical corticosteroids may be prescribed to help eliminate pruritus and inflammation. In most cases, they are useful when the inflammation is the primary manifestation of the contact dermatitis and the etiological agents have been dealt with concurrently. The anti-inflammatory activity of corticosteroids is based on the properties of vasoconstriction, the suppression of membrane permeability, and the immune response. This is expressed by the inhibition of the connective tissue response and by the control of reactive epidermal hyperplasia. The vasoconstrictor action of the corticosteroids decreases extravasation of serum into the skin and therefore inhibits swelling and discomfort.

In most cases, it is best to start treatment with a relatively mild topical corticosteroid, such as 1% hydrocortisone. The activity of the drug may then be enhanced by increasing its absorption, by applying it and overlying occlusive vehicles or dressings, or by applying it to previously hydrated skin. For increased medication activity, one of the more potent corticosteroids, such as fluocinolone acetonide or betamethasone dipropionate, may be applied. The most potent forms of topical corticosteroids are the fluorinated types (Table 10–2).

Systemic corticosteroids may be used to treat the more severe forms of contact dermatitis as long as no obvious contraindications are present. In almost all cases of contact dermatitis involving the lower extremities, a relatively short course of oral therapy is recommended. Systemic corticosteroid therapy is not recommended for patients with psychiatric disorders, diabetes mellitus, peptic ulcers, or hypertension, nor for pregnant women. It is also specifically contraindicated in the presence of acute infections and trauma.

Additional treatment may be provided by the application of antipruritic agents such as calamine and phenolated calamine lotions. One of the effective topical antipruritics is diphenhydramine (Benadryl); however, some patients exhibit additional contact allergic dermatitis to topical application of this medication. Secondary control of perspiration by using activated charcoal insoles may help control hyperhidrosis and bromhidrosis and reduce the amount of inflammatory response to a contact irritant on the feet.

TABLE 10–2 Common Topical Corticosteroids

I (High Potency)

Amcinonide ointment 0.1% (Cyclocort)

Betamethasone dipropionate ointment 0.05% (Diprosone)

Desoximethasone ointment, cream 0.25% (Topicort)

Desoximethasone gel 0.05% (Topicort)

Diflorasone diacetate ointment 0.05% (Florone & Topsyn Gel)

Fluocinonide 0.06% (Lidex)

Halcinonide cream 0.1% (Halog)

II (Potent)

Betamethasone benzoate gel 0.025% (Benisone)

Betamethasone dipropionate cream 0.05% (Diprosone)

Betamethasone valerate ointment 0.1% (Valisone)

Diflorasone diacetate cream 0.05% (Florone)

Triamcinolone acetonide cream 0.5% (Aristocort)

III (Mid-Potency)

Amcinonide cream 0.1% (Cyclocort)

Betamethasone valerate lotion 0.1% (Valisone)

Fluocinolone acetonide cream 0.2%, ointment 0.025% (Fluonid, Synalar)

Hydrocortisone valerate cream 0.2% (Westcort)

Triamcinolone acetonide ointment 0.1% (Aristocort, Kenalog)

IV (Low-Potency)

Aclometasone dipropionate 0.05% cream (Aclovate)

Betamethasone valerate cream 0.1% (Valisone)

Clocortolone pivalate cream 0.1% (Cloderm)

Fluocinolone acetonide cream 0.025% (Fluonid, Synalar)

Flurandrenolide 0.05% (Cordran)

Hydrocortisone valerate cream 0.2% (Westcort)

Triamcinolone acetonide cream 0.01%, lotion 0.025% (Kenalog, Aristocort)

V (Mild)

Desonide cream 0.05% (Tridesilon)

Flumethasone pivalate 0.03% cream (Locorten)

Fluocinolone acetonide 0.01% solution (Fluonid, Synalar)

VI (Least Potent)

Prednisolone 0.5% (Meti-Derm)

Methylprednisolone 1% (Medrol)

Fluorometholone 0.025% (Oxylone)

Dexamethasone 0.1% (Decadron Phosphate)

Hydrocortisone 0.25, 0.5, 1.0, 2.5% (Hytone, Nutraderm, Synacort)

From Kuwada GT, Dockery GL: Contact Dermatitis. Clin Podiatr Med Surg 3:551–561, 1986.

DRUG ERUPTIONS

Cutaneous rashes and dermal lesions are commonly observed as indications of an adverse reaction to systemic drugs. Drug eruptions may occur by means of allergic, toxic, pharmacological, or photosensitive mechanisms. They may occur in several different forms, and they may imitate numerous other skin conditions. When these reactions occur secondary to ingested or systemically administered medications, prompt recognition and intervention are necessary to prevent severe toxicity from developing.

Patients may have an immediate and acute reaction to a drug after only one dose, or they may have taken a particular drug for many weeks, or even years. Once sensitization occurs, a reaction may follow within 24 hours. Cross reactions to similar drug compounds may cause dermal reactions in sensitized patients. Once a skin reaction is reported, the pattern of the eruption should be determined. Maculopapular and urticarial patterns are the most common eruptions. They are usually generalized, evenly distributed, and severely pruritic. The drug or offending agents should be discontinued immediately. Symptomatic relief may be provided with oral antihistamines and topical corticosteroids. In more advanced reactions, systemic corticosteroid therapy may be necessary.

Clinical characteristics may include any of the following patterns: urticaria, maculopapular, eczema, erythema multiforme, erythema nodosum, acroexfoliative, exfoliative erythroderma, fixed drug reaction, lichenoid (lichen planus–like), photosensitivity, pigmentation, plantar keratotic, purpura, toxic epidermal necrolysis, or vesiculobullous. Because these morphological patterns related to drug reactions may be helpful in determining the causative agent, these specific reactions of the skin are discussed in more detail.

Urticarial reactions are usually produced as a result of an immediate-hypersensitivity reaction to some sensitizing agent. Urticaria is characterized by pruritic red wheals varying in size from a very small area to a large pattern (Fig. 10–29). Urticaria and pruritic and maculopapular (morbilliform) lesions are the most frequent types of skin eruptions secondary to drugs. A more involved version of urticaria, termed *angioedema*, occurs when both the dermal and subcutaneous tissues are involved. Any drug may elicit this response; however, aspirin, penicillin, and blood products are the most common agents implicated in urticaria.

Morbilliform (macular and papular) eruptions (Fig. 10–30) are more common drug-induced reactions than urticarial lesions. These dermal rashes are characterized by erythematous macules and papules that may become confluent. Fever may be present, and the general appearance and distribution are similar to those of viral exanthems. Common locations for this condition are the trunk, arms, legs, and feet. The palms and soles are usually spared. The eruption usually lasts for 1 or 2 weeks and may be associated with pruritus. Oral antihistamines decrease much of the pruritus. Ampicillin is a common agent that produces this reaction. Several other drugs also produce morbilliform eruptions, including barbiturates, diflunisal, phenytoin, gentamicin, isoniazid, meclofenamate, phenothiazines, quinidine, sulfonamides, thiazides, and trimethoprim-sulfamethoxazole.

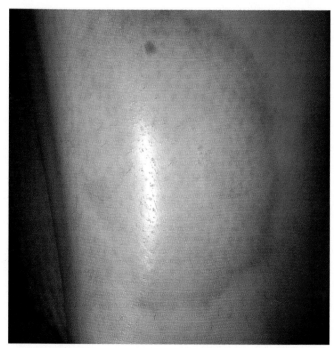

Figure 10–29 **Urticaria.** Note large pruritic wheal. The lesions appeared on the lower extremities and abdominal region 24 hours after oral administration of penicillin.

Eczematous dermatitis may follow systemic administration of drugs. These lesions are characterized by erythematous, pruritic vesicles and papules that may coalesce with continued use of the medication (Fig. 10–31). A patient who has developed contact dermatitis to a chemical agent may experience a flare or generalized skin reaction if given the same drug systemically.

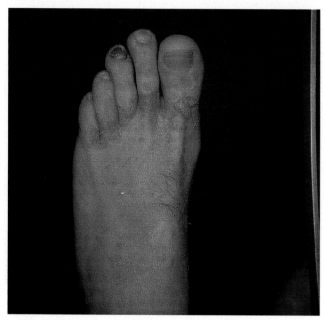

Figure 10–30 **Morbilliform eruption.** This reaction was secondary to therapy with a thiazide diuretic.

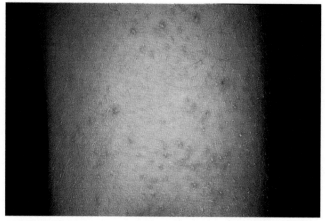

Figure 10–31 **Eczematous dermatitis.** Rash on the lower extremities occurred in a young woman taking dimenhydrinate tablets for vertigo.

Erythema multiforme is an acute reaction limited to the skin and mucous membrane with characteristic iris (target) lesions or bullae (Fig. 10–32). The onset of this rash is sudden, and there may be secondary symptoms of fever, malaise, sore throat, or muscular aches. A large group of drugs have been implicated in the formation of erythema multiforme such as barbiturates, codeine, phenytoin, furosemide, griseofulvin, ketoconazole, nonsteroidal anti-inflammatory agents, penicillin, phenothiazines, sulfonamides, sulindac, and tetracycline.

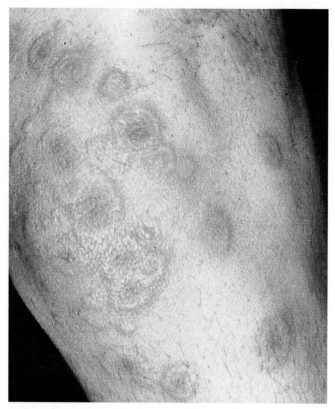

Figure 10–32 **Erythema multiforme.** Characteristic iris or target lesions are seen on the lower extremity.

Erythema nodosum is an acute reaction that occurs as erythematous, tender subcutaneous nodules on the lower extremities (Fig. 10–33). The nodules are usually symmetrically distributed on the front of the shins and are elevated, smooth, and very tender to touch (Fig. 10–34). They may occasionally be found on the thighs and on the dorsal surface of the foot (Fig. 10–35). The lesions may last for 1 or 2 weeks and range from 1 to 4 cm in diameter. They are bright red in the beginning and gradually turn purple and start to fade, similar to a bruise. The lesions usually appear in crops, and the process is over within 1 month. The patient may be ill with fever, malaise, arthralgia, or sore throat during the eruptions. The condition may recur for months or even years. Erythema nodosum in children is most commonly caused by an upper respiratory tract infection, especially from streptococci. In young adults, streptococcal infections are the most common causes. The condition is also frequently associated with a reaction to drugs. Many different drugs have been implicated, including birth control pills, barbiturates, sulfonamides, halogens, tetracycline, penicillin, and 13-*cis*-retinoic acid. Oral contraceptives are the most frequently responsible drugs. A prolonged search for systemic infection or causative drug may be required, and in many cases no cause can be determined.

Acroexfoliative dermatitis secondary to drug-induced reactions is characterized by generally mild exfoliative changes that occur principally on the hands and feet soon after beginning a medication (Fig. 10–36). No erythema is usually noted with this condition, and scaling occurs primarily on the palms and soles. The process occurs more frequently in males and is more common in the fourth decade. The hands may show mild lichenification or changes consistent with eczema, presumably due to rubbing or peeling of the scales. This self-limiting condition does not progress to more severe dermatitis. Drug reactions often undergo rapid resolution after withdrawal of the causative agent. Hydration

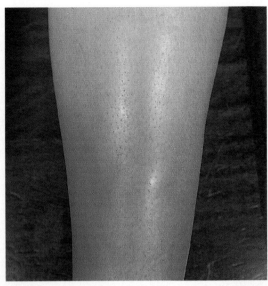

Figure 10–34   Erythema nodosum. The lesions are elevated, smooth, and red. Light touch reveals that the nodules are very tender. This 17-year-old girl had recently started using oral contraceptives.

of the skin followed by topical moisturizing creams affords symptomatic relief. Several drugs are known to cause this condition, including aspirin, barbiturates, codeine, cephalosporins, phenytoin, gold, iodine, isoniazid, penicillin, and sulfonamides.

Exfoliative erythroderma is a serious cutaneous reaction to drugs. The onset is generally acute, and the patient rapidly becomes very ill. Hospitalization is necessary, and treatment is immediate withdrawal of the causative medication, short-course systemic corticoster-

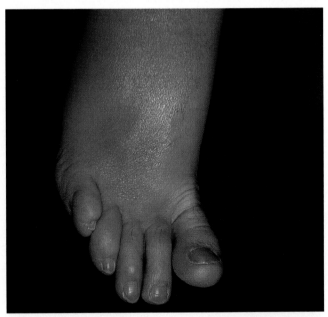

Figure 10–35   Erythema nodosum. Although most lesions are noted on the lower legs, they may also be seen on the dorsum of the foot. These lesions start as bright-red nodules that slowly become purple. They fade in a manner similar to bruises.

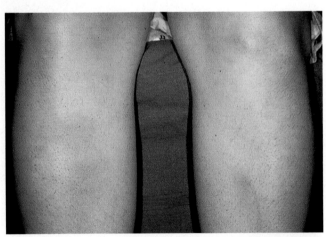

Figure 10–33   Erythema nodosum. Painful erythematous nodules occur mainly on the lower extremities. This 29-year-old woman had been taking barbiturates before the presentation of the condition.

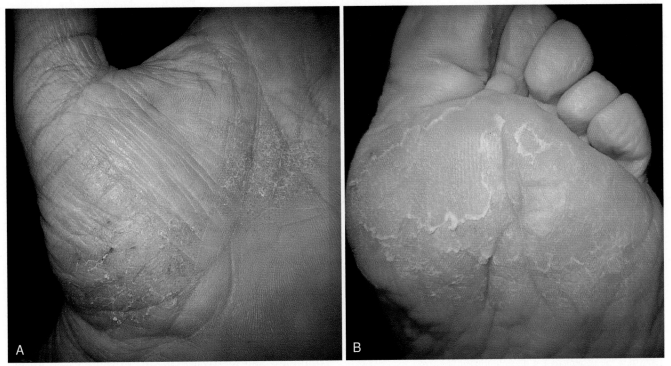

Figure 10–36 **Acroexfoliative dermatitis.** This dermatitis occurred in a 49-year-old man after systemic antibiotic therapy. *A,* Hand involvement shows typical pattern of exfoliative dermatitis in the distribution of the median nerve on the palm and thenar pad. *B,* Foot involvement shows almost complete loss of the upper epidermal layers.

oids, systemic antihistamines, hydration of the skin, topical emollients, and corticosteroids. Severe exfoliative dermatitis secondary to a drug-induced skin reaction is characterized by a very extensive obdurate scaling and pruritic erythroderma. This condition starts with erythema, swelling, and pruritus and progresses rapidly until the skin is completely involved. Desquamation is evident after a few days. The scales are thick, are cracked, and may occur in large sheets on the feet and hands (Fig. 10–37). The face is usually involved.

Figure 10–37 **Exfoliative erythroderma.** *A,* Hand involvement in a 64-year-old man with drug-induced reaction to phenytoin (Dilantin). *B,* Foot involvement in the same patient. Note the erythematous base with thick scaling and edema.

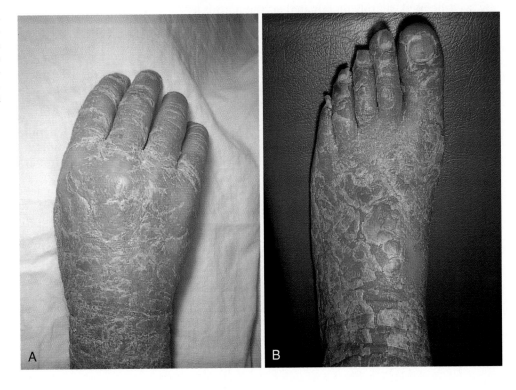

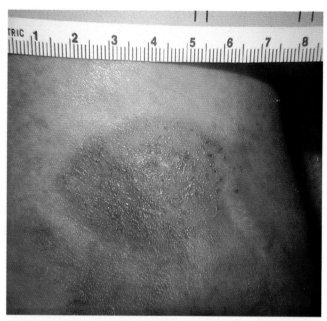

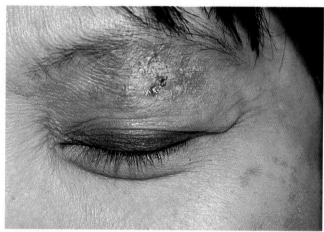

Figure 10-40   Fixed drug reaction. This reaction was secondary to oral griseofulvin therapy. (Courtesy of Dr. Jeffrey Christensen.)

Figure 10-38   Fixed drug reaction. The lesion is well-defined, reddish brown, and edematous. It occurs in the identical site each time the allergen is ingested. This condition recurred on the ankle each time the patient took a phenolphthalein laxative.

In more advanced cases there will be generalized involvement of the entire body. Secondary bacteria infections may complicate the course of this condition. Among the drugs known to cause this condition are allopurinol, arsenic, cefoxitin, cimetidine, phenytoin, gold, iodine, isoniazid, lithium, mercurial diuretics, penicillins, phenobarbital, and sulfonamides.

Fixed drug eruptions are characterized by solitary or few, well-defined, sharply marginated erythematous lesions that recur in the same location when the sensitizing medication is given. The lesions develop within hours of the ingested medication, leaving a character-

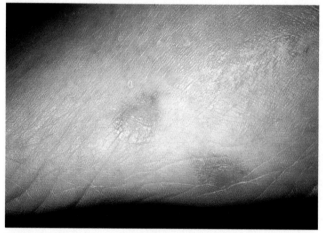

Figure 10-39   Fixed drug reaction. Two ovoid, sharply demarcated plaques appeared on the foot shortly after trimethoprim was given for a urinary tract infection.

istic hyperpigmented area on the skin (Fig. 10-38). These lesions may occur anywhere on the body but are very common on the back, mouth, hand, lower extremities, and feet (Fig. 10-39). In some cases, an eczematous fixed drug reaction occurs in limited areas, such as the eyelids (Fig. 10-40), earlobes, or fingers. Phenolphthalein in a laxative is one of the most common causes of the fixed drug reaction, but aspirin, barbiturates, griseofulvin, metronidazole, phenacetin, sulfonamides, tetracycline, and trimethoprim have all been implicated.

Lichenoid dermatitis mimics lichen planus both clinically and histologically. The lesions are secondary to several drugs, ingestion of heavy metals, and contact with photographic chemicals. The characteristic presentation is one of several polygonal, flat-topped papules of violaceous hue. They may form on the arms, legs, or feet (Fig. 10-41). Oral mucosal lesions do not form in this condition. The fine white lines and spots of idiopathic lichen planus (Wickham's striae) are also absent from the lesions that are drug induced. Gold ingestion is frequently associated with these lesions. Other drugs that may cause lichenoid dermatitis include arsenicals, beta-blockers, diflunisal, furosemide, methyldopa, nonsteroidal anti-inflammatory drugs, penicillamine, quinidine, and thiazides.

Photosensitivity reactions to drugs are characterized by the distribution of the dermatitis involving the exposed portions of the body, typically, the face, neck, distal arms, and lower legs (Fig. 10-42). Many drugs have the capacity to induce either a phototoxic or a photoallergic reaction. The most common photosensitivity eruptions are phototoxic. These reactions resemble a sunburn after brief sun exposure. The cause of photoallergy is less understood but appears to result from a radiation-induced alteration of the drug that sufficiently changes its antigenicity. The most common drugs causing photosensitivity reactions are thiazides,

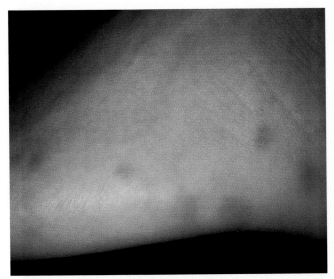

Figure 10–41   Lichenoid dermatitis. These lichen planus–like lesions on the foot had the same clinical appearance as idiopathic lichen planus. They developed shortly after this young woman began taking piroxicam, 20 mg daily, for knee pain.

griseofulvins, phenothiazines, tetracyclines, sulfonamides, and nonsteroidal anti-inflammatory agents.

Pigmentation due to drug-induced dermatitis may be secondary to stimulation of melanocytic activity or drug deposition in the skin leading to pigmentation. Pigmentary changes associated with medications are not a manifestation of an allergic reaction to the drug (as with a fixed drug reaction) but rather a function of the basic physiology of the skin and the bioactivity of the drug. Hyperpigmentation may also occur from a photoallergy during the healing process, and the distribution would be the same as those described in the previous discussion of photosensitivity. Pigmentary reactions that are not due to allergy and are not photosensitive form on nonexposed areas of the body in a generalized pattern or in a localized distribution with a propensity for changes in the hands, lower legs, and feet (Fig. 10–43). In many cases, the hyperpigmentation decreases or resolves after discontinuation of the drug; however, the condition is not necessarily reversible on stopping the medication. Drugs associated with increased pigmentation are arsenic, birth control pills, chlorpromazine, estrogen, fluorouracil, furosemide, gold, hydroquinone, mercurial compounds, minocycline, nicotinic acid, phenothiazine, silver, and thiazide.

Plantar keratotic lesions may form with the long-term ingestion of certain chemical compounds, especially arsenic (Fig. 10–44) and lithium (Fig. 10–45). The etiology of these lesions is directly connected with the ingestion of inorganic arsenic (1) from artesian well water in areas where arsenical herbicides and pesticides have been used, (2) from the intake of Fowler's solution or Asiatic pills containing arsenic, and (3) from the oral ingestion of lithium used to treat manic depression.

Clinically, these keratoses are punctate palmar and plantar lesions. A few to hundreds of lesions may be present, and they may take on a brown coloration (Fig. 10–46). Formation is usually symmetrical, and the le-

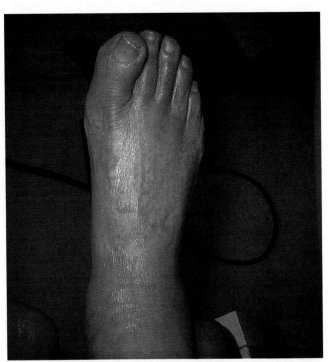

Figure 10–42   Photosensitivity reaction. This 60-year-old man had a phototoxic eruption on the lower legs, hands, and face shortly after being placed on a thiazide diuretic. The rash was seen only on the exposed areas of his body.

Figure 10–43   Drug-induced dermatitis. Increased pigmentary skin changes occur on both feet and lower legs after long-term treatment with generic form of furosemide.

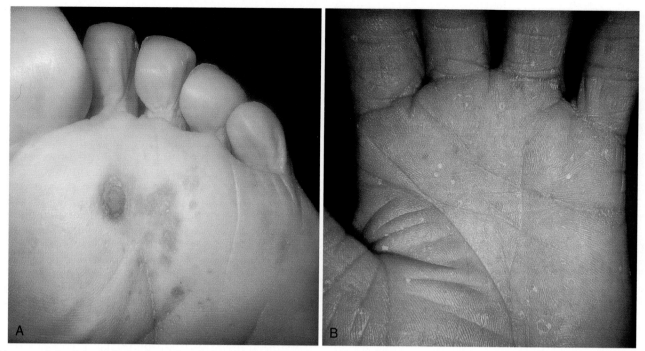

Figure 10–44   Palmar-plantar keratosis. *A,* Arsenical keratosis. Arsenical keratotic lesions appear on the sites of pressure and friction on the sole, with punctate keratosis of variable sizes. *B,* Typical punctate, hard, yellowish papules are present on the hands.

sions may grow or coalesce to form large areas of yellow or brown pigmented keratoses with a predilection for the lateral aspects of the soles (Fig. 10–47), palms, thenar eminences, and bases and lateral aspects of the fingers. The lesions of arsenical exposure may undergo malignant conversion to squamous cell carcinomas with the potential for metastases. In patients with large numbers of lesions, multiple basal cell carcinomas or multiple lesions of Bowen's disease may be present at the same time. Treatment of palmar plantar keratosis secondary to arsenic or lithium ingestion is difficult. Cryotherapy, curettage, and electrodesiccation are the preferred methods of treatment of lesions that are causing discomfort or have undergone a recent or rapid change.

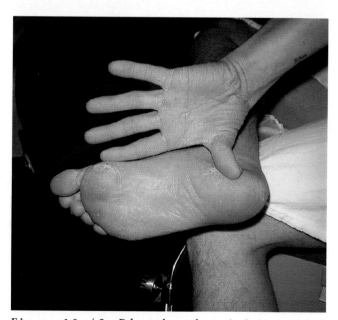

Figure 10–45   Palmar-plantar keratosis. Lesions were evident in a patient on long-term lithium therapy.

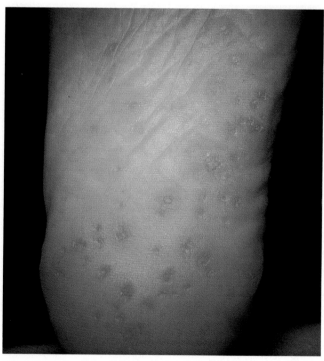

Figure 10–46   Palmar-plantar keratosis. Close-up of brown plantar punctate lesions on the sole of a patient on lithium therapy.

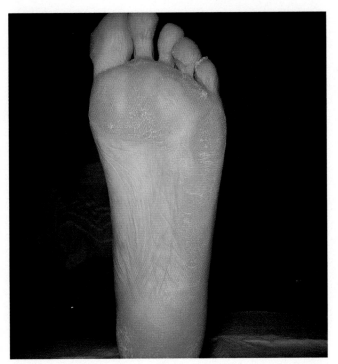

Figure 10–47 Palmar-plantar keratosis. Coalesced lesions occurred on the plantar sole of the foot in a patient who had been on lithium therapy for many years.

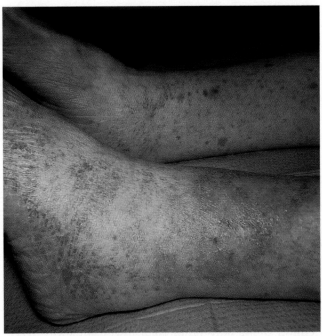

Figure 10–48 Drug-induced purpura. This 56-year-old man presented with a pigmented lichenoid rash on the lower extremity with adjacent purpura, edema, and intense pruritus after long-term treatment with quinidine for heart problems.

Purpuric eruptions secondary to drugs are usually found on the dependent areas, such as the lower extremities and feet. In bedridden patients, the dependent areas may be the buttocks or the back. Clinically, drug-induced purpura occurs as a pigmented purpuric lichenoid eruption with disseminated purpura and pruritus (Fig. 10–48). This condition may result from barbiturates, carbamides, chlorothiazide, chlorpromazine, gold, griseofulvin, iodides, quinidine, and sulfonamides. The condition usually resolves or greatly improves with withdrawal of the drug.

Toxic epidermal necrolysis is a very rare expression of a drug reaction. This condition is considered to be a variant of bullous erythema multiforme. It is characterized by extensive areas in which the skin becomes very tender with loose, thin bullae that begin to peel in sheets, leaving an erythematous, raw, and eroded surface (Fig. 10–49). Once peeling has occurred there may be very slow recovery of the skin. Weight-bearing and pressure areas, as well as the palms and soles, may be extensively involved. Mucous membranes are usually involved, and there may be sloughing of the fingernails and toenails. Other large areas of the skin may be totally uninvolved. This is a serious condition, and the mortality rate is relatively high. Causative agents are numerous and include allopurinol, ibuprofen, naproxen, penicillin, phenobarbital, phenytoin, phenylbutazone, streptomycin, sulfonamides, sulindac, and thiabendazole.

Patients must be hospitalized and the causative drug discontinued. Treatment consists of early administration of high doses of corticosteroids. Fluid and electrolyte therapy should be monitored closely. Complications such as infection, hemorrhage, and fluid and electrolyte imbalance are the leading causes of death.

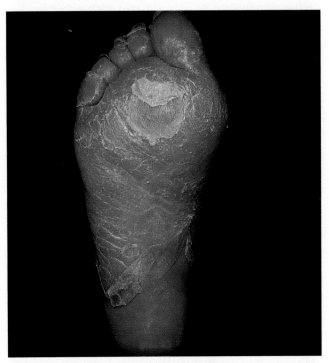

Figure 10–49 Toxic epidermal necrolysis. Skin is shedding from large areas of the hands, feet, and back in this 60-year-old woman being treated for pneumonia with penicillin.

Vesiculobullous eruptions may develop as single expressions of drug-induced reactions or they may be a part of other eruptions (erythema multiforme, fixed drug reactions, or toxic epidermal necrolysis). Nalidixic acid may produce a bullous eruption on an erythematous base, especially on the lower legs and feet (Fig. 10–50). The formation of vesicles and bullae may be part of several other drug reactions, or they may be present as isolated instances in patients who are not otherwise ill. Drugs that cause vesiculobullous lesions are barbiturates, furosemide, griseofulvin, iodides, nalidixic acid, nonsteroidal anti-inflammatory drugs, penicillamine, piroxicam, and sulfonamides.

The general treatment for all conditions diagnosed as a drug reaction is to discontinue the offending agent immediately if possible. Many of the drugs being used can simply be stopped, while others may be too necessary and no alternative medication may be available. In those instances, one may be forced to complete the entire course of the drug despite the secondary skin eruptions. Treatment of most drug eruptions is symptomatic. The mild and asymptomatic conditions may need no attention or therapy other than discontinuation of the drug, whereas the severe reactions as noted may require hospitalization and prompt medical intervention.

DYSHIDROTIC ECZEMA

Dyshidrotic eczematous dermatitis (pompholyx) is a recurrent cutaneous reaction that occurs as an acute phase and a chronic phase. In the acute phase the lesions are characterized by clear to pink, deep vesicles on the palms, soles, fingers, and toes with associated hyperhidrosis and pruritus (Fig. 10–51). The fluid found in the vesicles is not sweat, as the name would imply, but is clear, proteinaceous, and not associated with an inflammatory reaction secondary to an allergen. The chronic phase is characterized by scaling, fissures, and

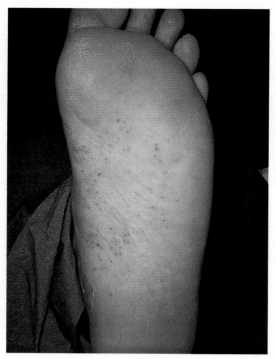

Figure 10–51   Dyshidrotic eczema. Acute dyshidrotic eczematous dermatitis was evident on the soles of the foot. Multiple firm, pink, and clear vesicles are located on the non–weight-bearing surface and are intensely pruritic.

erythema with thickening or lichenification of the skin (Fig. 10–52). Secondary bacterial infection is common during the chronic phase due to fissuring of the skin. In the acute phase, moderate to severe pruritus may

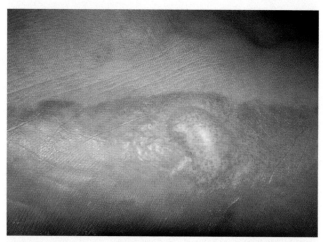

Figure 10–50   Bullous eruptions. An acute bullous reaction on an erythematous base occurred in a patient being treated with nalidixic acid.

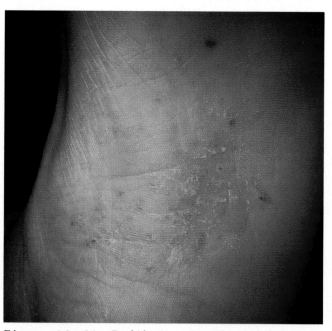

Figure 10–52   Dyshidrotic eczema. Chronic dyshidrotic eczematous dermatitis of the foot was accompanied by accentuation of skin lines and thickening of the skin due to rubbing and scratching.

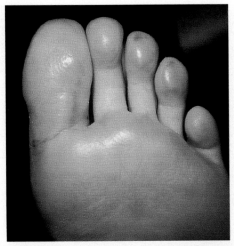

Figure 10–53   Dyshidrotic eczema. Erythematous plantar skin with hyperhidrosis and intense pruritus may precede the visual formation of vesiculation in acute dyshidrotic eczematous dermatitis.

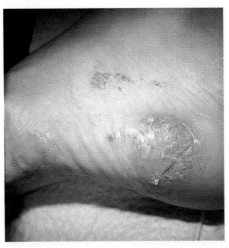

Figure 10–55   Dyshidrotic eczema. In the chronic form there may be hyperkeratosis, deep fissuring, and lichenification of the skin, especially over the medial plantar heel region.

precede the appearance of the vesicles on the hands and feet. The palms and soles may be erythematous and wet with perspiration before vesicle appearance (Fig. 10–53). Once formed, the vesicles resolve very slowly over 3 or 4 weeks and are replaced by small oval scales, which may coalesce. Because of the intense pruritus, scratching of the vesicles is a problem that results in worsening of the condition. Chronic eczematous changes may follow with increased erythema, scaling, and, ultimately, lichenification of the palms and soles (Fig. 10–54). The medial heel region of the foot is a common location for a large dyshidrotic eczematous lesion with hyperkeratosis and fissuring to occur (Fig. 10–55).

The cause of this condition is unknown, but it is frequently associated with hyperhidrosis and emotional stress. The condition is usually worse in the spring and summer months.

Treatment of dyshidrotic eczema includes using wet dressings or soaks to soothe the itching and burning during the acute stages. Burow's solution (aluminum acetate) in a 1:20 concentration is used for the dressings or soaks for 15 minutes twice a day. Topical corticosteroids such as 1% hydrocortisone should be applied after soaking. In most cases, fluorinated corticosteroids should be applied very sparingly, if at all. During the chronic phase, treatment is directed toward lubricating the skin. Topical corticosteroids are used to control the inflammation and pruritus. Occlusive plastic wrapping with topical 1% hydrocortisone may be applied at night for better absorption. This process should be done only for short periods of time to prevent excessive absorption of corticosteroids. Decreasing perspiration and stress also appears to be helpful in many patients.

EXFOLIATIVE DERMATITIS

Exfoliative dermatitis, which is not drug induced, is a noninflammatory disorder in which scaling and peeling of the skin occurs in a very localized manner to the palms and soles (Fig. 10–56) or is generalized to the hands and feet. This reactive dermatitis is sometimes referred to as keratolysis exfoliativa. The condition may occur as a result of an idiopathic process or in response to a systemic condition. It is probably just a variant of acroexfoliative dermatitis and exfoliative erythroderma. This exfoliative stage may be a part of the natural history of various cutaneous or systemic diseases or may follow exposure to certain drugs, as discussed previously.

The spectrum of clinical presentations is broad, and no exact morphological picture can be accurately produced. The condition may be seen with preexisting

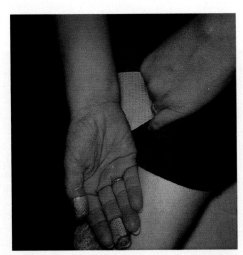

Figure 10–54   Dyshidrotic eczema. Lichenification of the skin on the hands and feet is secondary to chronic dyshidrotic eczematous dermatitis. The skin on the fingers and heels is fissured and painful.

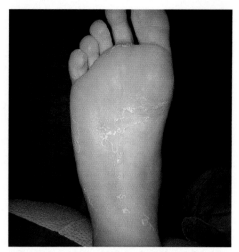

F i g u r e 1 0 – 5 6 Exfoliative dermatitis. Mild exfoliative dermatitis of the both feet and hands is present in this 35-year-old man with no underlying systemic conditions or preexisting diseases. No causative factors could be identified.

skin diseases such as atopic dermatitis, contact dermatitis, eczema, hereditary ichthyosis, psoriasis, seborrheic dermatitis, and stasis dermatitis. Systemic diseases implicated in exfoliative dermatitis include beta-streptococcal throat infections or viral infections with high fevers (Fig. 10–57) and internal malignancies (Fig. 10–58). In a large number of cases, no preexisting condition or underlying disease is found.

Treatment of this type of exfoliative dermatitis is supportive with symptomatic relief of pruritus, fluid loss, and inflammation. Hydration of the skin followed by moisturizing agents is helpful to reduce the dry scaling condition. In the severe forms, the patient should be hospitalized and the causative agent sought. Immediate therapy should be instituted as discussed earlier.

HAND AND FOOT DERMATITIS

Hand and foot dermatitis represents a variety of disease entities that involve inflammatory responses of the hands and feet to either endogenous or exogenous factors. The conditions may be keratotic or eczematous (Fig. 10–59). Many of these conditions can be attributed to preexisting diseases such as atopic dermatitis, nummular eczema, palmar and plantar hyperkeratosis, keratosis punctata and keratosis palmaris et plantaris, ingested allergens, internal malignancy, or irritant or allergic contact dermatitis. A variant of hand and foot dermatitis involves fingertip eczema with a similar eczematous dermatosis of the toes (Fig. 10–60). This condition occurs as erythematous, dry, cracked, and fissured skin on the fingers and toes. There may be associated keratotic eczematous dermatoses of the palmar and plantar surfaces. All or some of the fingers and toes may be involved. The condition is usually worse in the winter months but may improve with retirement or vacations.

F i g u r e 1 0 – 5 7 Exfoliative dermatitis. Moderate exfoliative dermatitis of both feet and hands occurred after a viral illness with a very high body temperature that lasted for 48 hours. The plantar and palmar skin almost completely exfoliated within several days.

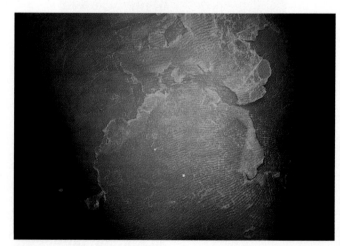

F i g u r e 1 0 – 5 8 Exfoliative dermatitis. This dermatitis occurred in an elderly patient with known liver cancer.

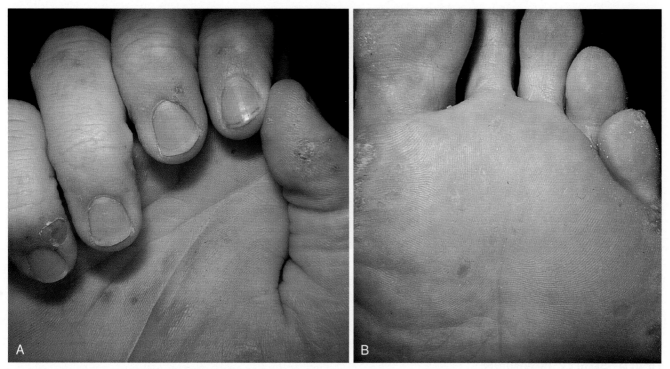

Figure 10–59 **Hand and foot dermatitis.** *A,* The hand lesions show palmar vesicles and eczematous eruptions on the fingers. *B,* The foot lesions are keratotic on the plantar surface and eczematous on the toes.

Treatment of hand and foot dermatitis involves avoidance of known irritants and allergens, wearing of protective gloves and foot gear when necessary, hydration and lubrication of the skin, and topical corticosteroid therapy as needed. Some of the foot lesions may be painful and require intralesional injection therapy with corticosteroids until control is maintained. In more severe cases, tar preparations may reduce ec-

zematous changes. Iodochlorhydroxyquin ointment may be combined with the tar or corticosteroid therapy to help reduce inflammatory and infectious conditions.

A similar condition, called chronic acral dermatitis, is usually found in middle-aged patients with elevated IgE levels who have no history of atopic dermatitis. This condition, unlike general hand and foot dermatitis, is intensely pruritic with a heavy hyperkeratotic eczema

Figure 10–60 **Hand and foot dermatitis.** *A,* Fingertip eczema involving all fingers is usually not allergic. There is diffuse keratotic eczematous dermatitis of the palmar surface of the hand. *B,* Toetip eczema is present on the hallux, and there is weight-bearing keratosis. No underlying disease or associated skin condition was identified.

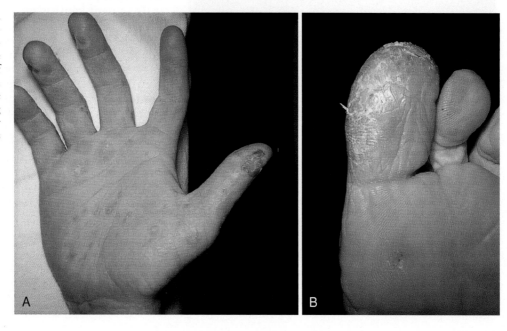

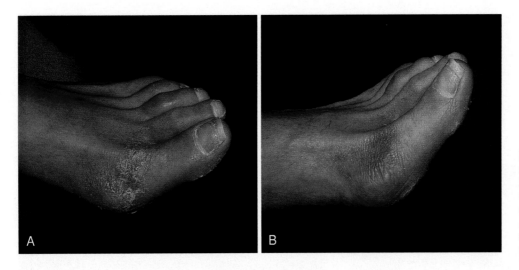

Figure 10–61 Chronic acral dermatitis. *A,* A large hyperkeratotic eczematous plaque over the first metatarsophalangeal joint of the foot was extremely pruritic. *B,* After 1 week of topical corticosteroid therapy the eczematous plaque was greatly improved.

that may form on the thenar aspect of the hand and first metatarsophalangeal joint region of the foot (Fig. 10–61). A clinical response is usually achieved with topical nonfluorinated corticosteroids.

LICHEN SIMPLEX CHRONICUS

Lichen simplex chronicus (circumscribed neurodermatitis) is a condition characterized by a localized and circumscribed thick area of the skin with lichenification secondary to rubbing and scratching. This eczematous eruption is created in a response to a variety of pruritogenic stimuli. The most common lower extremity lo-

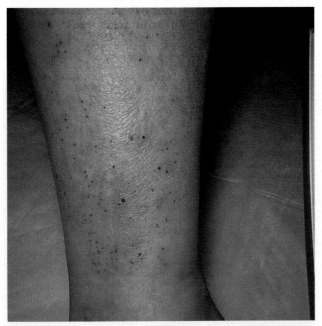

Figure 10–62 Lichen simplex chronicus. Note erythema, edema, and thickening of the skin with excoriated vesicles and papules from chronic rubbing and scratching of the lateral aspect of the lower leg.

cations are the outer lower portion of the lower leg and the ankle.

This condition is much more common in women, but it is also seen in men and children. Once the area becomes lichenified from rubbing or scratching there may be pleasure derived from additional rubbing or scratching of the pruritic area. This effect probably explains the high rate of recurrence of this chronic lesion. Clinical manifestations of lichen simplex chronicus show that patients have pruritus that is much greater than would be expected from the appearance of the lesion.

Initially, the area may be erythematous and edematous or present as coalescing pruritic vesicles and papules with small areas of excoriations noted (Fig. 10–62). The lesion then progresses to a thick lichenified plaque of red papules that coalesce to form a red, scaly, elevated lesion with accentuated skin lines (Fig. 10–63). The final presentation of the lesion is similar in appearance to Naugahyde.

Treatment consists of patient education into the nature of the condition. The patient should understand that the lesion will not resolve as long as he or she is rubbing or scratching the area. Because scratching may take place subconsciously or at night, the affected area may have to be covered to be protected. Topical corticosteroids and antipruritics (e.g., hydroxyzine, diphenhydramine, chlorpheniramine, and promethazine) usually control the itching problem. Cortisone-impregnated adhesive (Cordran Tape) will provide coverage, protection, occlusion, and topical corticosteroid therapy for the inflammation. In chronic recurrent eruptions, psychological consultations may be necessary to help resolve the condition.

NUMMULAR ECZEMA

Nummular eczema (discoid eczema) is defined by its clinical appearance as coin-shaped lesions. This common disorder of unknown cause occurs mostly in middle-aged and elderly patients and is more common

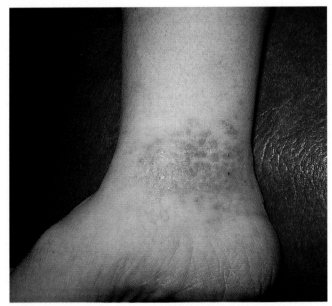

Figure 10–63   Lichen simplex chronicus. In later stages, red coalesced papules are evident within a lichenified plaque on the medial ankle.

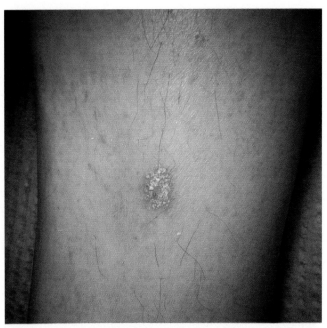

Figure 10–65   Nummular eczema. Eczema occurred on lower leg with increased thickness and formation of a thin scale after increased rubbing due to pruritus.

in men. Nummular eczema appears to be unrelated to atopic dermatitis and fixed drug reactions. It is associated with dry skin and is usually worse in the winter. The typical lesion is characterized by a coin-shaped erythematous plaque or patch that ranges from 1 to 5 cm in diameter (Fig. 10–64). This disorder may be singular or multiple and may progress from a small patch of dermatitis to a large confluent plaque. The lesions are pruritic, and chronic rubbing or scratching may increase the thickness of the plaque and fine scales may form (Fig. 10–65). The lower legs are the most common site

of involvement and the lesions may also be found on the back of the hands, on the upper extremities, and on the trunk. Nummular eczema may be more lichenified and be more difficult to distinguish in dark-skinned individuals (Fig. 10–66). Treatment of nummular eczema is aimed at hydration of the skin, topical emollients, topical corticosteroid therapy, and medications for relief of symptoms.

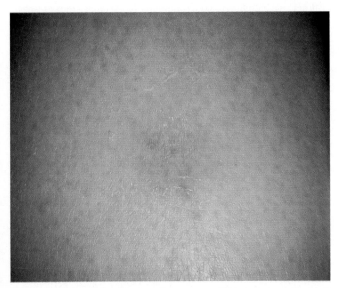

Figure 10–64   Nummular eczema. This acute eruption of minute vesicles forms a typical, discrete, erythematous, coin-shaped patch on the lateral aspect of lower leg.

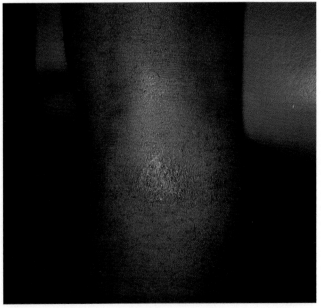

Figure 10–66   Nummular eczema. This may be difficult to identify in a dark-skinned patient.

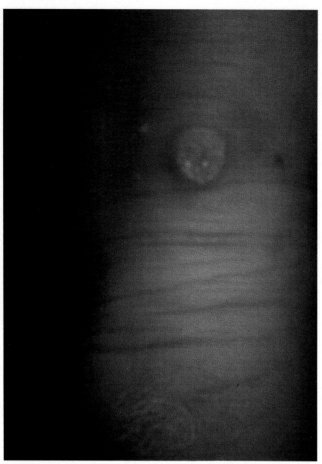

Figure 10-67 Prurigo nodularis. A thick, hard, elevated nodule is usually present on the extensor or flexor surfaces of the legs from chronic picking or isolated scratching.

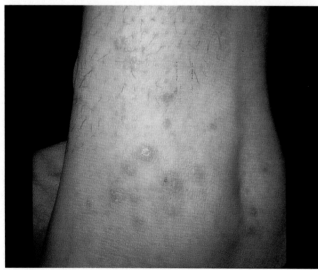

Figure 10-68 Prurigo nodularis. There may be multiple presentations of the erythematous, elevated nodules on the lower extremity secondary to picking and scratching.

PRURIGO NODULARIS

Prurigo nodularis is a variant of lichen simplex chronicus and is characterized by a discrete hyperkeratotic nodule that occurs mainly on the lower extremities as a single lesion (Fig. 10-67) or as multiple lesions (Fig. 10-68). The lesions may also be found on the extensor surfaces of the forearms, hands, and feet. As the name implies, pruritus is the predominant symptom. The lesions are created by repeated picking or scratching in an isolated area. The nodules are red or brown, hard, and dome shaped with a smooth, crusted, or warty central surface. They may reach a size of 2 cm in diameter.

Treatment is with patient education to refrain from picking at or rubbing the nodule. Cryosurgery or intralesional cortisone injections may reduce the pruritus and size of the lesion. In chronic recurrent cases, surgical excision of the lesion may be necessary.

BIBLIOGRAPHY

Baer RL, Ramsey DL, Biondi EL: The most common contact allergens. Arch Dermatol 74:108–111, 1973.

Baruch K: Acute contact dermatitis. J Am Podiatr Assoc 63:255–258, 1973.

Baruch K: Shoe dermatitis: A case report. J Am Podiatr Assoc 65:577–579, 1975.

Brady M: Hands and feet that blister and peel: Dyshidrosis. J Pediatr Health Care 7:37–38, 1993.

Caputo R, Carminati G, Ermacora E, Menni S: Keratosis punctata palmaris et plantaris as an expression of focal acantholytic dyskeratosis. Am J Dermatopathol 11:574–576, 1989.

Clark RA, Hopkins TT: The Other Eczemas. In Moschella SL, Hurley HJ (eds): Dermatology, 3rd ed, pp 465–504. Philadelphia, WB Saunders, 1992.

Cooper KD: Atopic dermatitis: Recent trends in pathogenesis and therapy. J Invest Dermatol 102:128–137, 1994.

Coskey RJ: Contact dermatitis caused by diphenhydramine hydrochloride. J Am Acad Dermatol 8:204–206, 1983.

DeLauro T: Pedal vesiculobullous diseases. In McCarthy DJ, Montgomery R (eds): Podiatric Dermatology, pp 188–197. Baltimore, Williams & Wilkins, 1986.

Dockery GL: Common skin conditions of the foot. Today's Jogger 2:54–56, 1978.

Dockery GL: Podiatric dermatologic therapeutics. In McCarthy DJ, Montgomery R (eds): Podiatric Dermatology, pp 311–335. Baltimore, Williams & Wilkins, 1986.

Dockery GL, Nilson RZ: Intralesional injections. Clin Podiatr Med Surg 3:473–485, 1986.

Epstein WL: Allergic contact dermatitis. In Fitzpatrick TB, Eisen AZ, Wolff K, Freedberg IM, Austen KF (eds): Dermatology in General Medicine, 3rd ed, pp 1373–1384. New York, McGraw-Hill, 1987.

Freedberg IM, Baden HP: Exfoliative dermatitis. In Fitzpatrick TB, Eisen AZ, Wolff K, Freedberg IM, Austen KF (eds): Dermatology in General Medicine, 3rd ed, pp 502–505. New York, McGraw-Hill, 1987.

Halevy S, Shai A: Lichenoid drug eruptions. J Am Acad Dermatol 29:249–255, 1993.

Hanifin JM: Atopic dermatitis in infants and children. Pediatr Dermatol 38:763–789, 1991.

Hanifin JM: Atopic dermatitis. In Moschella SL, Hurley HJ (eds): Dermatology, 3rd ed, pp 441–464. Philadelphia, WB Saunders, 1992.

de la Hoz B, Soria C, Fraj J, Losada E, Ledo A: Fixed drug eruption due to piroxicam (letter to the editor). Int J Dermatol 29:672 1990.

James WD, White SW, Yanklowitz B: Allergic contact dermatitis to compound tincture of benzoin. J Am Acad Dermatol 11:847–850, 1984.

Kavli G, Volden G: Phytophotodermatitis. Photodermatology 1:65–75, 1984.

Kuwada GT, Dockery GL: Contact dermatitis: A review. Clin Podiatr Med Surg 3:551–561, 1986.

Lahti A, Maibach HI: Contact urticaria syndrome. In Moschella SL, Hurley HJ (eds): Dermatology, 3rd ed, 433–440. Philadelphia, WB Saunders, 1992.

Lammintausta K, Maibach HI: Irritant contact dermatitis. In Moschella SL, Hurley HJ (eds): Dermatology, 3rd ed, pp 425–440. Philadelphia, WB Saunders, 1992.

Larsen WG, Maibach HI: Allergic contact dermatitis. In Moschella SL, Hurley HJ (eds): Dermatology, 3rd ed, pp 391–431. Philadelphia, WB Saunders, 1992.

Levy LA: Contact dermatitis and atopic dermatitis. In McCarthy DJ, Montgomery R (eds): Podiatric Dermatology, pp 178–187. Baltimore, Williams & Wilkins, 1986.

Marks JG: Allergic contact dermatitis to povidone-iodine. J Am Acad Dermatol 6:473–475, 1983.

Saha M, Srinivas CR, Shenoy SD, Balachandran C, Acharya S: Footwear dermatitis. Contact Dermatitis 28:260–264, 1993.

Saha M, Srinivas CR: Footwear dermatitis possibly due to paraphenylenediamine in socks. Contact Dermatitis 28:295, 1993.

Sampson HA: Atopic dermatitis. Ann Allergy 69:469–479, 1992.

Schultz Larsen F: The epidemiology of atopic dermatitis. In Burr ML (ed): Epidemiology of Clinical Allergy. Monogr Allergy 31:9–28, 1993.

Sehgal VN, Jain S: Atopic dermatitis: Clinical criteria. Int J Dermatol 32:628–637, 1993.

Stoll DM, Fields JP: Treatment of prurigo nodularis: Use of cryosurgery and intralesional steroids plus lidocaine. J Dermatol Surg Oncol 9:922–924, 1983.

Stoner JG, Rasmussen JE: Plant dermatitis. J Am Acad Dermatol 9:1–15, 1983.

Trevisan G, Kokelj F: Allergic contact dermatitis due to shoes in children: A 5-year follow-up. Contact Dermatitis 26:45–68, 1992.

Vance CE, Levy L: Recognizing arsenical keratosis. J Am Podiatr Assoc 66:91–93, 1976.

Veien NK, Hattel T, Justesen O, Nørholm A: Diagnostic procedures for eczema patients. Contact Dermatitis 17:35–40, 1987.

Webster GF: Pustular drug reactions. Clin Dermatol 11:541–543, 1993.

White SW: Palmoplantar pustular psoriasis provoked by lithium therapy. J Am Acad Dermatol 7:660–662, 1982,

Wishnie PA, Jenkin W: Uses of urea in podiatric medicine. J Am Podiatr Med Assoc 77:601–606, 1987.

Wilson BB, Deuell B, Mills TAE: Atopic dermatitis associated with dermatophyte infection and *Trichophyton* hypersensitivity. Cutis 51:191–192, 1993.

Zugerman C: Dermatitis from transcutaneous electric nerve stimulation. J Am Acad Dermatol 6:936–939, 1982.

11

PAPULOSQUAMOUS DISEASES

INTRODUCTION

The papulosquamous diseases are a heterogeneous group of disorders characterized by scaling papules or plaques. The etiology is primarily unknown. The classification of these diseases is based on a general descriptive morphology of clinical lesions that includes lichen planus and its variants (actinic lichen planus, annular lichen planus, atrophic lichen planus, bullous lichen planus, follicular lichen planus, hypertrophic lichen planus), lichen amyloidosis, lichen planus erythematosus, lichen nitidus, lichen spinosum, lichenoid dermatitis, vesicular lichen planus, and several forms of psoriasis. Because these lesions are characterized at some point by scaling papules, clinical confusion may occur during their diagnosis. Dermatopathological examination may be necessary in some cases for a more definitive differentiation.

LICHEN PLANUS

In 1869, Erasmus Wilson published the first definitive paper on lichen planus. He described lichen rubrous planus as an eruption of flat-topped, polygonal, violaceous papules of unknown cause. More than 125 years later, not much more is really known about its cause.

Lichen planus and its variants are papulosquamous diseases with a relatively common finding of elevated inflammatory papular lesions with scales or plaques. Some of these dermatoses and related conditions may be caused by adverse reactions to drugs, infections, or emotional stress; however, for the most part as mentioned, little is known about their cause. Oral lesions are found in approximately one third of patients with lichen planus. Characteristic papular lesions of lichen planus may range from discrete, individual lesions of 1 to 2 mm in diameter to larger, coalesced lesions of 4 to 5 mm in diameter. They may have a delicate white lace-like pattern known as Wickham's striae or small white or gray pinpoint spots (Fig. 11–1). Men and women are affected equally. Lichen planus usually affects persons between 20 and 60 years old. Cases of lichen planus are also reported in children and the elderly.

Multiple causes of lichen planus have been proposed, but there has been little to confirm or support these findings. Several reports have suggested that lichen planus is due to a bacterial agent, a viral agent, an immunological condition, a genetic-familial relationship, or a neurological condition. Several drugs have been reported to cause lichen planus and several of its variants. Emotional stress has also been implicated in this condition.

The two major types of lichen planus are the acute and the chronic forms. The acute version usually occurs rapidly over several days and may persist for up to 18 months. The condition may be extremely pruritic and may begin on the anterior aspect of the legs and the flexor surfaces of the forearms. A generalized dermatitis may ensue, involving the lumbar area, penis,

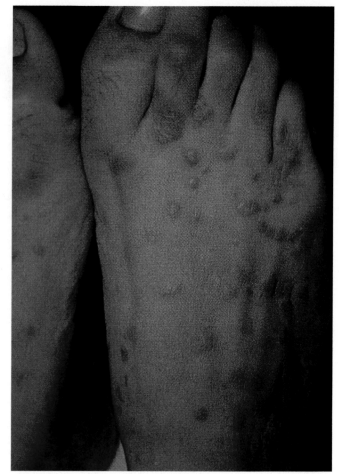

Figure 11–1   Lichen planus. Characteristic variously sized, irregularly shaped papules are evident on both feet. Wickham's striae may be seen on the superficial surfaces of some lesions.

hands, ankles, and feet. I have seen several patients with lichen planus who presented with only primary foot or ankle lesions.

The chronic form of lichen planus is characterized by a higher percentage of oral lesions, which may predispose the patient to oral squamous cell carcinoma. Chronic lichen planus may evolve slowly from generalized acute lichen planus or may occur insidiously and persist for many years. Hypertrophic lichen planus is usually of the chronic form, as is follicular lichen planus.

Lichen planus lesions may be individual, scattered, or grouped together into larger lesions. These papules are frequently pruritic and exhibit Koebner's phenomenon of spreading into an area that is scratched or injured (Fig. 11–2). Mucosal lesions are present in more than half of all patients and consist of white, lacy, reticulated streaks, papules, or plaques. These lesions may also become atrophic or ulcerative patches. The buccal mucosa and the tongue are involved in one third of the cases; however, the lips, gums, genitalia, and anus are also affected.

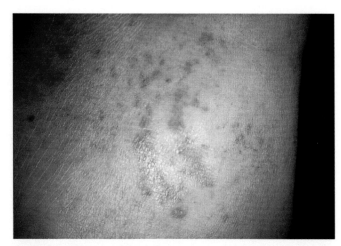

Figure 11-2   Lichen planus. Linear lichen planus is secondary to koebnerization along the lateral ankle due to scratching.

The toenails are involved in 10% of reported cases and may show atrophy, irregular ridging, and grooving of the nail plates. Complete loss of the great toenail is very common. Twenty-nail dystrophy (i.e., a syndrome in which the all of the nails of the hands and feet are dystrophic) is thought to be a variety of lichen planus nail involvement. Pterygium formation results from fusion of the posterior nail fold with the nail bed, causing splitting of the proximal nail plate.

Both acute and chronic lichen planus may involve the palms and soles with nonpruritic yellowish papules that may lack the distinct morphology of typical lichen planus lesions. There may be adjacent lichenification, with the familiar-appearing lichen planus in close proximity (Fig. 11-3). However, these palmoplantar papules may be difficult to diagnose if other, more typical, lesions are not present elsewhere on the body.

Distinct lichen planus variants are recognized, and each has its own characteristics and typical presentations. Pattern variations are altered in configuration, lo-

cation, or morphology. Additional descriptions of some of these variations follows.

ACTINIC LICHEN PLANUS. These mildly pruritic lesions occur on sun-exposed areas and on sunburned skin and may be pigmented, dyschromic, or similar in appearance to granuloma annulare. This is primarily due to Koebner's phenomenon in which ultraviolet light irradiation has aggravated an existing disease (Fig. 11-4). The scalp is rarely involved, and the nails are not affected in this condition. There is also a variety that seems to be a separate entity. It is seen in Middle Eastern and Mediterranean countries and involves the light-exposed areas of skin in children and young adults.

ANNULAR LICHEN PLANUS (NUMMULAR LICHEN PLANUS). These lesions form an annular pattern with a ring of small confluent papules with central clearing and peripheral spreading (Fig. 11-5). They may be seen in addition to the typical pattern of lichen planus, particularly on the lower extremities and penis. One variety occurs with only a few large, scattered, annular lesions that may involve the lower extremities or feet (Fig. 11-6). When these lesions are present, without any usual patterned lichen planus, the eruption may not be recognized clinically but the dermatopathology remains characteristic.

ATROPHIC LICHEN PLANUS. Atrophic lichen planus occasionally results as the active lesions begin to go into remission or resolution (Fig. 11-7). This change, from the typical elevated polygonal violaceous lesion to one that has an upper layer scaling crust and appears to be "melting" into the surrounding epidermis, is frequently mis-

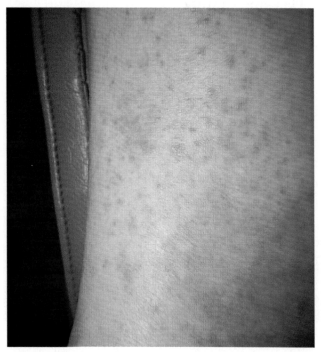

Figure 11-4   Actinic lichen planus. Lichen planus is evident on the sunburned skin of the lower leg and ankle.

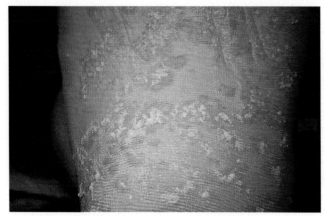

Figure 11-3   Lichen planus. Yellow asymptomatic lichen planus occurred on the plantar sole with more typical lesions found in adjacent areas.

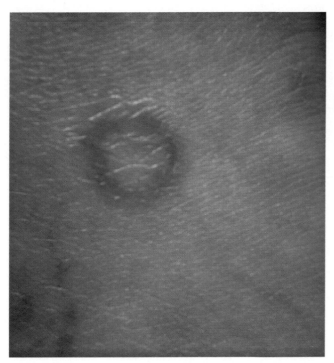

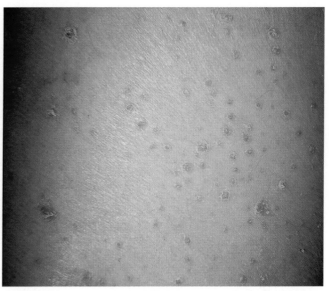

Figure 11–7   Atrophic lichen planus. The typical lichen planus lesions start to involute with a scaly top. The lesions also appear to be resolving, with some lesions becoming thinner with loss of pigmentation.

Figure 11–5   Annular lichen planus. Annular lesions usually form from a ring of typical lichen planus lesions that spread peripherally and produce central clearing.

diagnosed as psoriasis (Fig. 11–8). The atrophic form of lichen planus is commonly found on mucosal surfaces already affected with lichen planus. Atrophic lesions often appear during cortisone treatment of existing lichen planus, especially on the extremities. Atrophic white spots may form during the atrophic phase and should be distinguishable from lichen sclerosus et atrophicus.

BULLOUS LICHEN PLANUS. Tense bullous lesions may ap-

pear on unaffected skin or in areas of preexisting lichen planus. It is not uncommon for these lesions to be present on the lower extremities, particularly on the feet (Fig. 11–9). Once the blisters erupt, the resulting lesions may be more characteristic of typical-appearing lichen planus lesions. The bullous lesions of bullous li-

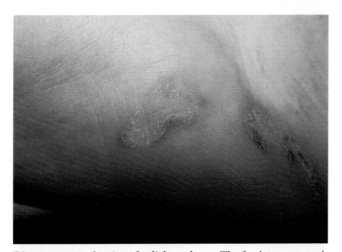

Figure 11–6   Annular lichen planus. The few large, scattered, annular lesions may present on the feet with no other typical lichen planus lesions noted. Diagnosis is often missed clinically and discovered only after biopsy.

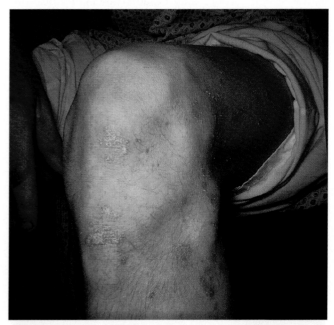

Figure 11–8   Atrophic lichen planus. Atrophy has occurred within some of these lesions of lichen planus. Several lesions have an upper-layer scaling crust and others appear to be "melting" into the surrounding epidermis. This stage may be clinically misdiagnosed as psoriasis.

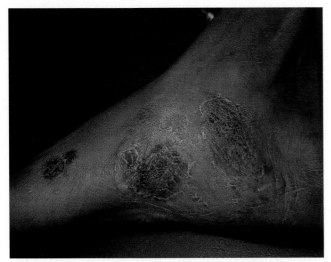

Figure 11–9   Bullous lichen planus. Blisters may occur during the course of lichen planus, especially on the lower extremities. Once the blisters break, the lesions may appear dry and dark and more characteristic of lichen planus.

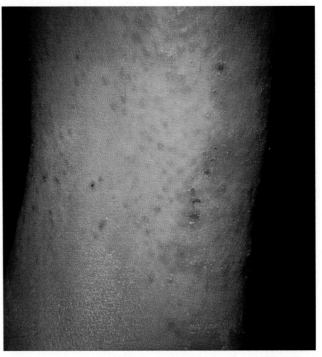

Figure 11–10   Follicular lichen planus or lichen planopilaris. Lichen planus predominantly involves the hair follicles with areas of postinflammatory pigmentation on the lower extremity.

chen planus are usually much larger than those of general lichen planus. The term *lichen planus pemphigoides* has been used to describe this condition, but most believe that these two conditions are separate entities. Routine histology results obtained from a punch biopsy demonstrate typical findings of lichen planus.

FOLLICULAR LICHEN PLANUS (LICHEN PLANOPILARIS). Follicular lichen planus may occur alone or in association with typical lichen planus. This form occurs as lichen planus of the hair follicles on any hair-covered area, especially the scalp and lower extremities (Fig. 11–10). These acuminate (sharp-pointed), keratotic, follicular papules may also exhibit scaling and atrophy as well as temporary alopecia. Scarring and permanent alopecia sometimes result. The direct immunofluorescence of follicular lichen planus is similar to that of typical lichen planus with the exception that the changes are found in the superficial follicular epithelium.

HYPERTROPHIC LICHEN PLANUS (LICHEN PLANUS VERRUCOSUS). These unique and highly pruritic lesions are composed of confluent, firm, lichenified, scaly, and violaceous or hyperpigmented plaques and occur mainly on the anterior shins, ankles, and soles (Fig. 11–11). The surface of the lesions often feels rough and raised and appears "warty." In dark-complexioned persons the violaceous color is easily discerned. Hypertrophic lichen planus may be heavily pigmented. The pigment may persist indefinitely after treatment. These lesions may be chronic (lasting more than 8 years) and the only manifestation of lichen planus. Because of their chronic nature and predisposition for irritation, the lesions of hypertrophic lichen planus may also show malignant degeneration. In the chronic stage, this condition may be difficult to distinguish from lichen simplex chronicus and a biopsy may be necessary to make a definitive diagnosis.

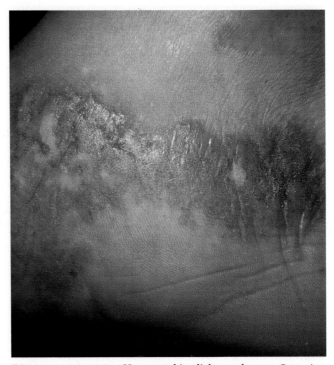

Figure 11–11   Hypertrophic lichen planus. Occurring primarily on the feet and legs, these lesions may be thickened, extremely difficult to treat, very persistent, and intensely pruritic.

Variants of Lichen Planus

Lichen Amyloidosus

Lichen amyloidosus occurs in all age and ethnic groups but has a predilection for dark-skinned middle-aged adults of Central and South America, the Middle East, and Asia. The condition usually occurs as an extremely pruritic collection of papules with diffuse atrophic changes around them on the anterior shins and ankles (Fig. 11–12). The lesions may range from yellow to brown and have the typical violaceous tinge. These lesions may coalesce to form large nonpainful spreading plaques onto the calves and ankles. The face, mucous membranes, and anogenital regions are typically spared. Differential diagnosis includes lichen simplex chronicus and hypertrophic lichen planus. A related form, macular amyloidosis, is moderately pruritic and appears as brown macules with areas of atrophy that may coalesce to form a wavy pattern or even larger hyperkeratotic plaques. These macular lesions may occur in symmetrical patterns over the anterior shins, thighs, or lower back (Fig. 11–13).

Lichen Planus Erythematosus

Lichen planus erythematosus usually occurs as soft, nonpruritic, round, erythematous papules, especially on the forearms and ankles of older women (Fig. 11–14). Other more typical lichen planus lesions may also be on other body areas. Mucosal and nail involvement

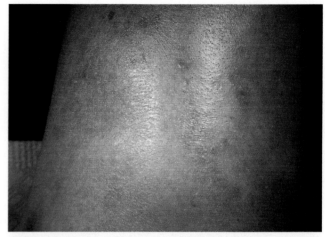

Figure 11–13   Macular amyloidosis. These lesions consist of macular hyperpigmented areas that may appear gray, brown, or blue and may be in a reticulate pattern with adjacent areas of atrophy.

may or may not be present. Histologically, the lesions appear to have characteristic features of lichen planus as well as degeneration of collagen and a marked vascular component. Differential diagnosis includes guttate psoriasis and perforating folliculitis.

Lichen Nitidus

Lichen nitidus is asymptomatic to mildly pruritic, flesh-colored to erythematous, tiny, discrete, sharply demarcated, round or flat-topped, shiny papules commonly located on the penis, arms, legs, ankles, back, and abdomen (Fig. 11–15). Papules may also be found on the palms, soles, and toes (Fig. 11–16). A hyperkeratotic

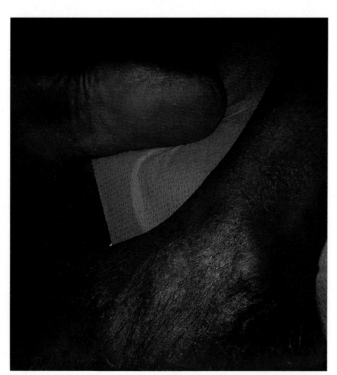

Figure 11–12   Lichen amyloidosus. The anterior and lateral ankle and shin region is often involved. The lesions tend to have a shiny surface of grouped, pigmented papules with diffuse atrophic changes around them.

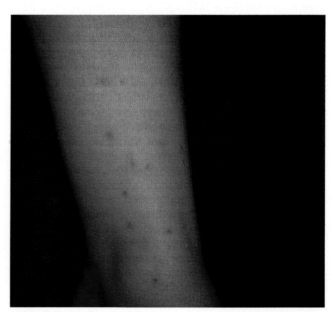

Figure 11–14   Lichen planus erythematosus. These small, nonpruritic, soft, red papules are seen in older women on the forearms and lower legs.

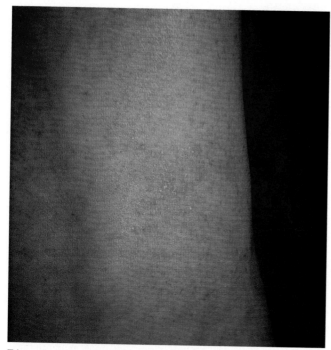

Figure 11–15 **Lichen nitidus.** The pinpoint lesions are small replicas of typical lichen planus. The shiny surface of the round and oval papules may be observed in the center of the grouped lesions on the lower extremity.

or parakeratotic scale is commonly seen on top of the affected epidermis, especially in confluent lesions. These lesions may show the Koebner phenomenon if scratched, although this is not a common occurrence since the lesions are usually nonpruritic. The transepidermal elimination of lichen nitidus inflammatory infiltrate from the upper dermis may result in perforation of the epidermis. Nail changes of pitting, ridging, and thickening with increased brittleness leading to fissures in the nail plate may be observed. The diagnosis is made clinically in most cases.

Lichen Spinulosus

Lichen spinulosus occurs primarily as small, spiny, firm papules that form circular patches over the thighs, lower legs, arms, and buttocks, especially in the flexural creases (Fig. 11–17). Differential diagnosis includes lichen planus, lichen planopilaris, and lichen nitidus. The lichen spinulosus lesions show an acuminate, sharp spiny apex that can readily be seen and felt, as compared with the smooth, flat, or round lesions of lichen planus and lichen nitidus (Fig. 11–18). The lesions may be differentiated from lichen planopilaris because they are located on the glabrous skin and no hair follicles are involved in most cases.

Lichenoid Dermatitis (Lichenoid Keratosis, Lichen Planus–like Keratosis)

Generally, lichenoid dermatitis is thought to be caused by several different types of medications and chemicals (see Chapter 10). At times, patients on medications may be seen with solitary or multiple symptomatic lichenoid papules varying in size from 3 to 10 mm in diameter (Fig. 11–19). These lesions may be round to polygonal and slightly raised with edges that slope gently downward to the periphery. Color changes from bright red to violaceous to rust brown. Most cases of lichen planus–like keratosis are in women as single lesions on the upper body and trunk or diffuse lesions on the arms and legs. I have seen four documented cases (all in women) with lower extremity presentations of lichen planus–like keratosis secondary to therapy with piroxicam (see Fig. 10–41). The cutaneous reaction was clinically and morphologically indistinguishable from that of lichen planus, with the exception that little pruritus was present in each case. These lesions all rapidly resolved when the drug was discontinued.

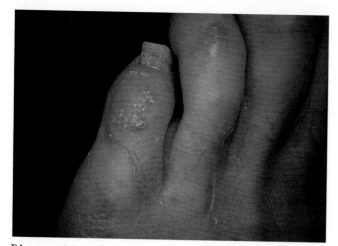

Figure 11–16 **Lichen nitidus.** The distribution of this disorder is similar to lichen planus, but it may occur on the dorsal aspect of the toes.

Figure 11–17 **Lichen spinulosus.** Small, spiny, firm papules on the lower extremities may form circular patches, as seen in this patient in the flexor space behind the knee.

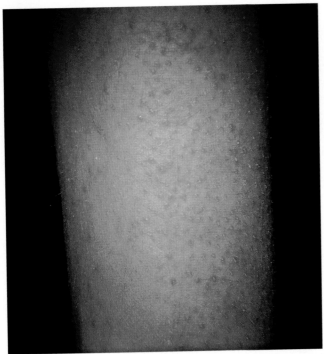

Figure 11–18　Lichen spinulosus. The small, spiny apex of the papules in this condition may readily be seen and felt, distinguishing it from lichen planus and lichen nitidus.

Vesicular Lichen Planus

Vesicular lichen planus may be a precursor or variant of bullous lichen planus. However, this is a very distinct and common variant form of lichen planus that occurs as small red to violaceous vesicles that are mildly to moderately pruritic (Fig. 11–20). These lesions may appear in direct relation to past or present patches of lichen planus, or they may be the primary presenting lesions. Frequently the vesicles are broken due to rub-

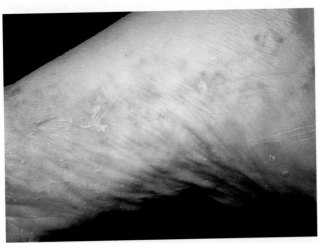

Figure 11–19　Lichenoid dermatitis. Lichen planus–like keratosis on the foot is secondary to systemic antibiotic therapy. Note the similar clinical characteristics and morphology of the lesions to typical lichen planus.

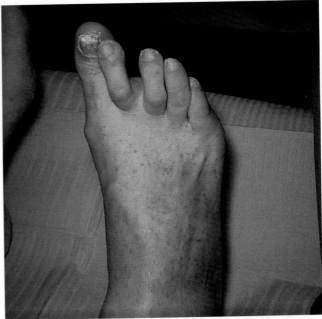

Figure 11–20　Vesicular lichen planus. These red to violaceous vesicles on the foot are very pruritic. They may appear in direct relation to past or present lesions of lichen planus.

bing, pressure, or scratching. This leaves an excoriated surface that will heal slowly (Fig. 11–21). Several cases of vesicular lichen planus have been seen involving the arms and legs or the feet only.

Treatment of Lichen Planus

Lichen planus tends to regress after varying amounts of time with 60% to 80% of patients showing spontaneous clearance within 1 year. For this reason only the patient's symptoms should be treated. Topical wet dressings reduce the pruritus and decrease the inflam-

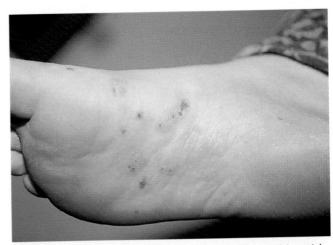

Figure 11–21　Vesicular lichen planus. The pruritic vesicles may be broken or excoriated, leaving an erythematous base that is slow to heal.

matory nature of individual lesions. Wet dressings may also augment other topical treatments. For acute lichenoid forms of lichen planus the importance of reviewing the patient's drug history cannot be overemphasized. The removal of the offending drugs or chemicals may be necessary to control the reaction.

For the most part, lichen planus is a corticosteroid-responsive disorder such that in the majority of patients only topical corticosteroids are needed. However, in mild cases and in children, therapy should begin with a trial of oral antihistamines, topical antipruritics, and soothing baths. In continuing cases, or moderately symptomatic cases, topical fluorinated corticosteroid compounds may be used. In severe, acute cases a tapered course of oral corticosteroids may be required for 2 to 4 weeks using prednisone 10 to 40 mg daily. An interesting phenomenon of "melting" may be seen during the early stages of oral corticosteroid therapy (Fig. 11–22). In chronic nonresponsive generalized lichen planus, intermittent megadose corticosteroid therapy may be warranted. Sometimes, topical fluorinated corticosteroids (flurandrenolide) with polyethylene occlusive dressing (Cordran tape [Dista Products, Indianapolis, IN]) may be very beneficial, particularly on the lower legs. Individual lesions may be injected with small amounts of dexamethasone or betamethasone sodium phosphate (Fig. 11–23). Other lesions such as hypertrophic lichen planus and nail lesions may also

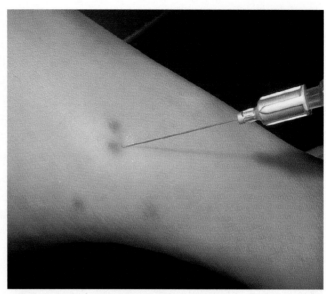

Figure 11–23   Lichen planus. Intralesional injection of individual pruritic lichen planus lesions may be very beneficial.

benefit from intralesional injections of triamcinolone acetonide, 10 mg/mL (Fig. 11–24). Flattening of the lesions should occur after one or two injections. These high-potency corticosteroids should be monitored closely and used for only a short time to prevent complications.

In severe, intensely symptomatic cases, which are unresponsive to the previously described treatments, oral 8-methoxypsoralen photochemotherapy (PUVA) may be added to the treatment regimen. Dapsone may be useful in severe resistant, bullous, or erosive cases of lichen planus.

Finally, a very important part of the management of lichen planus is rest and relaxation. Patients frequently show significant improvement of their skin condition when their emotional environment changes or when on vacation.

PSORIASIS

Psoriasis is a relatively common skin disease that affects an estimated 2% of the population. This papulosquamous disorder may occur with an extreme variability in its clinical expression and in its severity. Small patches of minimal psoriasis may be very disturbing to some patients, whereas other patients may tolerate large areas of involvement.

In general, psoriasis cannot be cured, only controlled. It is important for patients to understand that this condition is chronic and that long-term treatment will probably be necessary.

Clinically, psoriasis is characteristically red to brown, slightly raised, well-defined patches with silvery scales that involve the extensor surfaces primarily, but it may involve all body areas. The lesions vary from small pap-

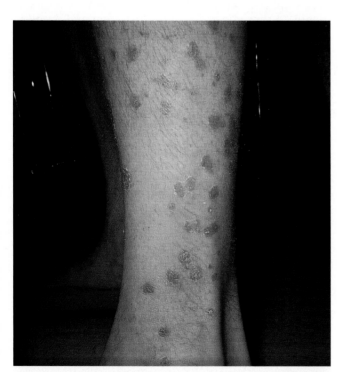

Figure 11–22   Lichen planus. Lesions may appear to be melting during the early stages of oral corticosteroid therapy. Inspection of the lesions shows that they are no longer elevated and the violaceous pigment appears to be spreading into the adjacent uninvolved skin (atrophic phase).

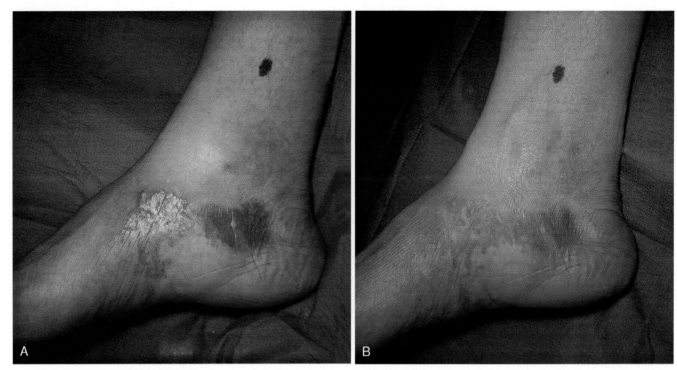

Figure 11–24   Lichen planus. *A,* Hypertrophic lichen planus on medial foot before treatment. *B,* Appearance after several injections of triamcinolone acetonide. The lesion was reduced in size, and the intense pruritus resolved.

ules to very large plaques. The lesions tend to heal centrally during treatment, giving the appearance of a ring. Gentle scratching of the lesion surface may cause pinpoint bleeding. Koebnerization after scratching is common.

Psoriasis is more common in fair-skinned persons with no predilection for sex or age. The condition may go through constant periods of remission and exacerbation. When psoriasis involves the lower extremities alone it may be easier to control than cases of total body involvement. Physical illness and emotional stress appear to make psoriasis worse, whereas rest and sunshine may cause significant improvement in the condition. Although this disorder is usually not difficult to diagnose on clinical examination, it may be helpful to consider certain forms of this disorder that have different therapeutic and prognostic implications. Several forms of psoriasis affect the lower extremities alone, and this presentation may give rise to a degree of diagnostic confusion.

ACUTE OR SUBACUTE PSORIASIS. This condition is generally one in which the preexisting area of psoriasis suddenly becomes inflamed, unstable, and sore (Fig. 11–25). There is frequently no apparent reason for this exacerbation or acute flare of the dermatitis. Treatment is with bland topical therapy using cool compresses or with topical corticosteroids until there is a return to a more stable state. In some instances, intralesional injection with a short-acting corticosteroid is beneficial.

PSORIASIS VULGARIS. This is the most stable form of cutaneous psoriasis. The patches are well defined and

raised and have a red base covered with a uniform silvery scale (Fig. 11–26). This form of psoriasis responds readily to topical corticosteroid treatment and, in more generalized conditions, to PUVA. The differential diagnosis includes nummular eczema, tinea corporis, and lichen simplex chronicus.

GUTTATE PSORIASIS. This form of psoriasis frequently follows a streptococcal throat infection in patients who are prone to psoriasis. The characteristic lesions are small, erythematous papules that appear suddenly over the body, especially the trunk, lower legs, and feet (Fig. 11–27). The size and presentation of the lesions differentiate it from psoriasis vulgaris. The condition is more common in younger, fair-skinned persons and usually

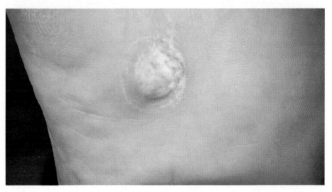

Figure 11–25   Psoriasis. In acute, unstable psoriasis, the lesion becomes inflamed, sore, and red at the base. Treatment is usually necessary to stabilize this active state.

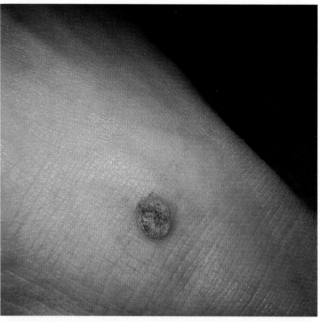

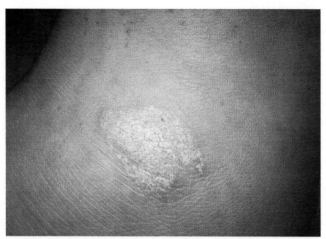

Figure 11–26 Psoriasis vulgaris. This is the most stable form of psoriasis with a red base that is well defined and is covered with a silver scale. This lesion must be differentiated from lichen simplex chronicus.

Figure 11–28 Guttate psoriasis. Occasionally, individual lesions remain and become chronic plaques with a general presentation similar to that of psoriasis vulgaris.

remits after 2 or 3 months. A few lesions may remain and eventually become larger, chronic plaques (Fig. 11–28). Differential diagnosis includes lichen planus, secondary syphilis, and pityriasis rosea. Treatment is usually not necessary except for chronic plaques, which may respond to topical corticosteroid therapy or PUVA.

PUSTULAR PSORIASIS. Localized pustular psoriasis of the palms and soles occurs as yellow pustules, which darken with time. They may appear on an erythematous base and be very intractable to treatment. This con-

dition is usually symmetrical and bilateral and involves the midportion of the soles with recurring crops of small pustules that dry up and form brown crusts (Fig. 11–29). An even more localized form of pustular psoriasis involves the toes, usually a single digit, with the formation of blisters or pustules around the distal phalanx

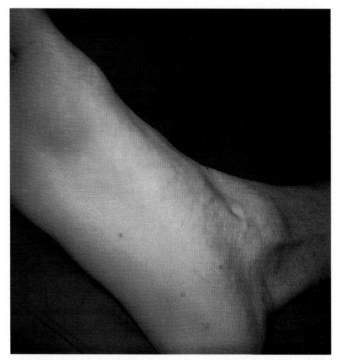

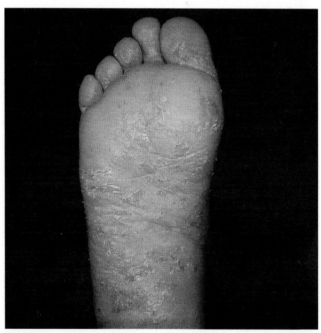

Figure 11–27 Guttate psoriasis. Tiny, red papules form suddenly on the trunk, legs, and feet after a streptococcal throat infection.

Figure 11–29 Pustular psoriasis. This condition of the sole is usually bilateral and symmetrical with small pustules that dry up and leave brown crusts.

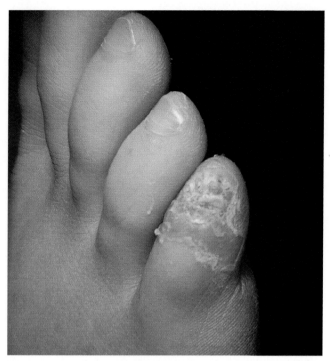

Figure 11–30   Localized pustular psoriasis. This condition begins on a single digit with small blisters or pustules forming adjacent to the nail that break and become crusted.

adjacent to the toenail. The blisters break and become crusted with peripheral scaling (Fig. 11–30). Eventually the nail becomes involved and may be lost. This condition is also known as acrodermatitis perstans and dermatitis repens. Both plantar pustular psoriasis and

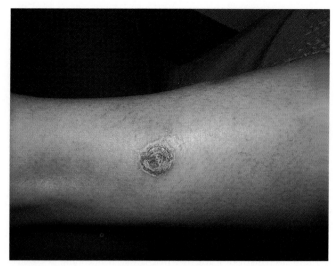

Figure 11–32   Psoriasis. An individual plaque is seen on the lower leg.

localized digital pustular psoriasis have periods of remission and exacerbation and are extremely resistant to treatment. Treatment usually consists of cool wet compresses and topical corticosteroids. Prevention of secondary bacterial infection is important. Systemic corticosteroid therapy should be avoided because it may precipitate the condition.

GENERAL FOOT AND NAIL PSORIASIS. Occasionally, the only presentation of psoriasis may be on the foot, ankle (Fig. 11–31), or lower leg (Fig. 11–32). In these instances there may also be toenail involvement (Fig. 11–33). These lesions usually respond to topical

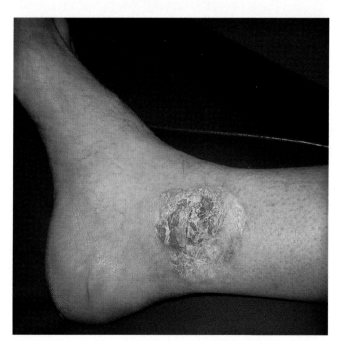

Figure 11–31   Psoriasis. A large psoriatic plaque at the medial ankle in an area of scar formation was the only dermal manifestation of the skin condition.

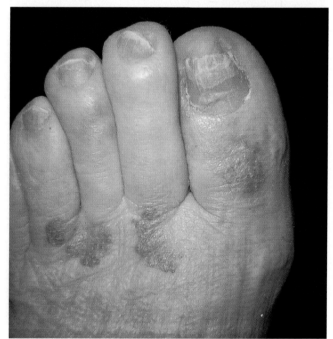

Figure 11–33   Psoriasis of the foot and toenail. In most cases, the presentation is consistent with psoriasis vulgaris. On the dorsum of the foot there may be no silver scaling seen on the plaques.

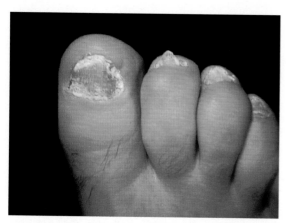

Figure 11–34 Psoriasis of the nails. Nail involvement is characteristically symmetrical, and considerable dystrophy may result. In this case, there was psoriatic arthropathy with prominent involvement of the distal interphalangeal joints.

corticosteroid creams or intralesional injections of short-acting corticosteroids. In generalized psoriasis, the nails may be involved. Usually there is onycholysis caused by separation of the nail plate from the nail bed due to subungual disease, and multiple small pits may be noted on the nail plate (Fig. 11–34). This disease may also involve the joints of the hands and feet, especially the fingers and toes. Skin involvement is usual when the joints are affected; however, it can be seen in patients with no skin presentation of psoriasis.

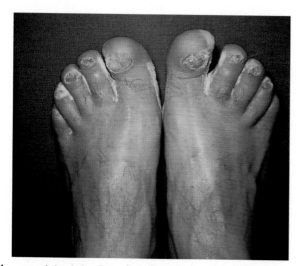

Figure 11–35 Interdigital psoriasis. Also called white psoriasis of the interdigital spaces of the toes owing to the distinct white color of the psoriatic plaques, this condition must be differentiated from candidal and fungal infections.

INTERDIGITAL PSORIASIS. This condition is also termed *white psoriasis* and is primarily seen between the toes (Fig. 11–35). Interdigital psoriasis might be suggestive of interdigital infections with bacteria, yeast, or fungus. All of these should be ruled out in the differential diagnosis. Treatment is difficult in this form of psoriasis because there are frequent recurrences once the condition appears to be responding.

BIBLIOGRAPHY

Cottoni F, Ena P, Tedde G, Montesu MA: Lichen planus in children: A case report. Pediatr Dermatol 10:132–135, 1993.

Fox BJ, Odom RB: Papulosquamous diseases: A review. J Am Acad Dermatol 12:597–624, 1985.

Friedman DB, Hashimoto K: Annular atrophic lichen planus. J Am Acad Dermatol 25:392–394, 1991.

Gardner SS, McKay M: Seborrhea, psoriasis and the papulosquamous dermatoses. Prim Care 16:739–763, 1989.

Heymann WR, Lerman JS, Luftschein S: Naproxen-induced lichen planus (letter to the editor). J Am Acad Dermatol 10:299–301, 1984.

Horn RT, Boette DK, Odom RB: Immunofluorescent findings and clinical overlap in two cases of follicular lichen planus. J Am Acad Dermatol 7:203–207, 1982.

Isaacson D: Summertime actinic lichenoid eruption (lichen planus actinicus). J Am Acad Dermatol 4:404–407, 1981.

Kanwar AJ, Kaur S, Rajagopalan M, Dutta BN: Lichen planus in an 8-month-old (letter to the editor). Pediatr Dermatol 6:358–359, 1989.

Lemont H, McGuire J: Lichen amyloidosis. J Am Podiatr Assoc 72:424–428, 1982.

Meola T, Soter NA, Lim HW: Are topical corticosteroids useful adjunctive therapy for the treatment of psoriasis with ultraviolet radiation? Arch Dermatol 127:1708–1713, 1991.

Miller RAW: The Koebner phenomenon. Int J Dermatol 21:192–197, 1982.

Oliver GF, Winkelmann RK: Treatment of lichen planus. Drugs 45:56–65, 1993.

Patterson JW: The spectrum of lichenoid dermatitis. J Cutan Pathol 18:67–74, 1991.

Pitlosh JP, Taubman MR, Tench W: Pedal pustular psoriasis. J Am Podiatr Assoc 72:429–435, 1982.

Rotstein H, Baker C: The treatment of psoriasis. Med J Aust 152:153–164, 1990.

Sanders LE: Psoriasiform disorders. In McCarthy DJ, Montgomery R (eds): Podiatric Dermatology, pp 106–121. Baltimore, Williams & Wilkins, 1986.

Shai A, Halevy S: Lichen planus and lichen planus–like eruptions: Pathogenesis and associated diseases. Int J Dermatol 31:379–384, 1992.

Taniguchi Y, Minamikawa M, Shimizu M, Ando K, Yamazaki S: Linear lichen planus mimicking creeping eruption. J Dermatol 20:118–121, 1993.

Tosti A, Peluso AM, Fanti PA, Piraccini BM: Nail lichen planus: Clinical and pathologic study of twenty-four patients. J Am Acad Dermatol 28:724–730, 1993.

Weiss RM, Cohen AD: Lichen nitidus of the palms and soles. Arch Dermatol 104:538–540, 1971.

Wilson E: On lichen planus. J Cutan Med 8:117–118, 1869.

Wise RD: Papulosquamous diseases of the lower extremities. Clin Dermatol 1:35–43, 1983.

12

METABOLIC AND INTERNAL DISORDERS

INTRODUCTION

Many patients with metabolic disorders and internal diseases first present with external cutaneous manifestations. The ability to recognize and diagnose systemic disorders by means of cutaneous signs is a great attribute for any physician. Abnormalities of the skin and its appendages offer the physician a wide opportunity to assess the nutritional status and general health of patients. By carefully scrutinizing a patient's skin, the physician may be able to confirm a suspected diagnosis or perhaps even recognize an undiagnosed systemic disease.

Examples of skin changes that may herald systemic disorders include jaundice, representing hepatic or biliary obstructive disease; vitiligo, reflecting thyroid disease; generalized pruritic dermatitis, preceding malignant disorders; and rheumatoid nodules, indicating systemic arthritis. Other dermal lesions that may represent underlying systemic or metabolic disorders are seen in cases of keratoderma in hormonal imbalance, xanthomatosis in hyperlipidemia, gangrene or ulcers in vascular disease, diabetic dermopathy or necrobiosis lipoidica diabeticorum in diabetes, and pigmentary changes in scurvy. Other conditions that may occur as dermal changes include gout, rheumatoid arthritis, neuropathy, dermatomyositis, and morphea. There may be some overlap of classification of dermal lesions with those presented in other chapters, and there is no attempt in this chapter to categorize each type with similar conditions.

DERMATOMYOSITIS

Dermatomyositis is a relatively rare inflammatory muscle disease. This condition may result from immune-mediated vessel injury in which complement is bound and activated to completion in the intramuscular arterioles and capillaries. Most patients are either children or adults (older than age 40). Associated underlying conditions include collagen vascular diseases and internal malignancy. Proximal muscle weakness is a common finding, but distal muscle function is usually well preserved. The affected muscles are weak and sore, and polyarthralgia may also be present. There are several dermal changes that may be present in dermatomyositis: violaceous discoloration around the eyes (heliotrope erythema of the eyelids), Gottron's sign or papules, photosensitive violaceous erythema over joints and legs, periungual telangiectasia, and poikiloderma. Gottron's sign consists of distinctive papular erythema, which occurs over the knuckles (Fig. 12–1). These smooth, flat-topped, violaceous-to-red lesions are considered to be a pathognomonic sign for dermatomyositis. They may range from 0.2 to 1.0 cm in diameter. This type of lesion may also occur on the elbows, knees (Fig. 12–2), or ankles.

Photosensitive violaceous erythema with or without

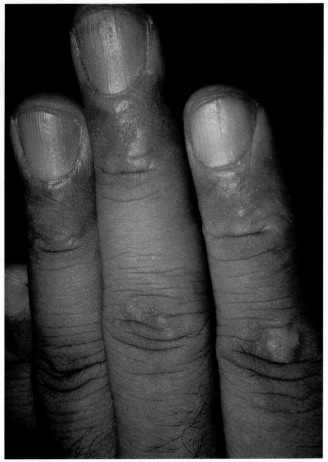

Figure 12–1 Dermatomyositis. Gottron's papules are a pathognomonic sign for dermatomyositis. These smooth, oval to round, violaceous-to-red, flat-topped papules occurred over the knuckles.

scaling may be present over bony prominences such as the knees (Fig. 12–3), elbows, feet, and interphalangeal joints (Fig. 12–4). The diffuse form of violaceous erythema begins as a patchy, diffuse, violet erythema that eventually becomes confluent, minimally raised, and slightly scaly (Fig. 12–5).

Periungual telangiectasia and erythema that are found in dermatomyositis may appear as generalized erythema of the digits with irregular red linear streaks most visible at the posterior nail fold (Fig. 12–6). This condition is not pathognomonic for dermatomyositis and can be very similar to that seen in other connective tissue diseases.

Poikiloderma is a descriptive term for the condition that consists of finely mottled white areas with adjacent brown pigmentation, telangiectasia, and atrophy (Fig. 12–7). This condition occurs late in the course of dermatomyositis when the erythematous rash fades and secondary skin changes become visible. It is sometimes referred to as poikilodermatomyositis. Poikiloderma may also occur in cases of mycosis fungoides and other systemic diseases.

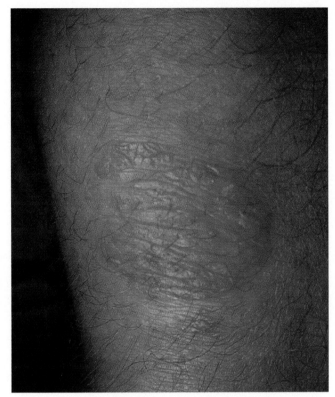

Figure 12–2 Dermatomyositis. Gottron's papules may also be seen on the knees and ankles.

Patients with dermatomyositis should be evaluated for internal malignancy and collagen vascular disease. Occasionally, the systemic condition may not be identified for many years after the development of the dermatomyositis; therefore, a search for malignancy should be repeated at 6-month intervals, especially in older patients. Treatment of dermatomyositis with oral corticosteroids is the treatment of choice for adults with dermal lesions. Topical corticosteroids may also improve the erythematous lesions. Exposure to sunlight should be minimized. Bed rest is important for those patients with active muscle disease, followed by physical

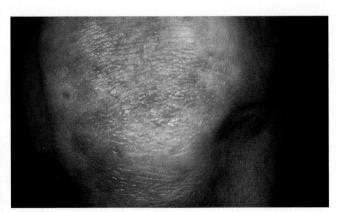

Figure 12–3 Dermatomyositis. Photosensitive violaceous erythema may affect the knees.

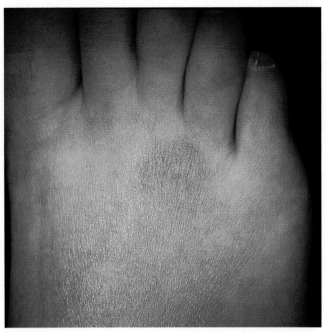

Figure 12–4 Dermatomyositis. The legs and feet may show a persistent erythematous rash with violaceous patches over the dorsal foot and interphalangeal joints. The lesions are worse after sun exposure.

therapy. A passive therapy program should be started early, followed by an active physical therapy exercise program. The patients should also be under the care of a medical specialist familiar with this condition.

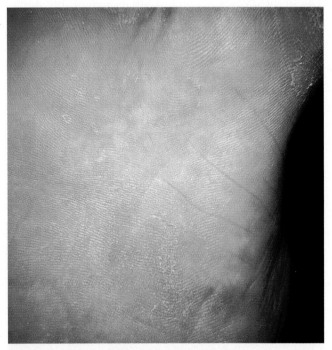

Figure 12–5 Dermatomyositis. A mauve-to-violet erythematous rash that is minimally raised and slightly scaly may occur in non–sun-exposed areas over a period of time. Other external dermal presentations are usually present as well.

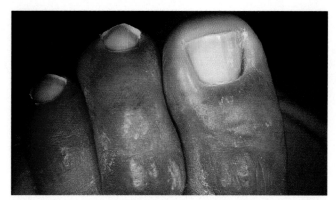

Figure 12–6   Dermatomyositis. Periungual erythema and telangiectasia may be seen on the fingers and toes.

DIABETES MELLITUS

Patients with diabetes mellitus often have cutaneous disorders. Approximately 30% of all patients with diabetes develop a skin complication at some point during the course of the disease. Many of these dermal conditions are present on the lower extremities. Some of these conditions are specific for diabetes (e.g., necrobiosis lipoidica diabeticorum and diabetic dermopathy), and others may be seen in unrelated conditions (e.g., granuloma annulare and ulcerations).

NECROBIOSIS LIPOIDICA DIABETICORUM. Necrobiosis lipoidica diabeticorum is a disease of unknown etiology; however, more than 50% of patients with this skin disorder have diabetes. Most of the patients are female, and in most cases the lesions are located on the anterior shins of the lower legs and dorsal aspect of the feet. The skin lesions may appear many years before the clinical onset of diabetes, and most patients with diabetes do not develop necrobiosis lipoidica. Initially, the lesions of necrobiosis lipoidica are well-circumscribed, oval, violaceous-to-red plaques that may have a fine scale, occurring on the anterior shin (Fig. 12–8) or dorsal aspect of the foot (Fig. 12–9). There is an advancing red border and a yellow-brown central area. The central area may have a waxy feel and undergo atrophic

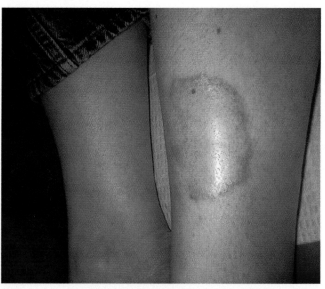

Figure 12–8   Necrobiosis lipoidica diabeticorum. Early lesions on the anterior shin are well-defined, slightly raised yellow plaques with a smooth waxy feel.

changes with increasing telangiectasia. Ulceration may occur in the central zone, especially after trauma. As lesions mature they may become thicker and more violaceous (Fig. 12–10). There is no specific treatment for this disorder because most cases remain asymptomatic. Topical corticosteroid cream will reduce the inflammation but may increase the atrophic dermal changes. Intralesional corticosteroids may reduce the inflammation and appearance of the lesions but may aggravate the systemic diabetes.

DIABETIC DERMOPATHY. Dermopathy is considered to be one of the most common skin problems associated with

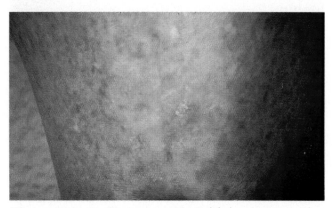

Figure 12–7   Dermatomyositis. Poikiloderma may occur late in the process in areas of previous erythematous scaling lesions of dermatomyositis.

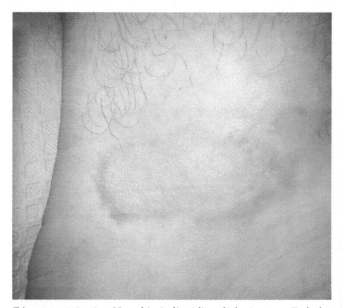

Figure 12–9   Necrobiosis lipoidica diabeticorum. Early lesions on the foot show an advancing red border with a yellow-brown central area.

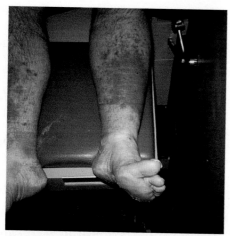

Figure 12–10 Necrobiosis lipoidica diabeticorum. Late lesions are thick, violaceous plaques on the anterior surfaces of the lower legs.

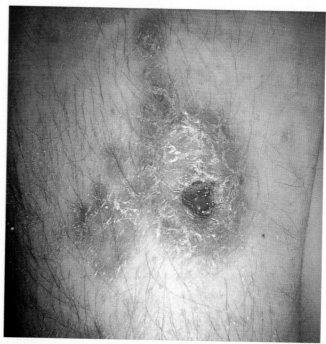

Figure 12–12 Diabetic dermopathy. The active lesions may become eroded or ulcerated in the central areas. Local treatment for ulcers is then recommended.

diabetes. This condition is referred to as "shin spots" because of its most usual location on the anterior shins of the lower extremities (Fig. 12–11). These asymptomatic, round-to-oval, flat-topped, red, scaly papules may become eroded or ulcerated in the central areas (Fig. 12–12). They may resemble a superficial dermatophyte infection. The lesions may clear with time, leaving multiple areas of epidermal atrophy or hyperpigmentation (Fig. 12–13). Many patients account for their lesions by reporting specific local trauma to the area of the shins. Because of this response, these lesions are frequently ignored by patients and disregarded by physi-

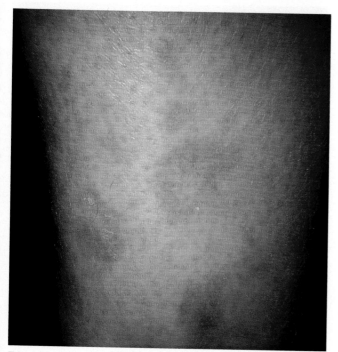

Figure 12–11 Diabetic dermopathy. The asymptomatic lesions on the anterior shin are round-to-oval, flat-topped, red, scaly papules.

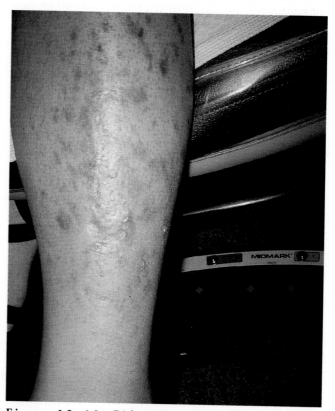

Figure 12–13 Diabetic dermopathy. Multiple small atrophic and hyperpigmented lesions (shin spots) may be seen on the anterior shin.

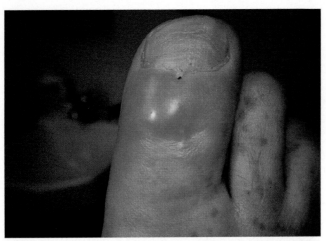

Figure 12–14   Diabetic bullae. Nonscarring, atraumatic, sterile blisters occur on the dorsal tips of the toes. A typical blister may have an erythematous base that heals within a few weeks with no scarring or atrophy.

cians. This condition may precede diabetes by many years and should alert the physician to the possibility of early diabetes.

DIABETIC BULLOSIS. Two different types of diabetic bullae may occur in diabetic patients. The most frequent is the spontaneous nonscarring type of acral bullae formation (Fig. 12–14) that occurs on the tips and dorsal aspects of the fingers and toes. Less frequently, the bullae may form on the dorsal or lateral surface of the foot (Fig. 12–15) or leg. A typical blister has an erythematous periphery, is not hemorrhagic, and heals spontaneously within a few weeks. The healed area does not show scarring or atrophy. There are usually no reports of trauma to the area before the presentation of the bullae. Patients with this condition are usually between the ages of 40 and 75 with long-standing diabetes and diabetic neuropathy. There may be recurrence of the blisters for a number of years. The second type of diabetic bullae differs from the first type in that the bullae heal with scarring and slight atrophy (Fig. 12–16). These blisters are occasionally hemorrhagic, and an inflammatory base is present. In both cases, protection of the intact blister is recommended. Extremely tense bullae should be aspirated using aseptic technique, and the roof of the blister left intact.

PIGMENTED PURPURA. Pigmented purpuric dermatosis is characterized by patches of orange or brown pigmentation and "cayenne-pepper" spots found on the lower extremities (Fig. 12–17). This condition results from the deposition of red blood cells into the skin that have extravasated from the superficial vascular plexus. Petechiae that occur on the lower legs and the dorsa of the feet transform into coexisting nonatrophic pigmented spots. Diabetic dermopathy may also coexist. Clinically, diabetic pigmented purpuric dermatosis may resemble the progressive pigmented purpuric dermatosis of Schamberg.

GRANULOMA ANNULARE. Generalized or disseminated granuloma annulare is found in as many as 33% of patients with diabetes. However, most patients with the more common localized form of granuloma annulare do not have clinical or laboratory evidence of diabetes.

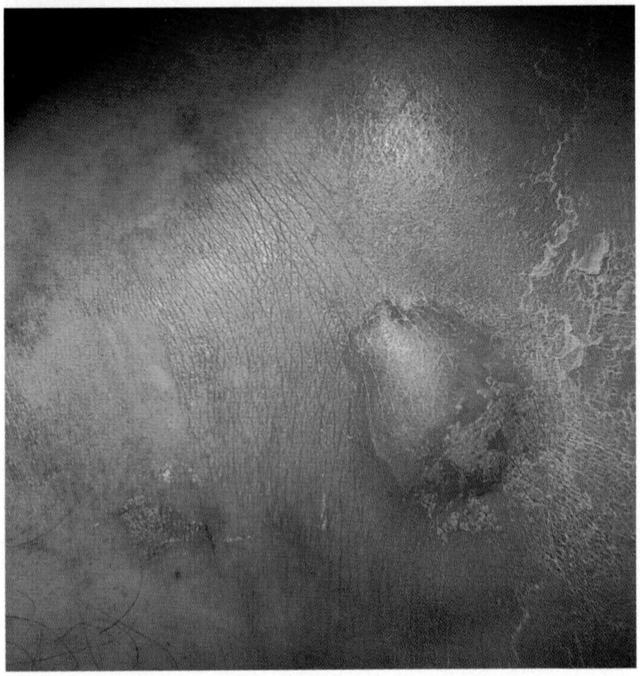

Figure 12–15   Diabetic bullae. Less common sites for the nonscarring blister formation are on the dorsal and lateral aspects of the foot or leg.

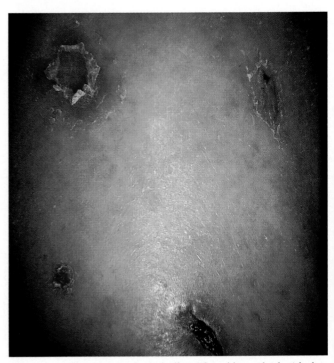

Figure 12–16   Diabetic bullae. These blisters heal with dermal scarring and atrophy. The bullae frequently take many months to heal once they are broken and the base remains inflamed.

This condition is characterized by a distinctive skin eruption consisting of a ring of firm, well-defined, small, pink-to-red papules (Fig. 12–18). The edge of the lesion may be raised or flat. The eruption occurs most commonly on the backs of the hands and fingers, as well as over the lateral and dorsal aspects of the feet, ankles, and legs. In the disseminated form, lesions may be present over the entire body. The annular lesions may range from 0.5 to 5.0 cm in diameter and may last for many years or may slowly undergo spontaneous involution without scarring. The lesions may be singular or become arranged in large annular or serpiginous patterns. Disseminated granuloma annulare occurs in adults, and the papules may be accentuated in sun-exposed areas.

Histopathological evaluation of biopsy specimens is characterized by areas of collagen degeneration, lymphohistiocytic infiltrate, deposits of mucin, and endothelial edema of the small blood vessels. Histological findings are similar to those seen in necrobiosis lipoidica and rheumatoid nodules.

Treatment is usually not necessary, but in the occasional symptomatic lesion or lesion that is a cosmetic concern to the patient, treatment may consist of intralesional injections of betamethasone sodium phosphate, 0.5 to 1.0 mL, with equal amounts of a local anesthetic agent. The solution should be injected only into the elevated advancing borders. Dapsone may be helpful in treating the disseminated form of granuloma annulare.

NEUROTROPIC ULCERS. The neurotropic ulcer with a characteristic punched-out central core surrounded by

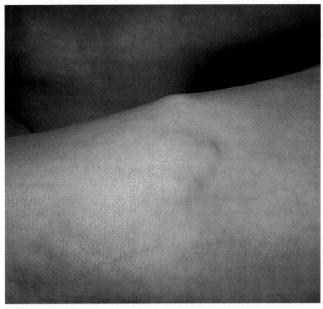

Figure 12–18 Granuloma annulare. The margin of the eruption is made up of individual flat-topped flesh-colored or red papules. The lateral and dorsal surfaces of the feet and ankles are a common site.

a thick peripheral callus may also be associated with diabetes (Fig. 12–19). The dermis surrounding the ulcer is usually anhidrotic even though the skin may be warm. The ulcer is frequently a result of increased pressure in an area that is insensitive due to peripheral neuropathy. Patients with diabetic ulcers on their feet

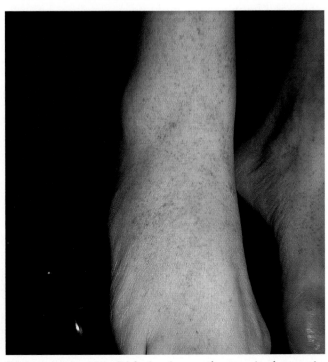

Figure 12–17 Diabetic pigmented purpuric dermatosis. Petechiae on the legs and dorsa of the feet in a patient with diabetes may resemble Schamberg's disease.

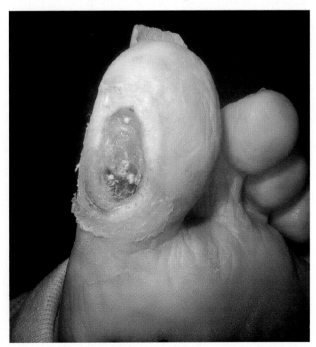

Figure 12–19 Diabetic ulceration. The weight-bearing aspect of the foot and toes is a common site for neuropathic ulcers in patients with diabetes.

may complain of deep pain, but examination of the ulcer usually shows that it is anesthetic. In some cases the condition is secondary to ischemia and small blood vessel disease. Treatment of the ulcer is outlined in the section on venous ulceration (see Chapter 9). It is very important that the hyperkeratotic callus be carefully debrided from around the ulcer rim and that the area be fully protected from additional trauma and pressure. Topical antibiotics may be necessary if superficial infection is present.

GANGRENOUS CHANGES. Small and large blood vessel disease results from the metabolic and lipid disorders of diabetes. Microangiopathy and premature vascular insufficiency may cause severe ischemia and, ultimately, tissue necrosis and gangrene. Foot gangrene is more common in diabetic patients older than the age of 40 than in nondiabetic individuals. Diabetic patients tend to develop digital gangrene as a manifestation of more peripheral small vessel disease (Fig. 12–20). Control of the diabetes is important, and many patients may benefit from revascularization surgery. Diabetic gangrene may be so extensive that amputation may be the only treatment, even in patients with palpable pulses. Regular skin care is essential for patients with diabetes because even minor injuries to the skin may lead to infection and gangrene (Fig. 12–21).

ERUPTIVE XANTHOMAS. Eruptive xanthomas (xanthoma eruptiva) develop in a small percentage of diabetic patients and are characterized by the sudden onset of firm, nontender, yellow papules with pink or red areolae. These lesions are common on the knees, elbows, back, buttocks, trunk, and heel (Fig. 12–22). They are associated with hyperlipidemia, hyperglycemia, and glycosuria. The lesions usually appear during the hypertriglyceridemic phase of uncontrolled diabetes. They usually clear with control of the diabetes and resolution of the elevated serum lipid levels. Histopathology of a typical lesion reveals dermal accumulation of foamy, lipid-

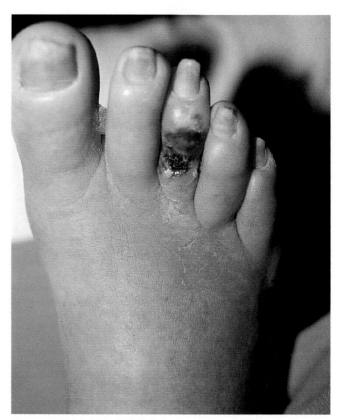

Figure 12–21 Diabetic gangrene. This diabetic patient sustained a relatively minor injury to the middle toe that resulted in infection and gangrene.

laden histiocytes and mixed inflammatory cell (neutrophilic and lymphocytic) infiltrate.

YELLOW SKIN AND NAILS. The yellow color of the skin on the soles, especially involving callus tissue (Fig. 12–23), was once thought to be secondary to carotenemia,

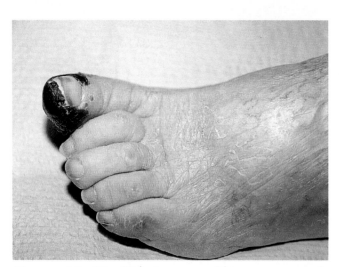

Figure 12–20 Diabetic gangrene. The toes are commonly involved in gangrenous changes in diabetic patients with peripheral small vessel vascular disease.

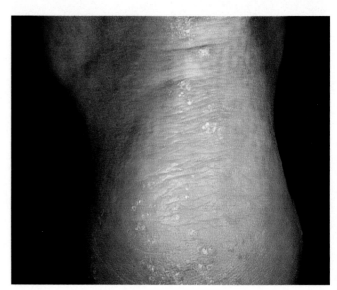

Figure 12–22 Diabetic eruptive xanthomas. Crops of yellow papules with red areolae are located on the posterior surface of the heel in a diabetic patient.

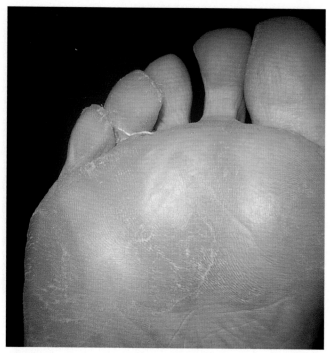

Figure 12–23 Diabetic yellow skin. The thicker or calloused layers of the soles and palms may show a distinct yellow coloration in patients with diabetes.

but this has not been confirmed. This condition is found in a large number of patients with diabetes, but the exact cause has yet to be elucidated. Yellow nails have also been recognized in more than 50% of patients with diabetes. The condition may occur as a very distinct yellow discoloration of all 10 toenails (Fig. 12–24). Alternatively, the yellow color may be more subtle and involve only the distal nail, especially the great toenail (Fig. 12–25). Diabetic patients with yellow nails have a tendency to present with other lower extremity cutaneous disorders, such as erythema, purpura, or diabetic dermopathy. The yellow discoloration may be due to

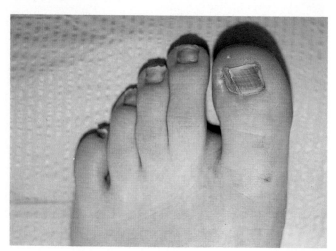

Figure 12–24 Diabetic yellow toenails. All toenails may show a distinct yellow discoloration in patients with diabetes.

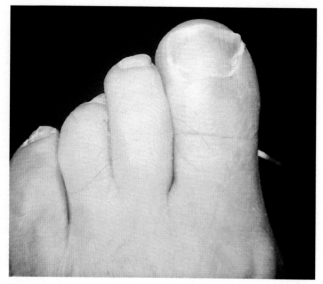

Figure 12–25 Diabetic yellow toenails. The great toenail, sometimes only distally, may show a subtle yellow coloration in patients with diabetes.

impaired circulation to the nail bed and matrix from microvascular disease. Other conditions that may also occur as yellow nails include lymphedema praecox and onychomycosis.

GOUT

Gout is secondary to a disorder of purine metabolism that is characterized by hyperuricemia. This condition may result from an increased production of uric acid, a decrease in uric acid excretion, or both. Persistent hyperuricemia may result in deposition of monosodium urate in various body tissues owing to limited solubility of uric acid and its salts in the tissue fluids. Gout is much more common in men, and the presenting pathological features almost always occur in the lower extremities.

The acute form of gout classically involves the first metatarsophalangeal joint of the foot (Fig. 12–26) and involves erythema, increased temperature, swelling of the area, and intense pain associated with the acute gouty attack. This condition may also involve the instep, dorsum of the foot (Fig. 12–27), ankle, and knee. Severe acute attacks of gout typically occur early in the morning before the patient gets out of bed and are precipitated by minor injury, increased alcohol intake (especially beer or wine), dietary indiscretion, emotional stress, intense physical activities, or medications.

Diagnosis is based on clinical presentation and demonstration of monosodium urate crystals in synovial fluid aspirate. Treatment of the acute episode is with oral anti-inflammatory agents, local infiltration injection of corticosteroids, and rest. Regression of the erythema, swelling, and pain is quick once treatment begins (Fig. 12–28). Exfoliation or peeling of the skin with generalized mild erythema in the area of inflam-

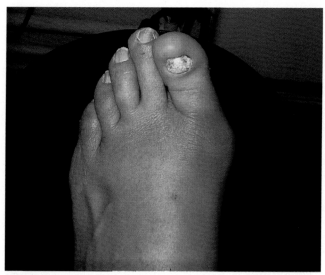

Figure 12–26   Acute gout. The first metatarsophalangeal joint is typically erythematous, hot, and exquisitely painful in the early inflammatory phase of gout.

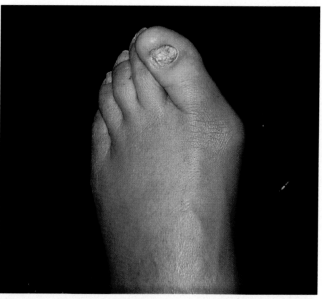

Figure 12–28   Acute gout. Resolution of the acute phase of gout may show a generalized mild erythema with superficial peeling of the skin. Same patient as in Figure 12–26.

mation may occur with resolution of the signs and symptoms.

Chronic gout may occur if the initial phase is not treated properly or the underlying precipitating condition is not controlled. Macroscopic monosodium urate crystals, or tophi, may appear in or around the joints, causing severe swelling and resulting in erosive joint deformation (Fig. 12–29). These deposits of urates tend

to develop in avascular areas and are seen in the ear, olecranon, and prepatellar bursae and in the tendons of the fingers, toes, heels, and ankles (Fig. 12–30). The overlying skin may become thin, vascular, and yellow or orange. The tophaceous deposits in the walls of bursae, capsules, tendon sheaths, and within the joints begin to cause destructive changes to these tissues. These

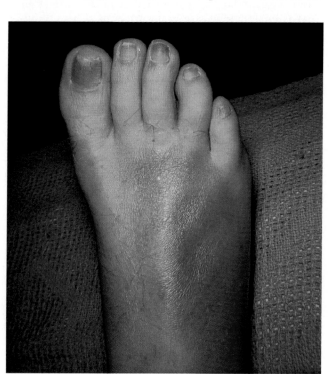

Figure 12–27   Acute gout. The dorsum of the foot may be involved in the acute phase of gout with a well-demarcated area of increased redness, heat, and pain.

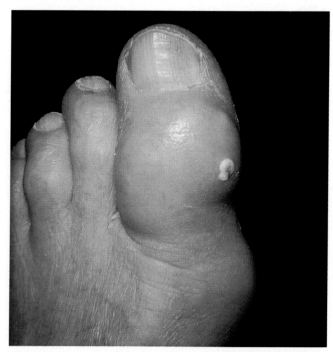

Figure 12–29   Chronic tophaceous gout. Deposits of macroscopic urate crystals within the capsule and joint may lead to ulceration with red, undermined walls and cheesy material filling the crater.

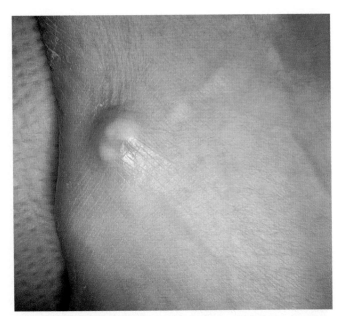

Figure 12-30   Ankle tophi. Tophaceous deposits may produce irregular asymmetrical tumescences over joints and tendons. The skin is frequently thin, vascular, and yellow or orange.

subcutaneous nodules may be easily injured, and a chronic ulcer may form with erythematous borders and' white cheesy material filling the base. Secondary cellulitis or frank infection may follow. Complete destruction of the joint may be seen in late or chronic cases of gout. Characteristic punched-out lesions in the subchondral bone of the joint may be seen on a radiograph (Fig. 12–31). Large tophi may be surgically removed, and joints that have been destroyed may be excised. The removal of urate deposits within ulcerations is usually necessary to heal the ulcers.

Treatment of chronic gout is similar to the treatment of the acute phase, with the addition of allopurinol, probenecid, or sulfinpyrazone. Referral to an internal medicine specialist or rheumatologist for medical evaluation of the cause of the gout and management of the chronic condition with medication is recommended.

HORMONAL IMBALANCE

Keratoderma Climactericum (Haxthausen's Disease)

The term *keratoderma* is frequently used synonymously with the terms *hyperkeratosis, keratoma, keratosis,* and *tylosis.* Palmoplantar keratoderma is characterized by excessive formation of keratin on the soles and palms. The congenital and the acquired forms may be present alone, or they may be a part of some syndrome or accompany other diseases. The acquired types include keratoderma climactericum and keratoma plantar sulcatum. Keratoderma climactericum was first reported by Brooke in 1891; however, in 1934 Haxthausen gave the first clear description of the condition presenting in women and described its association with the climacteric type, obesity, and hypertension. The condition is

described as circumscribed hyperkeratoses, mainly of the palms and soles in women, in association with the climacteric type and accompanied by various general signs and symptoms of which obesity, arthritis, and hypertension are frequently encountered. The cause of keratoderma climactericum is unknown. Because this disorder occurs only in women in association with menopause or after hysterectomy, estrogens and the role of endocrinological factors are usually implicated.

In the beginning of the disorder, the mild keratoses that form are sharply circumscribed, discrete hyperkeratotic plaques and papules without vesiculation or inflammation. Gradually, the papules and plaques increase in size, becoming scaly, and coalesce, resulting in diffuse palmar and plantar hyperkeratosis with fissures that may secondarily become infected. The keratotic patches are prone to form over weight-bearing areas and actively used surfaces such as the fingers and center of the palms (Fig. 12–32) and the ball and circumference of the plantar feet and heels (Fig. 12–33).

Histological examination reveals acanthosis with marked thickening of the stratum corneum. There is extensive parakeratosis without microabscesses such as are found in psoriasis, which it resembles clinically. The microscopic findings are nonspecific; however, acantho-

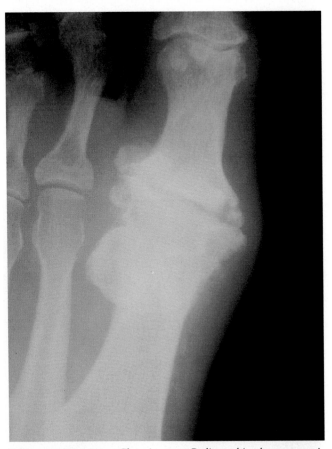

Figure 12-31   Chronic gout. Radiographic changes associated with chronic tophaceous gout show joint destruction of the first metatarsophalangeal joint, subchondral bone lesions, and extra-articular bone spur formation.

sis and dilated capillaries are seen in the upper dermis associated with a slight lymphocytic infiltrate.

Differential diagnosis of keratoderma climactericum includes congenital and other acquired hyperkeratoses of the palms and soles. The various types of congenital or hereditary keratodermas of the palms and soles are inherited as a mendelian dominant characteristic and are usually observed before the second decade. Acquired thickening of the skin of the palms and soles may be seen in psoriasis, pityriasis rubra pilaris, chronic contact dermatitis, occupational disorders, keratosis follicularis, porokeratosis, chronic eczema, and syphilis. Other conditions involving keratoderma of the palms and soles include esophageal carcinoma, ichthyosiform dermatoses, arsenical keratoses, and mycosis fungoides. On the sole the keratosis is diffuse and resembles the moccasin distribution of *Trichophyton rubrum,* and on the palms the disorder may resemble lichen simplex chronicus. In most cases, the disease can be differentiated by a complete history and physical examination, the distribution of the lesions, and the appropriate laboratory evaluations.

Treatment with local and systemic estrogens may be beneficial. The most appropriate form of treatment appears to be avoidance of contact irritants and drying agents; local palliative measures to remove excessive hyperkeratotic tissue either manually or with keratolytic agents; soaking the affected areas in warm water and pHisoHex soap to hydrate the tissue and cleanse the wounds; using a nonmedicated dermabrasive pad or pumice stone to help in desquamation; paring the lesions with a scalpel blade; applying a combination of 10% urea cream and 1% hydrocortisone to control dryness and secondary inflammation; and occasional painting of deep fissures with Castellani's paint. Cellulitis due to secondary infection of the deep fissures is treated with a course of appropriate antibiotics. This combina-

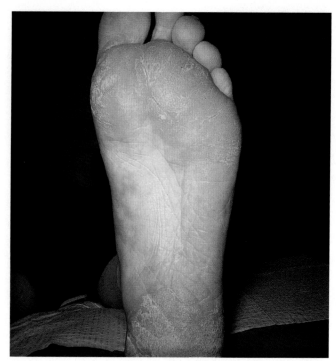

Figure 12–33   Keratoderma climactericum. This is a typical distribution of hyperkeratotic patches with thickening of the skin and deep fissures located on the weight-bearing plantar sole. The lesions seem to spare the longitudinal arch area.

tion of treatments appears to be satisfactory in the treatment of keratoderma climactericum when performed on a regular schedule. This condition will probably recur when the therapy subsides, and the patient should be properly instructed as to the chronicity of the disorder.

Thyroid Disorders

Cutaneous disorders of the lower extremities secondary to thyroid diseases are listed in three categories: (1) those with decreased level of thyroid hormone, (2) those related to an increased level of thyroid hormone, and (3) those not related to the presence of thyroid hormone.

DEFICIENCY OF THYROID HORMONE. Thyroid deficiency may occur when (1) there is a congenital absence of, or a small, thyroid gland; (2) there is loss or atrophy of thyroid tissue that results in decreased production of the hormone; (3) there is pituitary or hypothalamic failure (trophoprivic hypothyroidism); or (4) there is an impairment in biosynthesis of thyroid hormones (goitrous hypothyroidism). The most common cause is decreased or absent thyroid tissue caused by surgery or drugs. The skin in hypothyroidism appears cold, dry (xerotic) and rough, and pale or yellow (Fig. 12–34).

The coolness of the skin is secondary to cutaneous vasoconstriction and to a decrease in body core temperature. The dryness of the skin is due to a change in skin texture and absence of sweating. These lead to dif-

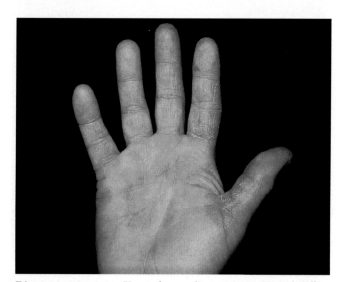

Figure 12–32   Keratoderma climactericum. Typical diffuse hyperkeratotic lesions are seen on the palm and fingers of the patient's right hand. The condition frequently spares the thenar eminence.

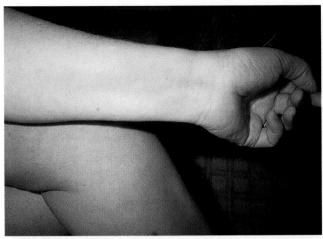

Figure 12-34 Hypothyroidism. The skin on the arms and legs may be cool, dry, pale to yellow, and coarse.

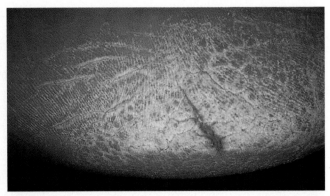

Figure 12-36 Hypothyroidism. Keratoderma with thick fissured plaques may form over the heels.

fuse dryness of the skin with scaling or ichthyotic changes with superficial fissuring of the skin (Fig. 12–35). The epidermis may become extremely thin and hyperkeratotic with fine wrinkling, which may give the skin a parchment paper–like quality. The skin may also be mottled and appear similar to the skin in cases of livedo reticularis. The pale color may be due to the increased content of mucopolysaccharides and water in the dermal layers, which change the refractive index of incidental light on the skin. There may also be a yellow presentation of the skin, which may be accentuated over the palms and soles, due to an accumulation of carotene in the stratum corneum. This condition (carotenemia) in hypothyroidism is probably due to a defective hepatic conversion of beta-carotene to vitamin A. Keratoderma of the feet with large, fissured hyperkeratotic plaques may appear on the heels (Fig. 12–36). The hair may be thick, dry, and very brittle with accentuated hair follicles. Generalized decreased body hair is frequently seen. Fingernails may be thin and

brittle, and toenails may become thick, brittle, and ridged, and grow very slowly (Fig. 12–37).

EXCESS THYROID HORMONE. Overproduction of thyroid hormone (thyrotoxicosis) is usually related to Graves' disease (exophthalmic or diffuse toxic goiter), multinodular goiter, thyroid adenoma, or excessive thyroid hormone administration. The cutaneous presentations are almost the complete opposite to those seen in hypothyroidism. The skin in hyperthyroidism is warm, moist, soft, pink or red, and smooth. The skin is frequently described as being fine, implying that it is thin; however, the skin is usually of normal thickness in patients with hyperthyroidism. The warmth of the skin is secondary to peripheral vasodilatation and increased blood flow. This effect causes a generalized flush of the face and erythema of the elbows, palms, and soles (Fig. 12–38). There is usually hyperhidrosis, but this is greatly accentuated on the palms and soles. Thyroid hormones appear to have an effect on pigmentation,

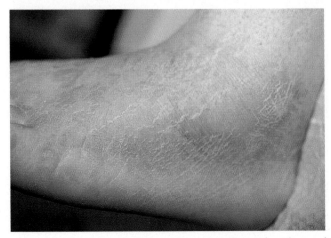

Figure 12-35 Hypothyroidism. Dry skin with scaling and diffuse fissuring may be seen on the extremities in patients with hypothyroidism.

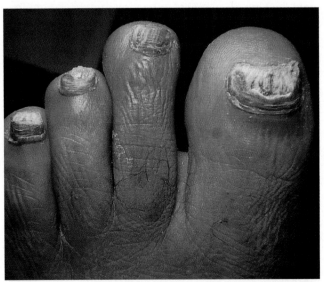

Figure 12-37 Hypothyroidism. The toenails may become thick, ridged, and brittle with an appearance similar to onychomycosis. The adjacent skin is usually thin and dry and shows accentuated skin lines. The hair may be coarse and show follicular plugging.

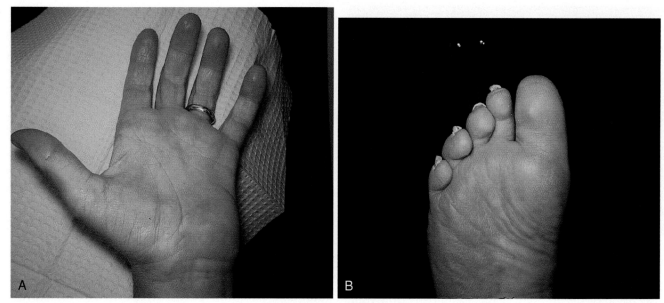

Figure 12–38   Hyperthyroidism. *A* and *B*, The palms and soles may be warm and erythematous and show signs of hyperhidrosis in cases of hyperthyroidism.

and both increased and decreased pigmentary changes are seen in hyperthyroidism. Hyperpigmentation of a patchy nature may be seen, especially on the face and lower legs. Vitiligo (hypopigmentation) may also occur on the face, knees, elbows, hands, or feet (Fig. 12–39). The precise nature of hyperpigmentary and hypopigmentary changes is not known but may be mediated in part through interactions of thyroid hormones with neurohumors.

CUTANEOUS FINDINGS NOT RELATED TO THYROID HORMONES. Not all cutaneous findings seen in thyroid disease can be attributed to a deficiency or an excess of thyroid hormones. Pretibial myxedema or generalized myxedema may develop in patients who are hyperthyroid, hypothyroid, or euthyroid. This condition may be seen with Graves' disease, after surgical or radioactive iodine treatment for thyrotoxicosis, or with Hashimoto's thyroiditis (struma lymphomatosa). It may also develop in the absence of hyperthyroidism. The condition is characterized by sharply circumscribed, flesh-colored, pink, or violaceous plaques or nodules over the anterior lower legs (Fig. 12–40). The lesions are bilateral but usually not symmetrical. These intradermal lesions may have a translucent or waxy appearance and are produced by large deposits of acid mucopolysaccharides

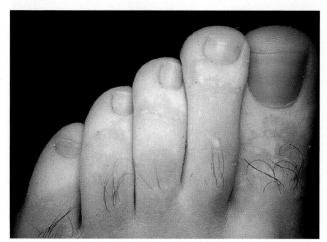

Figure 12–39   Hyperthyroidism. Vitiligo may occur on the hands and feet, especially the distal toes, in a small percentage of patients.

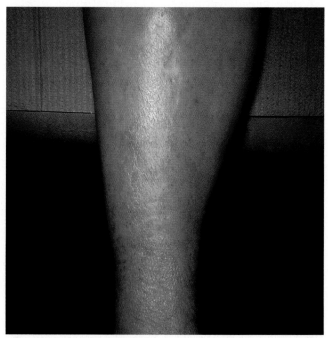

Figure 12–40   Pretibial myxedema. Skin of the entire leg is infiltrated with mucin to produce cylindrical legs with anterior shin plaques that are raised and nodular.

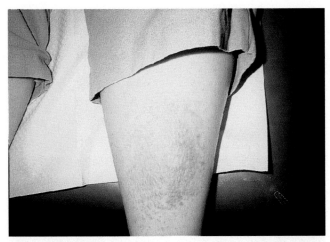

Figure 12–41   Pretibial myxedema. The anterior shin plaque may show exaggerated telangiectasia in acute cases.

(chondroitin sulfate and hyaluronic acid). As the mucin accumulates, the skin of the lower legs may take on a cylindrical appearance with the formation of shin nodules and plaques with prominent dilated follicular openings (orange-peel appearance). In a few cases, the pretibial plaques show exaggerated telangiectasia (Fig. 12–41). In addition to the typical lesions on the shins, some patients may exhibit massively swollen feet that are diffusely infiltrated by mucin (Fig. 12–42). The feet may be stony hard to palpation, and hyperpigmentation may be present. In rare cases, severe involvement causes large folds to overhang the ankles, simulating elephantiasis. Histologically, there is striking dermal thickening due to mucin deposition, which extends into the mid to deep dermis layer. At much higher magnification, the mucin widely separates the adjacent collagen bundles and appears as fine, branching streaks. Pretibial myxedema may spontaneously resolve in the mild and early stages. In the long-standing or chronic forms, treatment is not very successful, but pretibial myxedema may be improved with topical corticosteroids under occlusion when combined with compression dressings. If this approach is not successful, intralesional infiltration of triamcinolone acetonide (5 mg/mL) injected monthly may improve the condition. The longer the condition is present, the less effective are corticosteroid treatments.

HYPERLIPIDEMIA (XANTHOMATOSIS)

The xanthomatoses are a group of disorders that are characterized by deposition of lipids in the skin that results from hyperlipidemia. The lipid deposits are typified by flat, yellow plaques, papules, or nodules. Although certain types of xanthomas are characteristic of certain lipid abnormalities, none is specific because each form of xanthoma may be seen in many different disorders. Xanthomas may occur in an eruptive manner as a profusion of small yellow plaques or papules that appear quite suddenly (xanthoma eruptiva; see Fig. 12–22). Lipids may be deposited in the creases of the palms along with small planar papules (xanthomata planum; Fig. 12–43). Tuberous xanthomas may appear as slow-forming yellow papules or nodules that occur on the knees, elbows (Fig. 12–44), and extensor surfaces of the

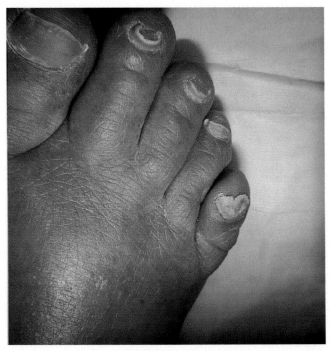

Figure 12–42   Pretibial myxedema. The feet may be infiltrated with mucin, be hyperpigmented, and be hard to palpation.

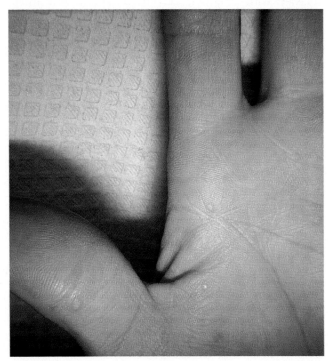

Figure 12–43   Hyperlipidemia. Xanthoma planum is characterized by small papules on the palms and the deposition of lipids in the palmar creases.

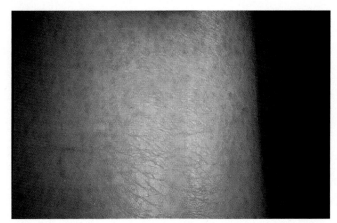

Figure 12–44   Tuberous xanthomas. Slowly evolving yellow papules may occur over the elbows and extensor surfaces in hyperlipidemia.

extremities. Tendinous xanthomas are smooth, deeply located nodules that are attached to tendons, ligaments, and deep fascia. They may be found on the dorsal aspect of the hands, especially at the metacarpophalangeal joint (Fig. 12–45), and most often on the Achilles tendons (Fig. 12–46).

LEUKOCYTOCLASTIC VASCULITIS

Leukocytoclastic vasculitis is associated with numerous diseases, including rheumatoid arthritis, internal malignancy, systemic lupus, polyarteritis nodosa, cryoglobulinemia, as well as other systemic illnesses. It is also associated with drug reactions, bacterial and viral infections, and certain connective tissue diseases. The clinical presentation is characteristic, with lesions referred to as palpable purpura.

The lesions originate as asymptomatic localized areas of cutaneous hemorrhage that eventually become palpable. They may coalesce, producing vast areas of purpura. Hemorrhagic blisters and necrotic ulcers may form in these purpuric areas on the lower legs (Fig. 12–47). Leukocytoclastic vasculitis has many systemic manifestations, which include kidney disease, peripheral neuropathy, gastrointestinal vasculitis, pulmonary vasculitis, and myocardial angiitis. Joint pain, swelling, and erythema are present.

This condition requires a complete evaluation to determine the underlying etiology of the problem. Identification and removal of the offending antigen (infection, chemical exposure, or drug) may be all that is necessary. Proper treatment of the arthritis or malignancy will cause an improvement in the condition. In those instances in which the cause is obscure, the vasculitis may be treated with short courses of prednisone, 40 mg/day. In patients with only cutaneous leukocytoclastic vasculitis, colchicine, 0.6 mg twice daily for 7 days, is given and then tapered and discontinued when the lesions resolve. Azathioprine, 150 mg/day, or dapsone, 100 to 150 mg/day, for 6 to 8 weeks may produce good clinical response in patients with skin involvement only.

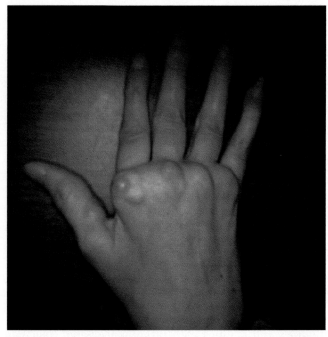

Figure 12–45   Tendinous xanthomas. Clinical manifestations of severe familial type II hyperlipoproteinemia involve the extensor tendons of the hands.

PEMPHIGOID (BULLOUS)

Localized bullous pemphigoid is a relatively rare, benign subepidermal blistering disorder of unknown origin that is questionably associated with internal malignancy. Drugs are often suspected of being the causative agents, and stopping or changing current medications

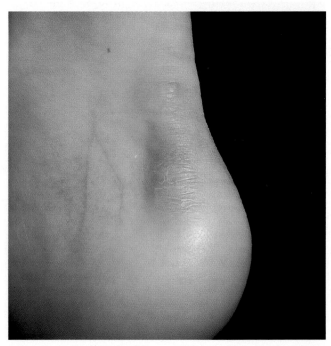

Figure 12–46   Tendinous xanthoma. The characteristic location for tendon xanthomas is at the posterior Achilles tendon.

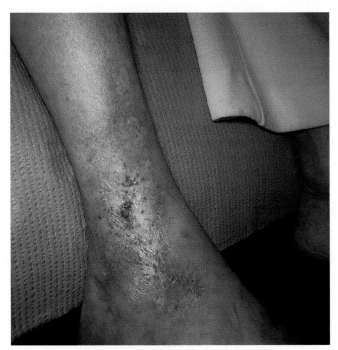

Figure 12–47 Leukocytoclastic vasculitis. This vasculitis occurred secondary to internal malignancy with an intense eruption on the lower leg and several areas of cutaneous necrotic ulcerations.

may be warranted. Pemphigoid is a disease of the elderly, with most patients older than the age of 60. Clinically, the lesions occur as extremely pruritic, tense blisters (bullae), often on an erythematous base, on the limbs, inner thighs, trunk, and feet (Fig. 12–48). They may be firm and full of clear fluid in the beginning of the presentation. Firm pressure on the blister will not cause an extension into normal skin lines (a negative Nikolsky's sign). The blister of bullous pemphigoid may be intact for several days because the roof of the lesion

consists entirely of epidermis. Later, the lesions become hemorrhagic and break down, resulting in erosions that may become secondarily infected. The skin heals quickly without scarring in most cases. Pruritus is treated with hydroxyzine, 10 to 50 mg, every 4 hours. Prednisone and an immunosuppressive drug may control pemphigoid effectively. Antibiotic therapy may be needed if secondary bacterial infection is present. Protection of the skin and prevention of dehydration should be considered.

PYODERMA GANGRENOSUM

Pyoderma gangrenosum is defined by its characteristic clinical appearance. Even though there is no true skin infection (pyoderma) or tissue gangrene (gangrenosum), the original name is still applied to this unique skin disorder. Pyoderma gangrenosum is a distinctive, cutaneous ulceration characterized by a painful pustule or nodule that breaks down to form a progressively enlarging ulcer with a raised, tender, undermined border on the lower legs and feet. The leading overhanging border may be dark purple or irregular with nodules and small pits containing purulent exudate (Fig. 12–49). Exuberant granulation tissue may form in more extensive cases (Fig. 12–50). Ulcers may expand rapidly over a few days and then progress slowly over many weeks. Adjacent lesions may appear as boggy blisters that may become confluent as they enlarge, producing new areas of ulcerations with irregular borders. These lesions have a tendency to heal in the center while continuing to spread peripherally.

An interesting clinical finding in pyoderma gangrenosum is a tendency of new lesions to form after minor trauma to the area or of existing lesions to worsen with manipulation. This phenomenon is known as *pathergy*.

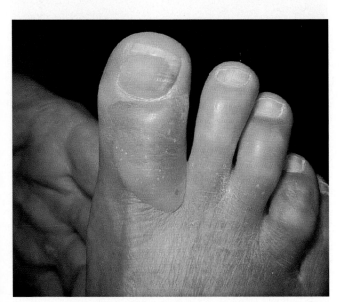

Figure 12–48 Bullous pemphigoid. Large tense blister formed over the dorsum of the great toe in a 66-year-old woman.

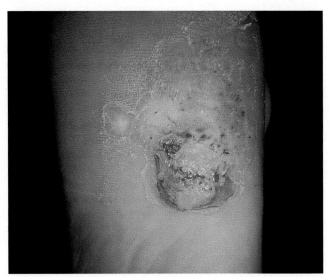

Figure 12–49 Pyoderma gangrenosum. This localized and rapidly progressive ulcer on the plantar sole of the foot shows a soggy undermined margin with clearing in the center in a 54-year-old man with ulcerative colitis.

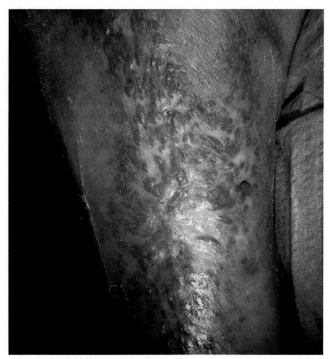

Figure 12–50   Pyoderma gangrenosum. An extensive indurated nodular plaque is ulcerated in several areas with exuberant granulation tissue on the lower extremity.

Pyoderma gangrenosum is frequently seen in patients with ulcerative colitis, Crohn's disease, chronic active hepatitis, rheumatoid arthritis, and hematological malignancies.

Because of the risk of pathergy, treatment involves the prevention of trauma or surgery (debridement or grafting) to the involved area. Early lesions may be resolved with intralesional injection of triamcinolone acetonide, 10 mg/mL. Systemic corticosteroids are effective in the treatment of larger active lesions. Oral prednisone, 40 to 80 mg/day, is required for control initially, and the dosage is then tapered and stopped. Dapsone, 100 mg/day, combined with the prednisone is also effective. In ulcers with a large amount of granulation tissue, silver nitrate (1/8 %) or Burow's wet compresses applied several times each day may help the condition. Other agents reported to be effective in the treatment of pyoderma gangrenosum include sulfasalazine, sulfapyridine, clofazimine, minocycline, rifampin, azathioprine, cyclophosphamide, cyclosporine, and potassium iodide.

RHEUMATOID ARTHRITIS

Cutaneous manifestations of rheumatoid arthritis include vasculitis, leg ulcers, erythematous and swollen knuckles, cutaneous (dermal) nodules, subcutaneous nodules, bursitic bunions, dermatitis, and periungual vasculitis referred to as Bywaters' lesions. The cutaneous lesions are not specific or pathognomonic for rheu-

matoid arthritis but are found frequently in patients who are afflicted with the condition. Many of these diseases precede the clinical presentation of rheumatoid arthritis by many months or even years.

Rheumatoid vasculitis (Fig. 12–51) is either an arteritis that involves the small arteries or a cutaneous venulitis. This condition is most often seen over the lower extremities and frequently occurs as palpable purpuric papules that do not blanch with diascopic pressure. Punched-out lesions may occur that are slow to heal. The vasculitis of rheumatoid arthritis is not related to the duration of the disease but to the severity of the arthritis. Ulcers of the lower extremities in patients with rheumatoid arthritis are often associated with stasis dermatitis and stasis ulcers, with vasculitis, or frequently with Felty's syndrome (rheumatoid arthritis with leukopenia and splenomegaly). In the latter case, the ulcer is commonly a pyoderma gangrenosum–like lesion (Fig. 12–52). Most patients with related ulcers show positive clinical and laboratory findings of rheumatoid arthritis.

Patients with rheumatoid arthritis typically have multiple joints with swelling, stiffness, and pain (Fig. 12–53). Joint edema is boggy, and the joints are tender. The joints may not be erythematous (although they can be), but they frequently feel warm. There may be ulnar deviation of the fingers and fibular deviation of the toes in patients with rheumatoid arthritis. Rheumatoid cutaneous nodules are visible external lesions that are usually present over joints in

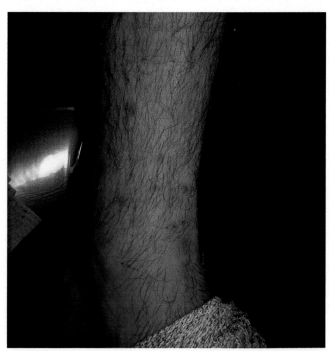

Figure 12–51   Rheumatoid vasculitis. Rheumatoid vasculitis is either an arteritis that involves the small arteries or a cutaneous venulitis. Most often seen over the lower extremities, it presents as erythematous papules that do not blanch under pressure.

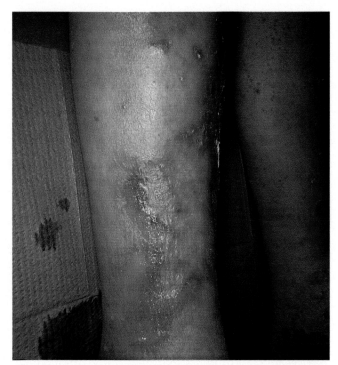

Figure 12–52 Rheumatoid pyoderma gangrenosum. Leg ulcers associated with rheumatoid arthritis are more common in Felty's syndrome (rheumatoid arthritis with leukopenia and splenomegaly). They may also represent stasis ulcers or vasculitis ulcers.

patients with seropositive rheumatoid arthritis (Fig. 12–54). Nodules may have a characteristic central necrosis and peripheral palisade. The patient may have no clinical symptoms during the early stages of cutaneous nodule formation. However, rheumatoid subcutaneous nodules are usually present in patients with significant clinical symptoms. These nodules are the most common type of skin presentation and are found in about 20% of patients with rheumatoid arthritis. They may also form in patients with systemic lupus erythematosus and scleroderma. The characteristic nodules typically form over bony prominences (Fig. 12–55) and are subcutaneous foci of necrobiotic material.

The patient with rheumatoid arthritis may also be prone to bunion and digital deformities (Fig. 12–56). Even though this condition is not specific for rheumatoid arthritis, it is a very common finding. The first metatarsophalangeal joint may be swollen and erythematous, and the underlying joint bursa may be inflamed. This condition may precede radiographic joint changes by many months or even years.

A high percentage of patients with rheumatoid arthritis also present with pruritic dermatitis involving the lower legs (Fig. 12–57). This skin condition may be an expression of the concurrent vasculitis, granuloma annulare, or stasis dermatitis. The dermatitis is cortico-

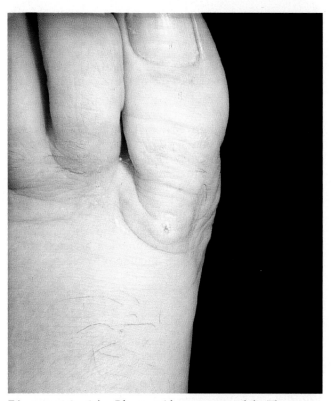

Figure 12–54 Rheumatoid cutaneous nodule. These external nodules over joints occur only in seropositive rheumatoid arthritis. They may have a characteristic central necrosis and peripheral palisade in a patient with no clinical symptoms.

Figure 12–53 Rheumatoid joints. Inflammatory edema of the joints (red, swollen knuckles) with ulnar deviation of the fingers or fibular deviation of the toes is common in the early stages of untreated rheumatoid arthritis.

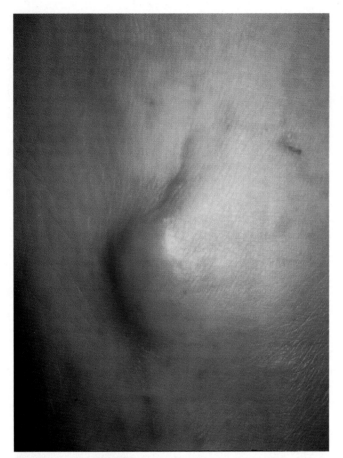

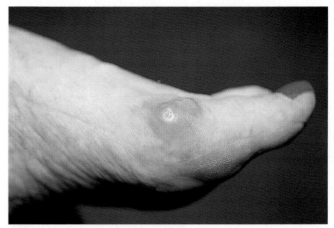

Figure 12–56   Rheumatoid bunion. Even though this condition is not specific for patients with rheumatoid arthritis, it is a common finding. The joint is swollen and erythematous, and the underlying bursa is inflamed.

Figure 12–55   Rheumatoid subcutaneous nodule. This is the most common type of skin lesion and is found in about 20% of patients with rheumatoid arthritis. These characteristic nodules typically form over bony prominences and are subcutaneous foci of necrobiotic material.

steroid responsive but may also regress during active treatment of the rheumatoid arthritis.

Another related dermatitis condition is Bywaters' lesion, which is a periungual, necrotic lesion that may form on the hand or foot in patients with rheumatoid arthritis (Fig. 12–58). This lesion may appear as a 1-mm black spot beside the nail or as several millimeters of dark, necrotic infarction adjacent to the nail. This condition is considered to be an expression of the vasculitis that is frequently present, and it may be seen in other small vessel vasculitides.

SCLERODERMA

There are three forms of sclerodermal lesions that may affect the lower extremity: generalized scleroderma, linear scleroderma, and localized scleroderma (morphea).
GENERALIZED SCLERODERMA. This is an uncommon condition of unknown cause that affects women more often than men, and it includes Raynaud's phenomenon, acrosclerosis (a combination of Raynaud's and scleroderma of the distal extremities) (Fig. 12–59), and in-

volvement of internal organs (gastrointestinal tract, heart, lungs, and kidneys). Edema of the hands and feet may precede the development of acrosclerosis. There may be severe arthralgia that may mimic rheumatoid arthritis. The course is usually slow but may progress within a few months, with sclerodactyly occurring with narrowing of the fingers and toes. There is loss of the skin lines and the creases in the hands and feet. Digital ischemia may lead to cutaneous infarction and ulcer-

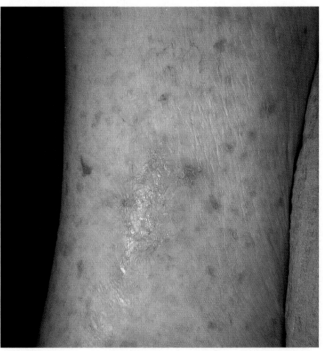

Figure 12–57   Rheumatoid dermatitis. A high percentage of patients with rheumatoid arthritis also present with a pruritic dermatitis involving the lower extremities. This may be an expression of vasculitis, granuloma annulare, or stasis dermatitis.

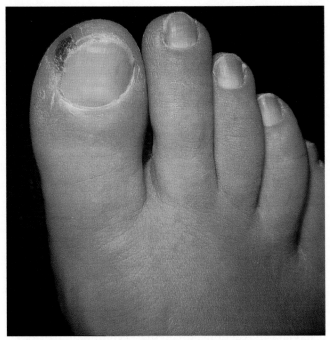

Figure 12–58 Rheumatoid vasculitis. Bywater lesion in a patient with rheumatoid vasculitis is evident as a 3-mm periungual, necrotic lesion on the hallux.

ation. The skin of the face is almost always involved, with loss of normal skin lines on the forehead, pinching of the nose, and tightening and narrowing of the mouth.

LINEAR SCLERODERMA. This condition has a slow and insidious onset and is seen in women four times more often than in men, and 83% of patients are younger than the age of 25 when the condition begins. The lesions of linear sclerosis involve a band-like induration, often with hypopigmented or hyperpigmented areas (Fig. 12–60). These linear lesions are often found on the lower legs but may be seen on the arms and face (en coupe

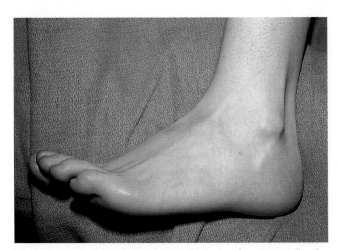

Figure 12–59 Scleroderma. There is often Raynaud's phenomenon, acrosclerosis with narrowing of the toes and fingers, and loss of the normal skin creases.

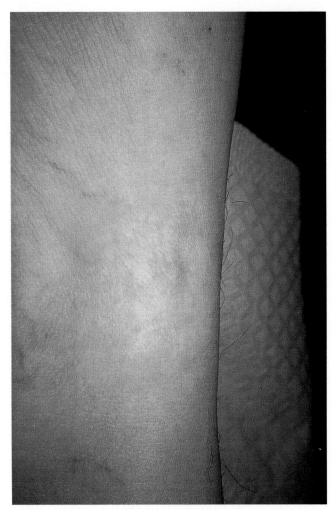

Figure 12–60 Linear scleroderma. Induration and irregular pigmentation are noted spanning the inner leg area in a 44-year-old woman.

de sabre). Two or more lesions may be present at the same time. When the linear sclerosis crosses a joint there may be mild to severe disability with joint contracture and stiffness. This condition may involve the underlying subcutaneous tissue and muscle, causing the fibrotic band to be more firmly anchored. High-potency topical corticosteroids may soften the firm fibrosis, and active and continued physical therapy is crucial to maintain joint motion.

LOCALIZED SCLERODERMA (MORPHEA). Morphea is also more common in women and in patients older than the age of 30. Morphea begins spontaneously and involves thickening or sclerosis of the skin. The primary lesion begins as an elevated circumscribed area of purplish induration. After several weeks the central portion of the discoloration becomes firm and thickened and turns an ivory color (Fig. 12–61). The central surface is smooth, waxy, and dull, and the active inflammatory border is lilac or violaceous. In some cases, multiple lesions form simultaneously (Fig. 12–62). These multiple small,

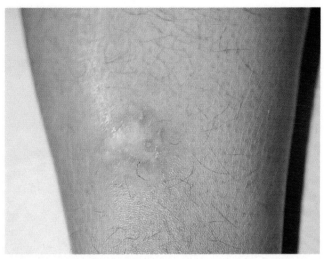

Figure 12–61   Localized morphea. A solitary sclerotic patch is present on the lower extremity. The skin of the lesion is tethered, and there is a violaceous border. Hair growth is absent in the lesion.

white, round-to-oval plaques have a predilection for the trunk and lower extremities. The active lesions frequently have the "lilac ring" borders that fade as the inflammation decreases. Hair loss and absence of sweat are characteristic in this condition. Transition to systemic sclerosis is rare. Treatment is usually not recommended, but topical corticosteroids may be applied to the active border with some results. Triamcinolone, 5 mg/mL, injected into the active border of solitary lesions may cause early regression, but most authorities recommend leaving these lesions alone to resolve spontaneously.

SCURVY

Scurvy is caused by a lack of ascorbic acid (vitamin C) and is probably the oldest recognized vitamin deficiency disease. In previous times, adult scurvy usually occurred in epidemic form. Currently, scurvy is rarely seen in the United States, and when it is, occurrence is usually in adult males living alone and on unbalanced diets. The exact incidence of scurvy is unknown, but an alert physician may see an occasional case in the susceptible members of his or her patient population. Adult scurvy, as mentioned, appears most often in those individuals who consume an unbalanced diet lacking in fresh vegetables or citrus fruits for one reason or other. Common causes include alcoholism or other substance abuse, psychoneurosis in individuals on bizarre diets, or lack of either the incentive or the financial resources on the part of elderly people (especially bachelors and widowers) to provide a proper diet for themselves. Scurvy may also occur in more affluent individuals who fall into poor dietary habits as a result of indifference or ignorance. It may also develop in patients who, as a result of chronic illness or anorexia, eat a vitamin-deficient diet or in patients with gastrointestinal disease, especially those on a special ulcer diet.

Scurvy is a reaction of a host in response to a lack of ascorbic acid in the diet. Most mammals, other than humans, can synthesize ascorbic acid from D-glucose or D-galactose. Ascorbic acid is found in high concentrations in citrus and other fruits, broccoli, raw cabbage, collards, green peppers, potatoes cooked in their skins, brussel sprouts, and tomatoes. Scurvy, then, is considered to be the result of a genetic defect because of the fact that susceptible species have lost their ability to synthesize ascorbic acid. The biochemical steps in the formation of the vitamin are well known:

$$\text{D-Glucuronate} + \text{NADPH} + \text{H}^+ \rightarrow \text{L-Gulonate} + \text{NADP}^+$$

$$\text{L-Gulonate} + \text{NAD}^+ \rightarrow \text{L-Gulonolactone} + \text{NAD}^+ + \text{H} +$$

$$\text{L-Gulonolactone} \rightarrow \text{L-Ascorbate} + \text{H}_2\text{0}$$

It is remarkable that a relatively simple hydrocarbon molecule such as L-ascorbic acid can be involved in such a wide variety of physiological processes and biochemical reactions. Ascorbic acid acts as the coenzyme in hydroxylation reactions involving tryptophan hydroxyphenyl pyruvate as well as hydroxylation of proline and hydroxyproline. Collagen is chemically composed of large amounts of glycine, proline, and hydroxyproline. The presence of these amino acids makes collagen unique because these hydroxyamines are not found in other proteins. Hydroxyproline is not synthesized in the absence of ascorbic acid, which appears to be needed for synthesis of an essential protein enzyme. Because exogenous hydroxyproline is not incorporated into collagen, it must be derived from the hydroxylation of proline in vivo.

The exact mechanisms by which ascorbic acid maintains the integrity of blood vessels and the coagulability of blood are still to be explained. The normal healthy adult total body level of L-ascorbic acid is approximately 1500 mg. This is used at about 3% of the existing

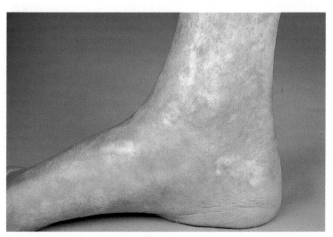

Figure 12–62   Localized morphea. Multiple sclerotic plaques are seen on the lower extremity. The lesions are tethered with lilac margins and loss of hair, and absence of sweat are common. (Courtesy of Dr. William Boegel.)

amount each day, or about 45 mg is used daily in an adult who has a fully saturated body pool. This means that it would take approximately a little over 1 month for the total body level of L-ascorbic acid to be depleted.

The onset of adult scurvy is seen 2 months or more after the depletion of ascorbic acid levels. The principal manifestations may begin slowly. The earliest sign, which could easily escape casual observation, is the appearance of a few petechial hemorrhages and small ecchymoses. These fade within a few days but are replaced by similar lesions. Large lower extremity ecchymoses begin to appear later and are accompanied by the petechiae, which become perifollicular (see Fig. 9–51). Follicular hyperkeratoses develop at the same time and are seen primarily on the thighs, calves, and ankles. These hyperkeratotic lesions contain coiled hairs and many demonstrate the classic lesion of scurvy: the hyperkeratotic follicular lesion with a red hemorrhagic halo. Multiple splinter hemorrhages may form a crescent near the distal ends of the nails and are more extensive than those seen in bacterial endocarditis (see Fig. 9–41).

The best prevention of adult vitamin C deficiency is a diet containing adequate amounts of ascorbic acid. Vitamin C tablets are stable for long periods and are relatively inexpensive. In adults, treatment involves administration of orange juice or ascorbic acid in divided doses up to 500 mg/day until signs have disappeared. It is also advisable to add one multiple vitamin capsule daily plus a normal well-balanced diet containing fresh vegetables and citrus fruits. Once treatment begins, hemorrhages and perifollicular hyperkeratoses usually disappear in 2 or 3 weeks.

TUBEROUS SCLEROSIS

Tuberous sclerosis (epiloia) is an autosomal dominant disease characterized by skin lesions, central nervous system lesions (hamartoma), and internal disorders.

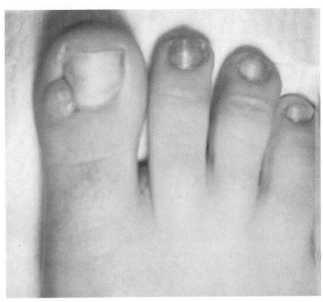

Figure 12–64 Tuberous sclerosis. Koenen's tumors are smooth, round periungual connective tissue tumors found on the digits. They are present from puberty or later and are similar to periungual fibromas seen in tuberous sclerosis.

There are also mental disorders and seizures (infantile spasms). Dermatological manifestations include adenoma sebaceum, shagreen patches, hypopigmented macules, periungual tumors (Koenen's tumors), and subungual and periungual fibromas.

Adenoma sebaceum consists of angiofibromas appearing during childhood (by age 2 or 3) on the face, particularly around the sides of the nose, and on the cheeks and chin area. The angiofibromas consist of numerous small red or yellow tumors measuring from 1 to 5 mm in diameter. These growths are benign hamartomas composed of fibrous and vascular tissue.

The *shagreen patch* is a highly characteristic lesion of tuberous sclerosis (Fig. 12–63). This connective tissue nevus is a soft, oval, elevated, flesh-colored to yellow plaque that is located on the lumbosacral region. There is usually only one lesion, and it has an irregular surface with a slightly pigmented border.

Hypopigmented macules (ash-leaf shaped, oval, or stippled) are the earliest sign of tuberous sclerosis and are found on the extremities and trunk. They are present in up to 90% of patients with this disease.

Koenen's tumors (Fig. 12–64) are round, smooth, connective tissue tumors that are periungual. These lesions are distinctive when present. They are usually asymptomatic and develop at puberty or later.

Periungual and subungual fibromas (Figs. 12–65 and 12–66) are smooth, flesh-colored, conical projections that emerge from the nail fold or nail bed of the toenail and fingernail. These lesions are present in 22% of patients with tuberous sclerosis. They usually appear late in childhood, at the time of puberty or later, and have the same pathology (angiofibroma) as adenoma sebaceum.

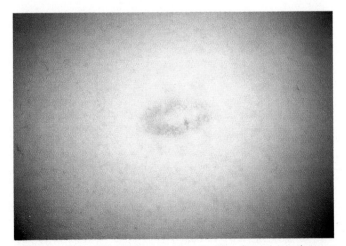

Figure 12–63 Tuberous sclerosis. The shagreen patch is an irregular, oval, elevated, flesh- to yellow-colored plaque located on the lumbosacral region.

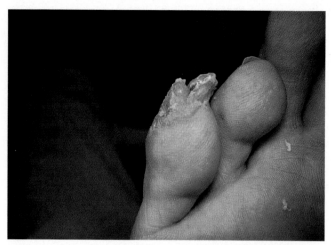

Figure 12–65   Tuberous sclerosis. Periungual fibromas are present on the fifth toe in a patient with tuberous sclerosis.

The diagnosis of tuberous sclerosis must be made early in infants with white macules or other previously described cutaneous lesions. Facial angiofibromas may be removed with dermabrasion. Digital fibromas and tumors may be surgically removed if they become symptomatic. Referral for genetic counseling is recommended.

VON RECKLINGHAUSEN'S DISEASE (NEUROFIBROMATOSIS)

This condition is an autosomal-dominant disorder of neural crest–derived cells characterized by changes in the skin (café-au-lait spots), the nervous system (mul-

tiple neurofibromas), Lisch nodules (pigmented iris hamartomas), bone (erosive changes, lordosis, kyphosis), and endocrine glands (causing cretinism, myxedema, acromegaly). Neurofibromatosis occurs in approximately 1 of 3000 births, and it affects males and females equally and with similar severity. Two forms of neurofibromatosis are recognized: classic von Recklinghausen's neurofibromatosis (type 1) and central or acoustic neurofibromatosis (type 2).

The pigmented "coffee with cream" colored patches (café-au-lait spots) develop first during childhood (usually during the first 3 years) but may be present at birth. These small pigmented macules occurring under the axillae and in the perineum (Crowe's sign) are considered to be pathognomonic of neurofibromatosis. The diagnostic criterion for generalized café-au-lait macules is five or more lesions measuring 5 mm in a patient before puberty and six or more lesions measuring 15 mm in a patient after puberty, when combined with two or more neurofibromas.

Neurofibromas, which are derived from peripheral nerves and supporting structures, develop during late childhood and adolescence. Most lesions are painless unless they are in a position of irritation or pressure. They may be dermal and consist of soft, sessile, dome-shaped nodules termed *molluscum fibrosa* (Fig. 12–67), which are usually less than 3 cm in diameter. Plexiform neurofibromas are characteristically seen only in von Recklinghausen's neurofibromatosis and are composed of cellular and hypertrophied nerve trunks, which ramify in a vermiform manner within the reticular dermis. Digital pressure on the neurofibroma may cause it to become invaginated or "button-holed." Subcutaneous neurofibromatosis consists of firm, discrete nodules that are often attached to a nerve. Histologically, neurofibromas are well-developed, nonencapsulated neoplastic lesions composed of small, variably cellular

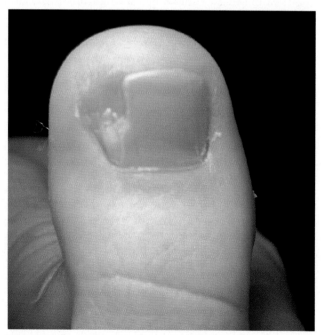

Figure 12–66   Tuberous sclerosis. Subungual fibroma with a typical appearance is noted on the hallux.

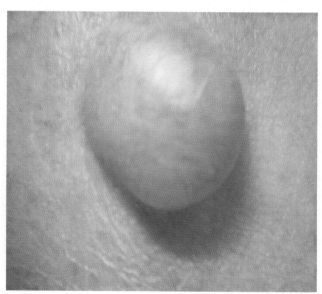

Figure 12–67   Neurofibromatosis. This dermal neurofibroma is a soft, dome-shaped nodule termed *molluscum fibrosa.*

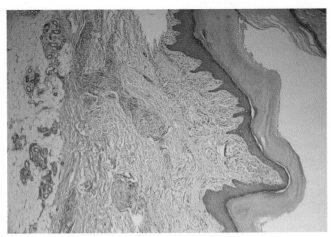

Figure 12–68 Neurofibroma. At low magnification, a sessile lesion shows a loosely arranged stroma partially surrounded by a diffusely hyperplastic epidermal layer with plexiform features.

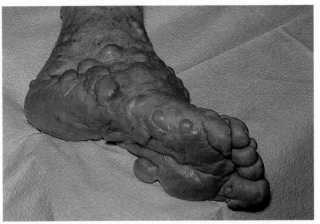

Figure 12–70 Neurofibromatosis. Multiple tumors are formed over the entire extremity, including the sole of the foot. (Courtesy of Dr. Richard Bouché.)

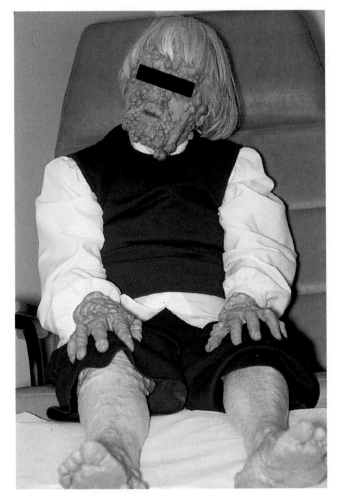

Figure 12–69 Neurofibromatosis. This adult patient had hundreds of grossly deforming lesions over the entire body. (Courtesy of Dr. Richard Bouché.)

aggregate of benign-appearing spindle cells embedded within a loose fibrillar, eosinophilic matrix (Fig. 12–68). Some patients have only a few small tumors, whereas others develop hundreds of tumors of various sizes over the entire body surface (Fig. 12–69), including the palms and soles (Fig. 12–70). The tumors may form anywhere on the body surface, including the oral cavity and ear canals.

In patients with severe involvement there may be systemic manifestation. Intracranial neurofibromatosis may develop in the optic, trigeminal, or acoustic nerves, or lesions may occur within the brain (astrocytomas, meningiomas). Other multiple systemic findings may include malignancy (Wilms' tumor, neuroblastoma, malignant schwannoma, rhabdomyosarcoma), pheochromocytoma, seizures, chronic headaches, kyphoscoliosis, pseudarthrosis, seizures, speech impediment, short stature, and constipation. Treatment involves referral for genetic counseling. Cutaneous tumors may be excised if they become symptomatic due to location.

BIBLIOGRAPHY

Baden HP: Keratoderma of palms and soles. In Fitzpatric TB, Eisen AZ, Wolff K, Freedburg IM, Austen KF (eds): Dermatology in General Medicine, 3rd ed, pp 529–533. New York, McGraw-Hill, 1987.

Bodman M, Friedman S, Clifford LB: Bullosis diabeticorum: A report of two cases with a review of the literature, J Am Podiatr Med Assoc 81:561–563, 1991.

Bollet AJ: The skin and mucous membranes in nutritional diseases. Resident Staff Phys 12:101–109, 1981.

Brooke HG: Notes on keratoses of the palms and soles. Br J Dermatol 3:19–22, 1891.

Brunsting LA, Goekerman WH, O'Leary PA: Pyoderma (ecthyma gangrenosum): Clinical and experimental observations in five cases occurring in adults. Arch Dermatol Syph 22:655–680, 1930.

Buchbinder MR, Brill LR, Louis JM: Lymphedema praecox and yellow nail syndrome: A literature review and case report. J Am Podiatr Assoc 68:592–594, 1978.

Bywaters EGL: Peripheral vascular obstruction in rheumatoid arthritis and its relationship to other vascular lesions. Ann Rheum Dis 16:84–89, 1957.

Callen JP, Fabré VC: Cutaneous manifestations of systemic diseases. In Moschella SL, Hurley HJ (eds): Dermatology, 3rd ed, pp 1682–1718. Philadelphia, WB Saunders, 1992.

Dahl MV, Ullman S, Gultz RW: Vasculitis in granuloma annulare: Histopathology and direct immunofluorescence. Arch Dermatol 113:463–467, 1977.

Dockery GL: Adult vitamin C deficiency: Scurvy: A case report. J Am Podiatr Assoc 71:628–631, 1981.

Dockery GL, Newell SG: Keratoderma climactericum: Haxthausen's disease. J Am Podiatr Assoc 68:595–597, 1978.

Habif TP: Cutaneous manifestation of internal disease. In Habif TP (ed): Clinical Dermatology—A Color Guide to Diagnosis and Therapy, 2nd ed, pp 639–664. St. Louis, CV Mosby, 1990.

Hardwick N, Cerio R: Superficial granulomatous pyoderma: A report of two cases. Br J Dermatol 129:718–722, 1993.

Harland CC, Millard LG: Pyoderma gangrenosum: A complication of chronic venous leg ulceration? Clin Exp Dermatol 18:545–547, 1993.

Haxthausen H: Keratoderma climactericum. Br J Dermatol 46:161–163, 1934.

Hilton L, Simpson RR, Simpson RR: Differential diagnosis of plantar palmar keratoderma. J Am Podiatr Assoc 68:578–584, 1978.

Hofbauer MH, Puleo D: Idiopathic diabetic bullosum. J Am Podiatr Med Assoc 81:613–617, 1991.

Huntley AC: The cutaneous manifestations of diabetes mellitus. J Am Acad Dermatol 7:427–455, 1982.

Jorizzo JL, Daniels JC: Dermatologic conditions reported in patients with rheumatoid arthritis. J Am Acad Dermatol 8:439–457, 1983.

Kissel JT, Mendell JR, Rammohan KW: Microvascular deposition of complement membrane attack complex in dermatomyositis. N Engl J Med 314:329–334, 1986.

Lerner J, Lerner M, Pasternack WA: Pyoderma gangrenosum. J Foot Surg 32:569–572, 1993.

Levine N: Cutaneous signs of life-threatening conditions. Cross Section 10:4–10, 1982.

Margolis DJ: Dermatology of the lower extremity: Three unusual diseases that cause ulcers. Ostomy Wound Manage 39:36–39, 1993.

Martin JE, Harkless LB: Pyoderma gangrenosum: A literature review and case report. J Am Podiatr Assoc 76:416–419, 1986.

Nelder KH: Vitamins, trace elements, and the skin. In Moschella SL, Hurley HJ (eds): Dermatology, 3rd ed, pp 1605–1628. Philadelphia, WB Saunders, 1992.

Parker F: Disorders of metabolism. In Moschella SL, Hurley HJ (eds): Dermatology, 3rd ed, pp 1629–1681. Philadelphia, WB Saunders, 1992.

Perry HO: Pyoderma gangrenosum. South Med J 62:899–908, 1969.

Pirotta SS, Johnson JD, Young G, Bezzant J: Bullosis diabeticorum. J Am Podiatr Med Assoc 85:169–171, 1995.

Port M: Diabetic dermopathy: A controversy in dermatology. J Am Podiatr Assoc 72:418–423, 1982.

Port M, Ottinger ML, Fenske NA: Connective tissue disorders. In McCarthy DJ, Montgomery R (eds): Podiatric Dermatology, pp 264–282. Baltimore, Williams & Wilkins, 1986.

Rabinowitz AD: Cutaneous manifestations in the diabetic foot. In Brenner MA (ed): Management of the Diabetic Foot, pp 120–130. Baltimore, Williams & Wilkins, 1987.

Richardson JB, Callen JP: Pyoderma gangrenosum treated successfully with potassium iodide. J Am Acad Dermatol 28:1005–1007, 1993.

Rosenberg FW: Cutaneous manifestations of internal malignancy. Cutis 20:227–234, 1977.

Shore RN: New look at pyoderma gangrenosum. Cutis 20:209–219, 1977.

Vander Ploeg DE: Skin markers of internal disease. Diagnosis 9:85–93, 1981.

Witkowski JA: Cutaneous manifestations of systemic diseases: Metabolic diseases. Clin Dermatol 1:77–87, 1983.

Witkowski JA: Cutaneous manifestations of systemic diseases: Collagen vascular disease and vasculitis. Clin Dermatol 1:88–101, 1983.

13

Benign Tumors, Cysts, and Lesions

INTRODUCTION

Benign skin tumors, cysts, and pigmented lesions make up a large segment of lower extremity dermatology. The number of different conditions that affect the dermis and epidermis far exceeds conditions in all other body organs. The benign conditions that are presented in this chapter must be differentiated from similar-appearing malignant lesions. Deciding which entities are benign and which are malignant may be extremely challenging. Benign lesions are usually slow growing and expansile, pushing aside the supporting stroma. The tissues typically consist of well-differentiated cells with a high degree of structural differentiation. Metastases do not occur in benign tumors and cysts. Proper diagnosis and treatment of benign skin lesions depend on the level of suspicion of the clinician and his or her basic knowledge of the clinical presentations of these conditions. Small tumors and cysts may simply be excised, allowing full material collection for histopathological identification as well as resolving the condition. Larger lesions may require incisional wedge or punch biopsy to examine the tissue properly. Some of the benign tumors and cysts known to exist on the lower extremities have already been discussed in other chapters and are not reviewed again.

ACROCHORDONS

Acrochordons, or skin tags, are very common, benign, polyp-like, skin-colored to pigmented skin tumors that are seen equally in male and female patients. They are soft and frequently multiple. They begin as small brown to skin-colored oval lesions attached by a short stalk. The darker lesions may have irregular borders and give the general appearance of small soft raisins (Fig. 13–1).

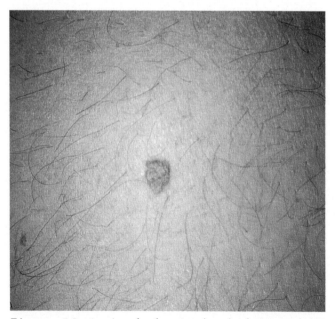

Figure 13–1   Acrochordon. A pedunculated pigmented skin tag with a broad stalk is seen on the lower leg.

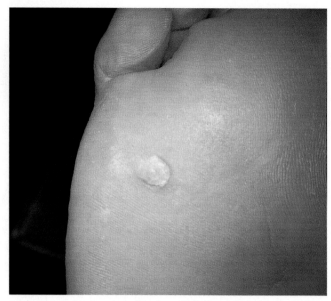

Figure 13–2   Acrochordon. A flesh-colored skin tag with a narrow stalk on the plantar foot has an atypical clinical appearance simply due to pressure of weight bearing.

The lighter or skin-colored lesions tend to be smooth but may also be irregular or pedunculated. On the weight-bearing areas of the foot the skin tag may take on a different appearance as it is flattened by pressure (Fig. 13–2).

These lesions are usually asymptomatic unless there is external pressure or irritation from clothing. As they mature, the size may increase up to 1 cm and the stalk may become long and slender. Treatment is simple with lifting of the skin tag and cutting of the stalk close to the skin level. The attachment point is then touched with the electrocautery tip. Local anesthesia is usually not needed. Recurrence after treatment is rare. Histologically, these polypoid structures are covered with epidermis that is hyperplastic and may resemble seborrheic keratosis. The dermis shows loose edematous collagen and dilated vessels. In pigmented lesions there may be nests of nevus cells, and some lesions contain fat cells.

ACQUIRED DIGITAL FIBROKERATOMAS

These uncommon flesh-colored lesions of unknown cause may resemble cutaneous horns, acrochordons, or fibromas and occur on the fingers, palms, toes (Fig. 13–3), and plantar heels (Fig. 13–4). The growth is solitary and occurs as a nodular to dome-shaped fibrotic or keratotic lesion that may be warty or pedunculated. Fibrokeratomas may be surrounded by a collarette of elevated skin. Microscopic evaluation shows centrally located, thick interconnecting collagen bundles oriented along the vertical axis of the lesion. A short projection of collagen and capillaries may be covered by epithelium and retained keratin. The epidermis shows variable hyperkeratosis and acanthosis. Treatment of ac-

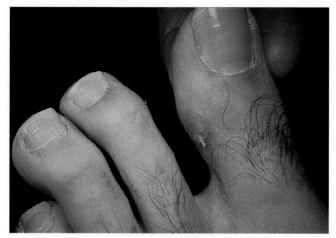

Figure 13–3   Acquired digital fibrokeratoma. This uncommon lesion on the medial hallux resembles a cutaneous horn, the base of which is surrounded by a collarette of elevated skin.

quired digital fibrokeratoma is with simple shave excision and cautery or with surgical excision and suture closure. Recurrence after treatment is rare.

ACQUIRED FIBROEPITHELIAL POLYPS

Acquired fibroepithelial polyps (squamous papilloma) are typically benign connective tissue tumors of the dermis. They are essentially enlarged skin tags with unusual shapes that may occur on the lower leg (Fig. 13–5) or foot (Fig. 13–6). The larger polyps appear as soft, cerebriform, skin-colored to slightly pigmented tumors. They are frequently pedunculated with an irregular surface. These polyps occur most often in menopausal women. Most polyps are asymptomatic unless they have been irritated or the pedicle becomes twisted, causing infarction of the mass. Histologically, examination of this lesion shows epithelial hyperplasia with an irregular, convoluted surface. There is loose areolar

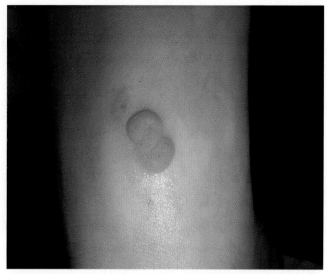

Figure 13–5   Acquired fibroepithelial polyp. Typical lesion with convoluted dome is found on the lower extremity.

connective tissue with dilated blood vessels in the dermal layer. Within the core, mature adipose tissue and occasionally nerve fibers may be observed. If necessary, treatment is excision of the lesion and cautery of the base. Recurrence is minimal.

CUTANEOUS HORNS

The cutaneous horn is a conical hyperkeratotic lesion of varying size composed of keratin and resembling an animal horn. It occurs commonly on the ears, hands, and feet (Fig. 13–7). Occasionally, a cutaneous horn arises from the weight-bearing plantar sole (Fig. 13–8). Viral warts, seborrheic keratoses, stucco keratoses, actinic keratoses, solar keratoses, basal cell and squamous cell carcinomas, and keratoacanthomas may all retain keratin at their base and produce horns. Malignancy at the base of a cutaneous horn is more common in the

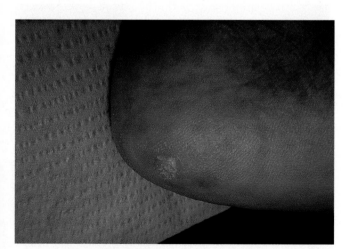

Figure 13–4   Acquired digital fibrokeratoma. A solitary, circular, dome-shaped nodule on the heel, with a raised hyperkeratotic collarette, is characteristic.

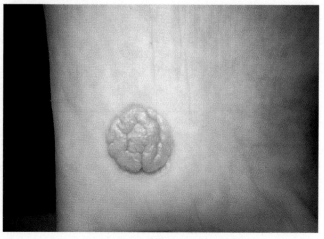

Figure 13–6   Acquired fibroepithelial polyp. Large cerebriform lesion is located on the foot.

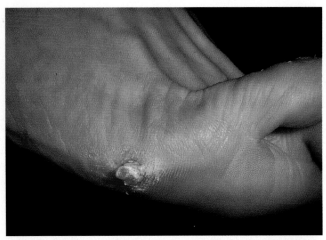

Figure 13–7 Cutaneous horn. This hard conical projection composed mostly of keratin located on the lateral foot would extend outward for many millimeters if not trimmed regularly.

older patient. A biopsy should be performed if malignancy is suspected. Microscopic evaluation shows compacted keratin layers with a base characteristic of one of the previously listed conditions. Treatment is by cryotherapy or curettage of the base after the horn has been removed. Surgical excision of the horn and underlying base is curative in most cases.

DERMATOFIBROMAS

Dermatofibromas (solitary fibrous histiocytomas) are common, benign tumors that are usually asymptomatic

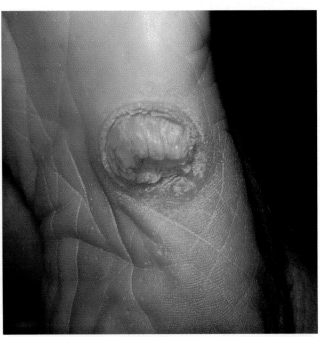

Figure 13–8 Cutaneous horn. This keratin horn was located on the plantar weight-bearing surface of the sole and had an appearance similar to a ram's horn. The base was a preexisting plantar wart.

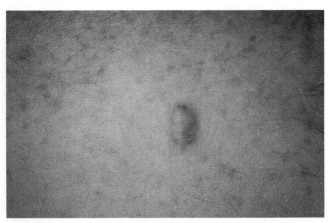

Figure 13–9 Dermatofibroma. The lower leg is a common location for this round-to-oval, elevated, and pigmented lesion.

to slightly pruritic. They are frequently found on the lower legs (Fig. 13–9) and occasionally on the toes (Fig. 13–10). These firm, raised, round-to-oval, elevated, pigmented lesions retract beneath the skin surface when they are squeezed from either side (Fig. 13–11). Dermatofibromas are adherent to the overlying skin but are easily moved in the underlying tissue plane. The lesions vary from a few millimeters to 2 cm in diameter. The surface of the lesion is usually smooth but may be hyperkeratotic or velvety or show slight scaling. The cause of these lesions is unknown, but many believe that there is a connection between minor trauma or insect bites. Microscopically, this lesion has a variable histological appearance depending on the relative proportions of histiocytes, fibroblasts, and collagen fibers. It is a spindle-cell neoplasm that occupies the reticular dermis (Fig. 13–12). Treatment is usually not indicated. Surgical excision frequently leaves a hyperpigmented scar that is often less cosmetically acceptable than the original lesion. The elevated lesions may be removed with shave biopsy

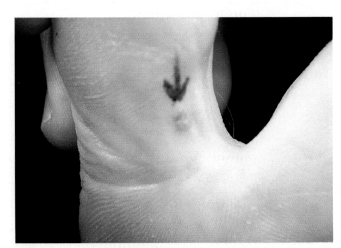

Figure 13–10 Dermatofibroma. Early lesions may be small and have a well-defined border, with an elevated irregular red surface. The pigmentation occurs at the periphery but almost never reaches the center of the lesion.

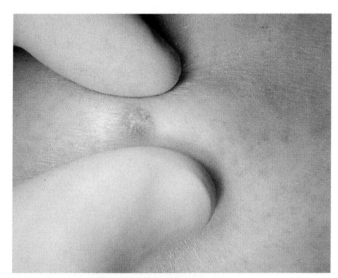

Figure 13–11 Dermatofibroma. Dermatofibromas will retract beneath the skin in the center (dimple sign) when they are compressed from the sides. (Same patient as Figure 13–5.)

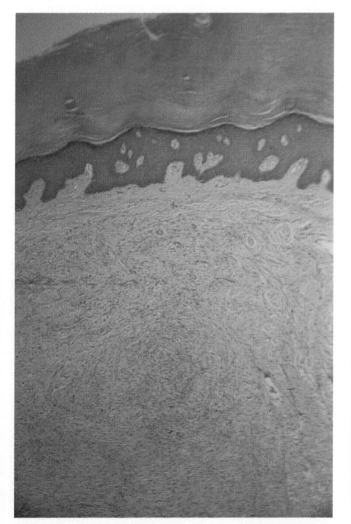

Figure 13–12 Dermatofibroma. At scanning magnification, there is a subtle spindle cell proliferation within the mid and deep dermis. The overlying epidermis is generally hyperplastic.

with the wound allowed to granulate in, healing by secondary intention. Cryosurgery may eliminate much of the color and size of the lesion but will not usually remove the entire lesion. Intralesional injection of short-acting cortisone (dexamethasone sodium phosphate, 4 mg/mL) may be helpful.

EPIDERMAL INCLUSION CYSTS

The common epidermal inclusion cyst occurs secondary to traumatically or surgically implanted epidermis within the dermis (Fig. 13–13). This grafted epidermis then grows in the dermis, with accumulation of keratin within the cyst cavity. Epidermal inclusion cysts may range in size from a few millimeters to several centimeters. They may have a thin epidermal cover with small blood vessels visible in the dome (Fig. 13–14) or a very thick epidermal cover with overlying hyperkeratotic tissue (Fig. 13–15). The lesion usually grows very slowly and may spontaneously drain. If the lesion drains or is opened, the extruded thick, white keratin material may have a very foul odor (Fig. 13–16). Cultures may show pathogenic bacteria. Treatment is not necessary unless the condition is cosmetically or symptomatically bothersome to the patient. Simple excision of the entire lesion is preferable to aspiration or incision and drainage, which has a high recurrence rate.

FIBROMAS

Formation of plantar and palmar fibromas results from proliferation of the aponeuroses of the palms and soles. Plantar fibromatosis tends to affect younger patients when compared with palmar fibromatosis. The nodules may be singular (Fig. 13–17) and found on the lateral peripheral surface of the plantar foot, or they may be

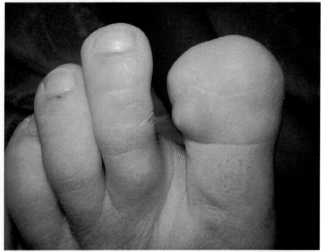

Figure 13–13 Epidermal inclusion cyst. The large nontender inclusion cyst resulted after implantation of epidermis following a terminal distal hallux Syme's amputation.

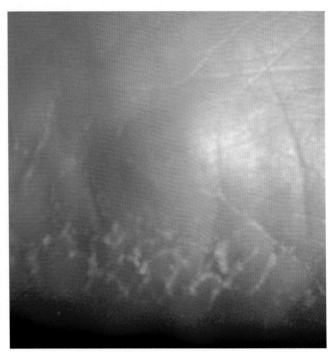

Figure 13 – 14   Epidermal inclusion cyst. This dome-shaped lesion has a thin overlying epidermis, and small blood vessels are visible through the top.

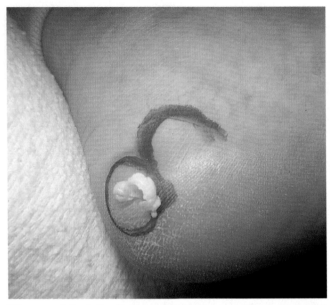

Figure 13 – 16   Epidermal inclusion cyst. This large dermal nodule contained a thick, dense, white keratin material with a foul, putrefied odor.

multiple (Fig. 13–18) and found more centrally located on the plantar foot, usually on the medial sides of the soles. The cause of these lesions is unknown, but trauma seems to play a role in many patients.

On microscopic evaluation, plantar fibromatous lesions have multiple small nodules of fibroblasts and blood vessels. In early tumors, the fibroblasts are densely packed and the amount of collagen is minimal

(Fig. 13–19). Later, the lesions show diminished cellularity and greater deposition of collagen.

Treatment of this benign lesion consist of one or two intralesional injections of triamcinolone acetonide, 10 to 40 mg/mL. Plantar fibromas may also be injected with 0.5 to 1.0 mL of 4% sclerosing solution directly into the central portion of the lesion. Subsequent injections may be infiltrated throughout the mass, and the

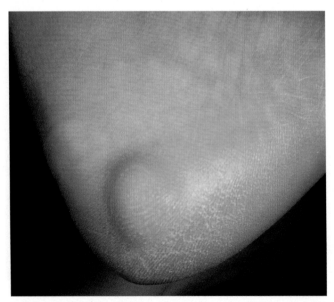

Figure 13 – 15   Epidermal inclusion cyst. This large painful cyst had a thick epidermal covering with hyperkeratosis.

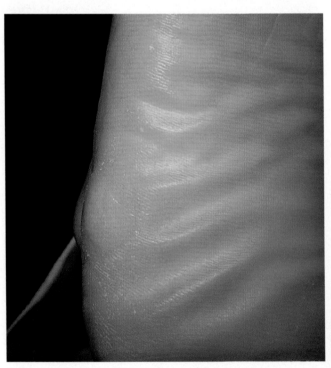

Figure 13 – 17   Plantar fibroma. Single lesions may occur and are more common on the sides or periphery of the plantar foot.

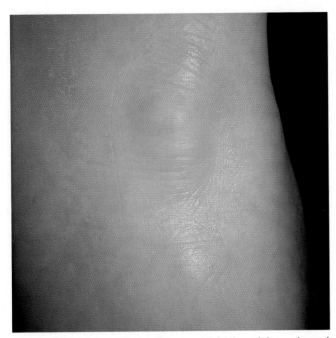

Figure 13–18 **Plantar fibroma.** Multiple nodules are located within the plantar fascia of the foot.

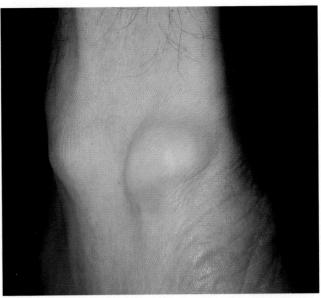

Figure 13–20 **Ganglion cyst.** A large, soft, fluctuant, ganglion cyst is located adjacent to the posterior Achilles tendon on the heel.

injection is followed by a 5- to 10-minute ultrasound treatment. This treatment is repeated weekly for up to five visits, and additional softening and shrinking of the fibroma may be expected for several months after the final injections. Surgical excision of the plantar fibroma with partial fasciectomy is sometimes necessary for relief of this condition. Recurrence after incomplete resection is common, and the procedure may have to be repeated or a total plantar fasciectomy may be required.

GANGLION CYSTS

These chronic, soft-to-firm, fluctuant, painless cystic swellings usually occur over the ankle, heel, or dorsum

of the foot (Fig. 13–20). Each cyst contains fluid that is thought to result from leakage of synovia through the tendon sheath or joint capsule. This fluid is then encapsulated by fibrous tissue, and a fluid-filled cyst results. Aspiration of the lesion usually demonstrates mucinous fluid. Most ganglion cysts remain intact with activity and normal external pressures; however, occasionally they spontaneously erupt and the clear, thick fluid disperses in the tissues (Fig. 13–21). Treatment is not necessary unless the lesion becomes symptomatic owing to its location. Intralesional injection with a 4% alcohol sclerosing solution after aspiration of the synovial fluid may be successful. Surgical excision is frequently necessary to resolve the condi-

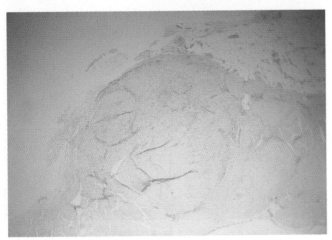

Figure 13–19 **Plantar fibroma.** Scanning microscopic view shows densely packed, multiple small nodules of fibroblasts and blood vessels.

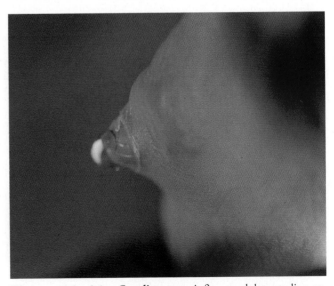

Figure 13–21 **Ganglion cyst.** A firm, nodular ganglion on the hallux began spontaneous leakage of thick mucinous fluid.

tion. Recurrence is common if the cystic lining is not completely excised.

HEMANGIOMAS

Vascular hemangiomas are usually located on the trunk, lower legs (Fig. 13–22), or toes (Fig. 13–23). These lesions are well defined and raised and have a smooth dome-shaped surface. They are frequently bright red to purple, which suggests the diagnosis. Cherry hemangiomas (senile hemangiomas), also known as Campbell de Morgan spots, are found commonly in elderly patients, but there may be onset early in adult life. Multiple lesions are usually present, ranging from 1 to 3 mm in diameter. Lesions on the digits may be larger than those found on the trunk and lower legs. Microscopic evaluation reveals multiple dilated blood vessels lined by flattened endothelial cells supported by an edematous and fibrous stroma. Cherry hemangiomas do not usually require treatment, but smaller lesions may be removed with electrodesiccation, cautery, or excision.

KERATOACANTHOMAS

These relatively common, benign, epithelial tumors, possibly of viral origin, are seen most often on the head and neck in the elderly but may be seen anywhere on the body. The malignant potential for keratoacanthoma is unknown, but it has been known to convert to a squamous cell carcinoma.

Keratoacanthoma is not common on the lower extremity, but two forms are seen there. The more typical smaller lesion of the solitary keratoacanthoma begins as a smooth, dome-shaped, red papule that resembles a large lesion of molluscum contagiosum. In a few weeks the lesion may expand to 1 or 2 cm in diameter and develop a central keratin-filled plug that

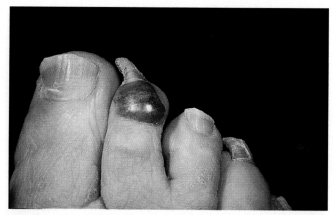

Figure 13–23   Cherry hemangioma. This large red lesion on the second toe is often termed a *senile hemangioma.* This long-standing lesion may persist indefinitely and in this case has caused deformity of the toenail.

may crust over (Fig. 13–24). This solitary form of keratoacanthoma frequently regresses slowly over a period of 2 to 8 months and often heals with fibrous scarring. The less common form is the giant keratoacanthoma, which may form on the weight-bearing surface of the foot (Fig. 13–25). Giant keratoacanthomas tend to continue to increase in size with time and become more necrotic in the center. These rare variants resist treatment and are very unlikely to undergo spontaneous regression.

Treatment has been approached conservatively in the past with the view that the lesion may regress over time. However, the potential of a lesion to convert to a more aggressive and even malignant condition dictates more aggressive treatment. There are many advantages of surgical excision of solitary and giant keratoacan-

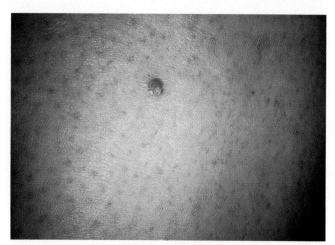

Figure 13–22   Cherry hemangioma. This lower extremity lesion is also known as a Campbell de Morgan spot.

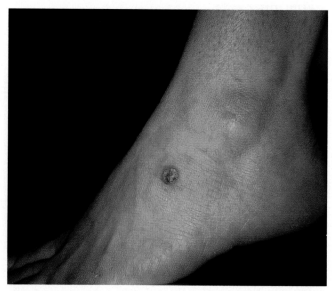

Figure 13–24   Solitary keratoacanthoma. This early dome-shaped well-circumscribed tumor on the lateral foot is raised well above the surface and has a crusted center.

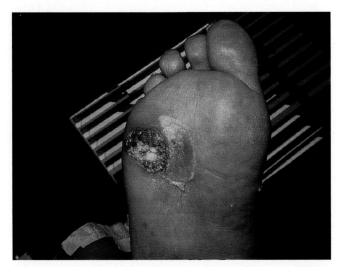

Figure 13–25 Giant keratoacanthoma. A 70-year-old man presented with a nonhealing ulcerous lesion on the plantar aspect of the foot.

thoma with only a few disadvantages. Biopsy is necessary in all cases; however, an accurate diagnosis is difficult with a superficial biopsy. For this reason, an excisional biopsy is mandated. Solitary keratoacanthomas, which have been surgically excised, have a better-appearing scar than lesions that are allowed to spontaneously regress. Lesions on the plantar aspect of the foot should be aggressively addressed, owing to the possibility of painful scar formation after regression. The main disadvantage to surgical excision is that the resulting scar may be larger than would be seen if the lesions were allowed to resolve. Other treatment options include intralesional 5-fluorouracil, curettage, cryosurgery, and electrodesiccation. The best treatment, however, is complete removal with total excision, thus allowing an optimum biopsy specimen and improved scar.

The microscopic pathology of keratoacanthoma is characterized by invagination of the epidermis forming a cup-like structure with a keratin-filled core (Fig. 13–26). Keratoacanthoma is both exophytic and endophytic compared with squamous cell carcinoma, which is only endophytic and often ulcerates. There is epidermal proliferation at the base and the sides of the keratoacanthoma lesion. The depth of the base extends to but not beyond the sweat glands. The base of the lesion has an irregular border but is not infiltrative like squamous cell carcinoma. Keratoacanthoma normally extends more lateral than downward and has intraepidermal abscess formation.

LEIOMYOMAS

Leiomyomas are defined as benign tumors derived from cutaneous smooth muscle. Most of these lesions arise from the arrector pilorum muscle, whereas some arise from vascular smooth muscle and are termed *vascular leiomyomas* or *angiomyomas*. Leiomyomas derived from the arrector pilorum muscle are usually multiple, whereas angiomyomas are usually solitary. Characteristically, leiomyomas occur over the face, trunk, and extremities and are seldom clinically diagnosed correctly. Leiomyomas are smooth, firm nodules that are fixed to the underlying skin and range in size from just a few millimeters to 2 cm in diameter. The color may vary from skin colored to pink to brown. The nodules may have a translucent or waxy appearance and are generally very painful. The pain usually occurs spontaneously and may be paroxysmal, with sharp, stabbing, or pinching qualities. The tumor impinges directly on cutaneous nerves to produce the pain.

Figure 13–26 Keratoacanthoma. *A,* Photomicrograph shows a well-demarcated, cup-shaped mass filled with keratinous debris that is surrounded by hyperplastic squamous epithelium. *B,* The deep margin of the lesion has a blunt, rounded contour and discontinuous nest of squamous epithelium that appears to be superficially invasive and associated with an inflammatory infiltrate, consistent with keratoacanthoma. (*A* and *B,* hematoxylin and eosin, ×40.)

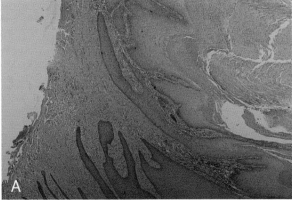
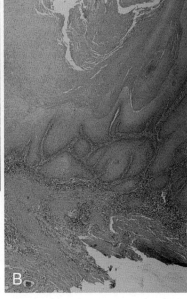

The extensor surfaces of the extremities and anterior surface of the trunk are the most common areas for this lesion. It is also found on a regular basis on the toes (Fig. 13–27). Solitary lesions arising from smooth muscle are usually larger than the nodules of the multiple type and tend to show no familial tendency. Angiomyomas arise later in life as solitary nodules over the extremities, with the majority occurring over the lower extremities. The majority of vascular leiomyomas are usually more deeply situated than those that arise from the arrector pilorum muscle. Most lesions on the lower extremity are solitary.

Leiomyomas are encapsulated lesions with numerous blood vessels of various sizes with thick muscular walls composed of poorly defined proliferation of smooth muscle fibers that interlace and merge into the surrounding collagen. The muscle fibers also run tangentially from the blood vessels and enter the intervascular muscular fascicles. Most of the vessels involved appear to be veins rather than arteries. Microscopic evaluation of the nodular fragments show that it is composed of bundles of smooth muscle arranged in a whorled pattern. Within the smooth muscle fibers are multiple small vascular spaces (Fig. 13–28). The preferred treatment of leiomyoma and angiomyoma consists of surgical excision.

MUCOID CYSTS

Synonyms for the digital mucoid cyst include cutaneous synovial (myxoid) cyst, focal cutaneous mucinosis, digital synovial cyst, and dorsal digital ganglionic cyst. All of these conditions appear to be descriptive names for the same clinical entity. These soft, dome-shaped, smooth, oval to round, translucent, white to pink structures occur intradermally on the dorsal surface of the

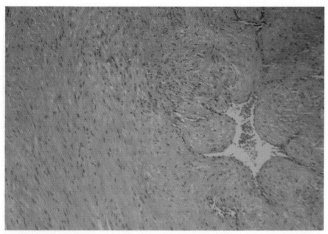

Figure 13–28   Leiomyoma. Photomicrograph scanning view of leiomyoma-angiomyoma shows complete replacement of the dermis by broad, interlacing fascicles of eosinophilic spindle cells with blood vessel present.

distal phalanx of the fingers and toes (Fig. 13–29). This condition is most common in middle-aged and elderly patients. There is a greater frequency in females (3:1 ratio), and the condition is uncommon in younger patients. The slow-growing and well-localized lesion is almost always solitary and favors the distal interphalangeal joint and periungual areas. The lesion is firm to soft and fluctuant and contains a clear viscous jelly-like substance that exudes if the cyst is incised (Fig. 13–30). The cyst usually refills within 8 weeks after puncture. Some cysts may become painful, or the adjacent toenail may develop a longitudinal depression or ridging as a result of pressure (Fig. 13–31).

There are two types of digital mucoid cysts, those located at the proximal nail fold and those located over the dorsal interphalangeal joint. Although they are formed separately, the lesions have a similar clinical appearance. The cysts on the proximal nail fold result from localized fibroblast proliferation and are not usually directly connected to the joint space or tendon sheath. Cysts located on the dorsolateral or medial digit at the distal interphalangeal joint are probably caused by herniation of tendon sheaths or joint linings and are

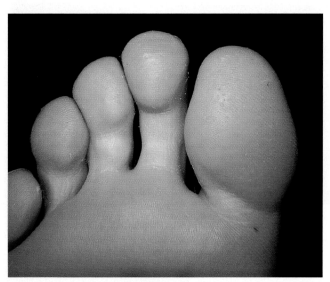

Figure 13–27   Leiomyoma. A typical location for this lesion is on the plantar or lateral surface of the lesser toes. This lesion on the plantar third toe was very painful.

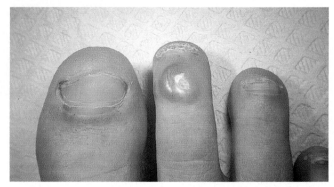

Figure 13–29   Digital mucoid cyst. A typical location of the mucoid cyst is over the dorsal aspect of the distal phalanx of the toe.

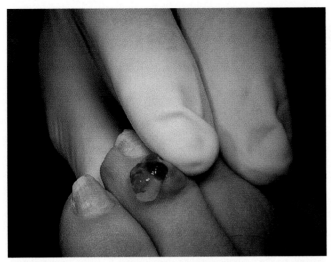

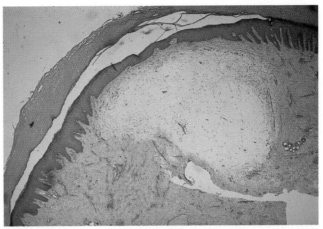

Figure 13–30 Digital mucoid cyst. When incised, the cyst will extrude a thick, clear viscous jelly-like substance.

Figure 13–32 Digital mucoid cyst. This cross-sectional microscopic view of an intradermal mucoid cyst shows a nodular area with irregular angulated stellate-shaped fibroblasts dispersed in a myxomatous stroma with adjacent normal tissue (hematoxylin and eosin, ×40). (Courtesy of Dr. Harvey Lemont.)

related to ganglia and synovial cysts. The two types may be differentiated with the Newmeyer test, which involves injecting a radiopaque dye mixture into the interphalangeal joint and observing its distribution under fluoroscopy or radiography. If there is a connection between the joint and the cyst, it will be visualized at that time.

The mucoid cyst is associated with irregular angulated (stellate-shaped) fibroblasts dispersed in a myxomatous stroma surrounded by normal dermis (Fig. 13–32). The basic pathogenesis of these lesions appears to be an alteration of fibroblast function from the usual collagen production to the elaboration of mucin, a normal but usually subsidiary function. Microscopically,

there is replacement of dermal collagen by a basophilic amorphous or stringy material. The fibroblast numbers increase and are roughly proportional to the degree of mucinous change. Histochemical studies identify the mucin as hyaluronic acid.

A variety of treatments have been recommended for the relief of digital mucoid cysts, from cortisone injections or incision and drainage to complete excision of the lesion. Recurrence rates are very high for injectional and incisional procedures. The best overall results (greater than 95% success) come from complete excision of the digital mucoid cyst, with or without bone removal, and a rotational skin flap for final closure. This combination of skin, cyst, pedicle, tendon sheath, capsule, and possibly bone removal with final rotational flap closure has given the best cosmetic results and the least amount of recurrence in long-term follow-up. The Schrudde skin flap is a single-lobed flap that is a combination of a rotational flap and a transpositional flap in which the flap employed to close the defect and the defect itself are cut to a round shape. This flap is created so that the pedicle or base of the flap has the incoming blood supply and the resultant scar gives the best cosmetic appearance (Fig. 13–33).

NEVI

BLUE NEVI. Blue nevi are acquired, benign, firm, slightly elevated, oval, sharply defined papules that contain a large amount of pigment that appears dark-blue to gray-black (Fig. 13–34). This common nevus is found on the hands, feet, and buttocks most often but may occur at any site. It is usually first noticed during late adolescence and is usually less than 1 cm in diameter. Giant blue nevi (greater than 1 cm in diameter) are more common on the scalp and buttock area. The pigment is located within the dermis and is brown. The brown pigment absorbs the longer wavelengths of light

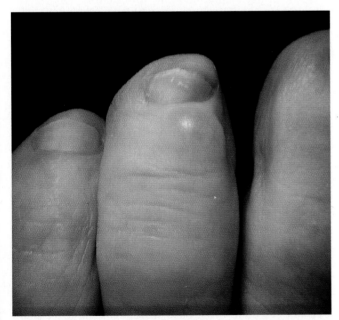

Figure 13–31 Digital mucoid cyst. Tumefaction or pressure results in longitudinal nail depression or nail growth disturbances. These are usually resolved after proper treatment.

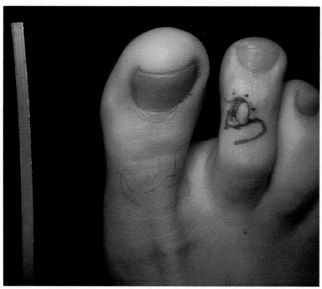

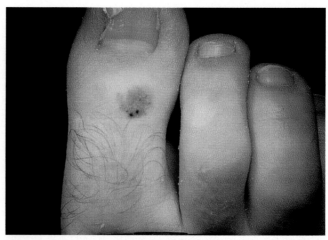

Figure 13–35   Compound nevus. The center is elevated, and the lesion is less pigmented than usually seen. Confirmation is by excisional biopsy.

Figure 13–33   Digital mucoid cyst. The lesion has been excised, and the adjacent rotational skin flap has been designed to rotate into the defect area on the second toe.

and scatters blue light, giving the lesion its typical appearance. Occasionally, this lesion has a target-like or star-like pattern of pigmentation on the dome. Histological evaluation shows that the lesion occurs as excessive fibrous tissue production in the upper reticular dermis. Melanin-containing fibroblast-like dermal melanocytes are grouped in irregular bundles admixed with melanin-containing macrophages. Except in those instances in which a coexistent epidermal derived melanocytic nevus (combined nevus) is present, the epidermis is normal. There is no association of malignant conversion. Treatment of this lesion is usually not necessary unless there are strong cosmetic concerns or the lesion shows any appearance or color change. Shave or punch biopsy is not recommended for confirmation of this lesion. Simple surgical excision is satisfactory.

COMPOUND NEVI. Compound melanocytic nevi are slightly elevated, flesh-colored to dark-brown, smooth to rough-surfaced lesions commonly seen on the hands and feet, but not on the palms or soles (Fig. 13–35). These nevi may be round or slightly irregular, and they may become more elevated with increasing age. The typical lesion is nodular, smooth, and uniformly pigmented. Occasionally, lesions are flat, warty, and irregular in shape and color, making the clinical diagnosis more difficult. Hair may be present in the compound nevus, and a white halo may appear at the periphery of the lesion (halo nevus). Histological evaluation of the compound melanocytic nevus shows collections of nevocytes within the dermis and the junctional zone (Fig. 13–36). Superficially, melanin production may be retained, but the deeper layers of the nevus show little to no pigmentation. Mitotic activity is not present in this lesion. There may be prolific squamous epithelial proliferation that may result in a warty appearance on

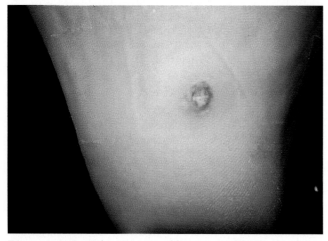

Figure 13–34   Common blue nevus. This is a solitary, asymptomatic, blue-gray nevus on the weight-bearing foot with a small peripheral callus from pressure.

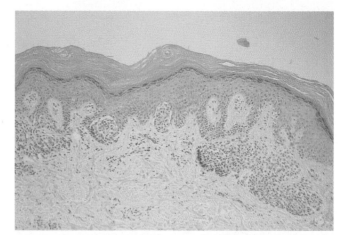

Figure 13–36   Compound nevus. Photomicrograph shows that the nevus is composed of both junctional and dermal nevus cell nests. The dermal nevus nests are routinely smaller than those located at the dermoepidermal junction (hematoxylin and eosin, ×40).

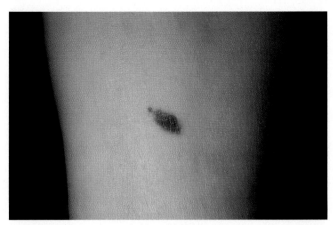

F i g u r e 1 3 – 3 7   Congenital pigmented nevus. This lesion has been present since birth and has not changed in color or appearance. The pigment is evenly distributed.

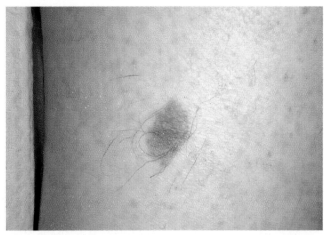

F i g u r e 1 3 – 3 8   Hairy nevus. This congenital macular nevus had irregular borders with thick coarse hair growth from the center.

gross examination. Treatment is usually not necessary unless there are changes in appearance or size of the lesion; then it may be widely excised for microscopic identification.

CONGENITAL PIGMENTED NEVI. These uniformly pigmented, irregular shaped nevi are present at birth and may range from a few millimeters to several centimeters in diameter (Fig. 13–37). They may be light brown to very dark brown, and they may have areas of hair growth. These lesions may appear at any site and are common on the trunk and lower extremities. After many years the larger nevi may convert to malignant melanoma, although this is not very common. Congenital pigmented nevi tend to involve the deeper aspects of the reticular dermis. The melanocytic spread is into the fibrous septa and adipose tissue of the subcutaneous fat. These lesions involve the adnexae—sebaceous glands, hair follicles, arrector pili muscles, and eccrine glands. There may also be nevocytic permeation of nerves, lymphatics, and blood vessels. This invasive infiltration should not be regarded as having any sinister implication (i.e., not precancerous). Treatment is not necessary in most cases of congenital pigmented nevi unless there is a change in appearance or color of the lesion.

HAIRY NEVI. Many different types of pigmented nevi contain hair. Two common types are the congenital pigmented nevi and Becker's pigmented hairy nevus. When hair is present on a nevus, it is usually coarse. Such nevi are generally uniformly pigmented, with various shades of brown or black predominating (Fig. 13–38).

INTRADERMAL NEVI. The nevocytes are within the dermis, and the lesions occur as flesh-colored to lightly pigmented, raised nodules. Intradermal nevi may have streaks or flecks of brown pigment scattered throughout the lesion (Fig. 13–39). They may be found on any body part but are common on the face. These are very benign lesions that appear in the second or third decade and have no propensity for malignant conversion. As the dermal nevus matures the junctional component

is lost, leaving an entirely intradermal nevus. The nevocytes become progressively smaller, with darkly staining nuclei with little cytoplasm, in the deep layers of the lesion. The epidermis is flattened over the surface of the lesion (Fig. 13–40). In a regressing lesion the pathology of the specimen may show marked neural features including a number of "Meissner-like corpuscles" (neurotization). Giant cells are also frequently a feature of involuting nevi. Smaller intradermal nevi may be removed by shaving them off flush with the surface and cauterizing the base. Most lesions do not require treatment.

JUNCTIONAL NEVI. Junctional nevi are flat, macular, or slightly elevated, light brown to brown-black and hair-

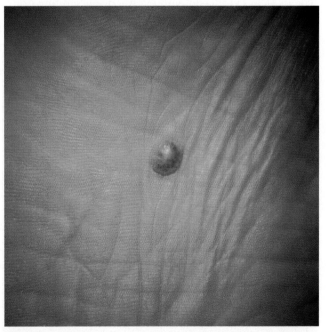

F i g u r e 1 3 – 3 9   Intradermal nevus. The lesion is raised, regular in outline, and smooth surfaced. There are lacy pigmented streaks and flecks within the lesion.

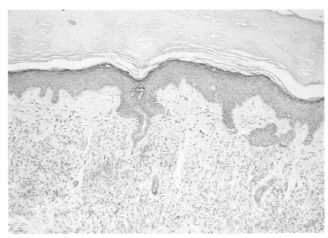

Figure 13–40   **Intradermal nevus.** Photomicrograph shows nevus cells growing in superficial nests, mid-dermal cords, and relatively small spindle cells exhibiting neural differentiation (hematoxylin and eosin, ×40).

less, with uniform pigmentation that may be slightly irregular. Junctional nevi vary in size from 0.1 to 0.6 cm in diameter and are found commonly on the soles (Fig. 13–41), lower extremities, hands, trunk, and face. This is a common nevus, and it is estimated that the average white person has at least 25 of these lesions. Junctional nevi are rare at birth and generally develop after 2 years of age. These nevi may change into compound nevi after childhood but remain as junctional nevi on the palms and soles. Malignant degeneration is extremely rare. Melanocytes proliferate to form discrete nests of nevocytes in the lower epidermis, usually within the epidermal ridges. The uniform cells have pale or clear cytoplasm with evenly dispersed fine granules of melanin pigment with regular oval nuclei with

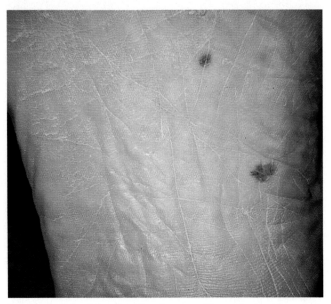

Figure 13–41   **Junctional nevus.** These pigmented macular lesions commonly occur on the sole of the foot.

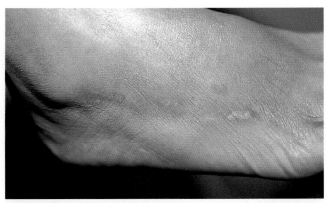

Figure 13–42   **Linear verrucous epidermal nevus.** This lesion is usually unilateral and is commonly seen on the side or dorsum of the foot.

prominent nucleoli. In the darker pigmented lesions, melanin may be seen within the cytoplasm of the histiocytes within the papillary dermis. Treatment is usually not necessary.

LINEAR VERRUCOUS EPIDERMAL NEVI. These lesions consist of pruritic erythematous verrucous papules arranged in a linear pattern. They are frequently seen unilaterally and commonly involve the lower extremities (Fig. 13–42). Females are affected more often than males, and the lesions may be present at birth or appear before puberty. Variants of this lesion are linear epidermal nevus, nevus unius lateris, nevus verrucosus, ichthyosis hystrix, and zosteriform lentiginous nevus. Differential diagnosis includes linear psoriasis, linear lichen planus, linear lichen simplex chronicus, lichen striatus, and linear seborrheic keratosis. Microscopically, the lesion is psoriasiform and inflammatory, with alternating orthokeratotic and parakeratotic hyperkeratosis accompanied by focal spongiosis and edema. The lesions may respond to topical and intralesional corticosteroids.

NEVI DEPIGMENTOSUS (ACHROMIC NEVI). This is a congenital, stable, hypopigmented lesion located randomly, segmentally, linearly (Fig. 13–43), or in a whorled pattern (Fig. 13–44). It is frequently present at birth and commonly seen as an isolated circular lesion on the lower extremities. The defect (hypopigmentation) is the result of a defect in melanosome transfer from melanocytes to keratinocytes. However, melanocytes are always present histologically. Because some pigment is present in these nevi, they should probably be termed *nevi hypopigmentosus*. Wood's light may accentuate these lesions. Owing to the decreased level of pigmentation, this nevus should not be exposed to ultraviolet sunlight.

PIEZOGENIC PEDAL PAPULES

Piezogenic pedal papules are skin-colored, palpable, soft herniations of fat that appear at the medial, lateral, and posterior aspects of the heel (Fig. 13–45) or over the medial longitudinal arch of the foot (Fig. 13–46) with

Figure 13–43   Nevus depigmentosus. The linear pattern of this lesion became much more noticeable during the summer after tanning occurred.

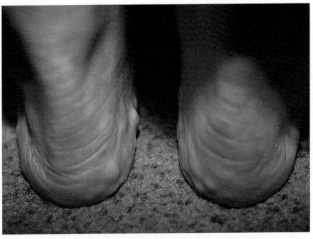

Figure 13–45   Piezogenic pedal papules. The most common location for these fat herniations is around the periphery of the heels during weight bearing.

weight bearing. The term *piezogenic* (*piezo* = pressure and *genic* = caused by) has been applied to these papules because they are typically seen only with manual pressure or weight bearing.

This condition is common in the majority of the population. The herniations are viewed as protrusions of fatty subcutaneous tissue through small connective defects in the dermis. Most papules are asymptomatic, but painful pedal piezogenic papules do occur. The extrusion of fat with its associated neurovascular structures may cause anoxic pain and entrapment symptoms in cases of obesity, repeated trauma, and long periods of standing.

Piezogenic papules range in size from several milli-

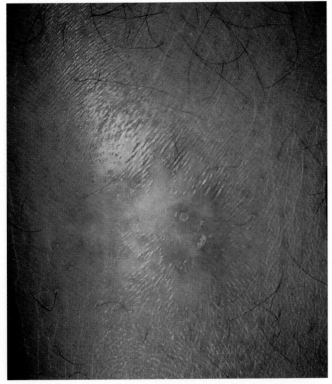

Figure 13–44   Nevus depigmentosus. The whorled pattern of this lesion had been present on the lower leg since childhood and had not changed in size or appearance.

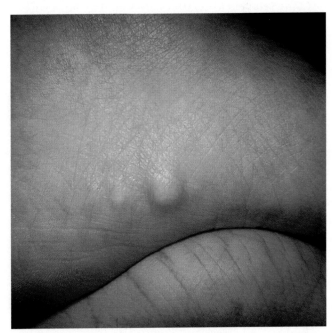

Figure 13–46   Piezogenic pedal papules. A less common site for fat herniations is over the medial longitudinal arch of the foot.

meters to 2 cm. They are more common in females than in males. Histological examination reveals a sharply circumscribed focus of subcutaneous fat with a conglomeration of normal fat chambers.

Treatment is usually not necessary, unless the papules are painful. Weight loss, avoidance of prolonged standing, orthotic devices, and plastic heel cups may alleviate pressure and therefore decrease pain in the papules. In cases that are resistant to conservative measures, the area of the painful pedal papules may be incised surgically. The fatty lobules are excised, and the defect is closed in layers.

SEBORRHEIC KERATOSIS

Seborrheic keratoses are very common, hereditary, pigmented, benign growths that originate in the epidermis. These brown, stuck-on, waxy, warty-appearing papules or plaques occur in the majority of adults after age 30. They range from 1.0 mm to 6.0 cm in diameter. The border may be round and smooth or irregular and notched. The early type is usually a barely elevated plaque with or without pigment (Fig. 13–47). The surface shows fine stippling with an irregular border. Early lesions commonly show variations in the pigment, with the majority being light in color with visible pink or red spots. The late type is usually a larger plaque with a warty surface and a "stuck on" appearance (Fig. 13–48).

In older lesions, white or black pearls of keratin (1 mm in diameter) may be seen embedded in the surface of smooth, dome-shaped keratoses. These *horn cysts* are easily seen with a magnifying hand-held lens. The presence of horn cysts on the surface of a lesion helps to confirm the diagnosis and rule out malignant melanoma on visual examination.

Many seborrheic keratoses are found in sun-exposed areas and are very common on the arms and legs. Although these lesions are generally asymptomatic, they can be pruritic and they may become irritated if rubbed or scratched. When inflamed, they may become slightly

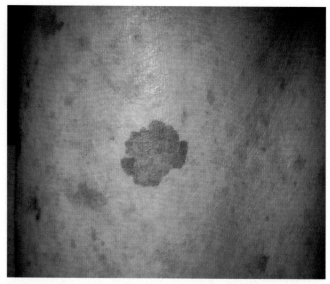

Figure 13–48   Seborrheic keratosis. In the late stage, the larger, darkly pigmented plaque has a waxy stuck-on appearance.

swollen and develop an erythematous ring around the periphery of the lesion. With continued inflammation, the seborrheic keratosis may lose most of its characteristic appearance and become a red, ulcerated lesion with a friable surface that itches intensely (Fig. 13–49). At this stage the only treatment is protection of the lesion from additional scratching, removal of inflamed tissue, and topical administration of corticosteroids.

Treatment of noninflamed lesions is usually not necessary unless they have become a cosmetic problem. They may be frozen, curetted, shaved, excised, or simply ignored. The sudden appearance of multiple seborrheic keratoses or an increase in the number and size of these lesions on noninflamed skin may herald the presence of internal malignancy. The most common type of associated malignancy is adenocarcinoma, espe-

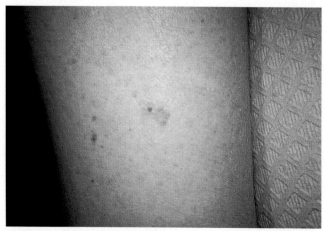

Figure 13–47   Seborrheic keratosis. In the early stage, this small plaque occurred with light pigmentation, an irregular border, and a small red spot.

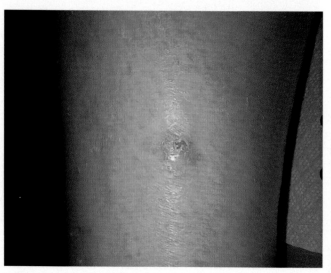

Figure 13–49   Seborrheic keratosis. This irritated lesion occurred as a red, ulcerated mass with a very friable surface that was extremely pruritic.

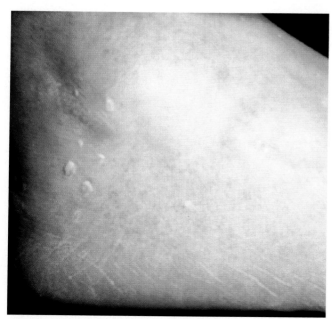

Figure 13–50   Stucco keratoses. Multiple small, white hyperkeratotic papules scattered on the heel and side of the foot in an older man is characteristic of this condition.

cially of the gastrointestinal tract. This sign of internal malignancy is termed the *Leser-Trélat* sign.

STUCCO KERATOSIS

Stucco keratoses (keratoelastoidosis verrucosa) are seen in patients (predominantly men) older than 40 and are commonly seen in the elderly. These lesions are found on the forearms and lower extremities, especially on the dorsum of the feet and Achilles tendon area. They are never seen on the palms or soles. Multiple small, white, dry scaly lesions may occur as 1- to 6-mm, oval or round discrete papules (Fig. 13–50) or as larger (up to 1 cm) scaly plaques (Fig. 13–51). These lesions are sometimes referred to as "barnacles of life" because they are seen primarily in the elderly. They are very dry and

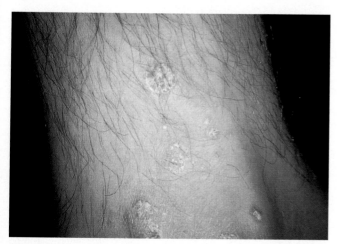

Figure 13–51   Stucco keratoses. Larger, round, white plaque-like keratoses are seen on the ankles and dorsa of the feet.

appear to be "stuck-on" lesions that can simply be peeled off the skin. Most patients are unaware of these lesions and consider them to be a manifestation of dry skin. When the lesions are removed intact from the skin there is no bleeding, however, the lesions will quickly re-form. Histologically, the picture is that of an epidermal nevus and is not unique. Treatment is usually not necessary, but topical emollients will soften the lesions so that they may be easily removed. For a more permanent resolution, curettage or cryotherapy may be performed.

BIBLIOGRAPHY

Banik R, Bubach D: Skin tags: Localization and frequencies according to sex and age. Dermatologica 174:180–183, 1987.

Barrett C, Weaver TD, Schaffer SG: Ganglion cyst of the hallux: An aberrant presentation. J Foot Ankle Surg 34:57–60, 1995.

Bart RS, Kopf AW: Techniques of biopsy of cutaneous neoplasms. J Dermatol Surg Oncol 5:979–983, 1979.

Chin FE, McCarthy DJ: The cytological and biomechanical implications of periungual fibroma. J Foot Surg 31:486–497, 1992.

Dockery GL: Digital mucoid cysts: Diagnosis and treatment. J Foot Ankle Surg 33:326–333, 1994.

Dockery GL: Hypertrophic and keloid scars. J Am Podiatr Med Assoc 85:57–60, 1995.

Dockery GL: Single-lobe rotation flaps. J Am Podiatr Assoc 85:36–40, 1995.

Dockery GL, Diana JL: Painful piezogenic papules. J Am Podiatr Assoc 68:703–705, 1978.

Dockery GL, Nilson RZ: Intralesional injections. Clin Podiatr Med Surg 3:473–485, 1986.

Dockery GL, Wendel RE: Vascular leiomyoma-angiomyoma: A case report. J Am Podiatr Assoc 69:438–439, 1979.

Habershaw GM, Hurchik JM, Nasser I: Pedal leiomyoma. J Foot Ankle Surg 33:260–265, 1994.

Hale D, Dockery GL: Giant keratoacanthoma of the plantar foot: A report of two cases. J Foot Ankle Surg 32:75–84, 1993.

Harvey CK, Park E: Multiple dermatofibromas in patients with autoimmune disease: A case report. J Am Podiatr Med Assoc 84:523–531, 1994.

Kint A, Baran R, De Keyser H: Acquired (digital) fibrokeratoma. J Am Acad Dermatol 12:816–821, 1985.

Kocsard E, Ofner F: Keratoelastoidosis verrucosa of the extremities (stucco keratoses of the extremities). Dermatologica 133:225–235, 1966.

Laine W: Benign neoplasia of the foot. In McCarthy DJ, Montgomery R (eds): Podiatric Dermatology, pp 219–234. Baltimore, Williams & Wilkins, 1986.

Lemont H: Common myxoid cysts of the foot. Lower Extrem 2:263–265, 1995.

Novicki DC, Anselmi SJ: Fibrous histiocytoma. J Am Podiatr Assoc 68:606–612, 1978.

O'Keefe RG: Surgical management of soft tissue tumors. In Oloff LM (ed): Musculoskeletal Disorders of the Lower Extremities, pp 626–638. Philadelphia, WB Saunders, 1994.

Pontius J, Lasday S, Mele R: Piezogenic pedal papules extending into the arch. J Am Podiatr Med Assoc 80:444–445, 1990.

Port M: Rounds in podiatric dermatology. Clin Podiatr Med Surg 3:413–425, 1986.

Saeva JT, Kaye MR: Presentation of an intermetatarsal ganglion. J Podiatr Med Assoc 85:274–276, 1995.

Schrudde J, Petrovici C: The use of slide-swing plasty in closing defects: A clinical study based on 1308 cases. Plast Recon 67:467–481, 1981.

Sperry K, Wall J: Adenocarcinoma of the stomach with borrheic keratoses: The sign of Leser-Trélat. Cancer 4 1980.

Spitalny AD, Lavery LA: Acquired fibrokeratoma of Surg 31:509–511, 1992.

Visalli AJ, McCarthy DJ: Podiatric considerations J Foot Surg 31:372–377, 1992.

m

g skin

str Surg

ruptive se-
:2434–2438.

the heel. J Foot

f angioleiomyoma.

14

PREMALIGNANT AND MALIGNANT SKIN TUMORS

INTRODUCTION

Premalignant and malignant skin tumors are much rarer than benign lesions but are of significantly more concern. The first section of this chapter on premalignant lesions shows that many of these conditions may evolve into invasive cancer. Histologically, most of these conditions might be viewed as squamous cell carcinoma, that is, the microscopic changes are confined to the epidermis. Those lesions that are typically labeled "premalignant" are those that may show pathological changes in the tissue layers that, without actually being cancer, show the tendency to develop into cancer. Many types of benign lesions have been known to convert to malignant lesions with the right combination of time, environmental exposure, external and internal chemicals, sun exposure, and lesion irritation. The most common lesions that are termed *premalignant* are discussed in this chapter and include actinic keratosis, arsenical keratosis, Bowen's disease, chronic cicatricial keratosis (Marjolin's ulcer), radiation dermatitis, and verrucous carcinoma. The malignant tumors that are discussed include basal cell carcinoma and squamous cell carcinoma. In the final section the focus is on Kaposi's sarcoma and malignant melanoma.

ACTINIC KERATOSIS

The most common epithelial premalignant lesion among white individuals is actinic keratosis. This condition is also called solar dermatitis and senile keratosis, because there is an increase in this condition on sun-exposed skin and in the elderly. Light-complexioned individuals, with a propensity for sunburn, are more susceptible than those who are dark complexioned. Actinic keratoses are well-defined, raised, red papules or plaques with a rough surface of adherent scales (Fig. 14–1). The lesions vary from 1 mm to several centime-

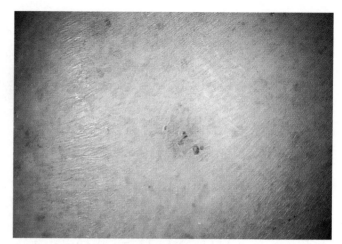

Figure 14 – 2   Actinic keratosis. Early lesion on lower leg has typical excoriated area due to scratching.

ters in diameter and frequently are first identified by feel rather than by appearance. The head, neck, face, and upper extremities are most susceptible to solar damage, but close evaluation of patients with this sun injury reveals that there are lesions on the lower extremities as well.

Actinic keratoses may undergo spontaneous remission during the winter or with decreased sun exposure. Many patients relate that the skin condition began after a sunburn and is worse during the summer months. Actinic keratoses begin as an area of increased vascularity, with the skin surface becoming slightly rough. During this stage, there may be mild pruritus or irritation. The patient may excoriate the upper layer with rubbing or scratching (Fig. 14–2). Gradually, over long periods of time, an adherent yellow scale or crust forms (Fig. 14–3). The removal of the adherent scale may cause bleeding of the base. Several lesions are usually seen in the same area that may represent all of the vari-

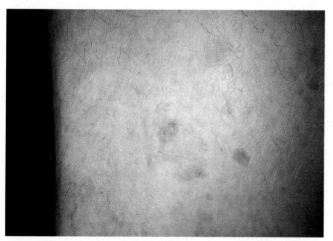

Figure 14 – 1   Actinic keratosis. The lesion is a well-defined, raised, red plaque with an adherent scale commonly found on sun-exposed surfaces of the skin.

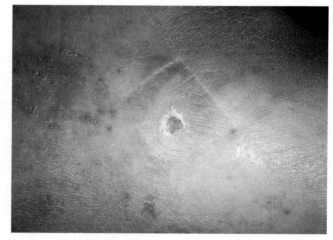

Figure 14 – 3   Actinic keratosis. A more advanced lesion with yellow adherent scale is located adjacent to a large plaque of intense sun damage with a red base and the typical rough surface.

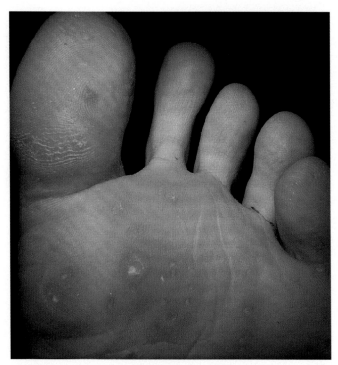

Figure 14–4 Arsenical keratoses. Multiple, discrete, wart-like keratotic lesions occurred on the soles in a patient who was treated for psoriasis with inorganic arsenic many years earlier.

ous stages of lesion development. Actinic keratoses may gradually degenerate into squamous cell carcinomas. Induration, inflammation, increasing size, and oozing of an old actinic lesion may suggest malignancy.

The patient should be counseled about the importance of reduction of further sun damage by using sunscreens and protective clothing. Treatment is accomplished with cryotherapy. Curettage and electrodesiccation may also be performed for larger lesions. Topical 5-fluorouracil can be used on larger areas of involvement.

ARSENICAL KERATOSIS

Arsenical keratosis is another precancerous lesion that may be seen on the lower extremities. These frequently form at sites of irritation, friction, or trauma, such as on the palms and the plantar soles (Fig. 14–4). Usually 20 or more discrete, yellow, round-to-oval, punctate, wart-like lesions are present. They may become confluent to form verrucous plaques. On the foot, the lesions almost always spare the non–weight-bearing portion of the arch. Exposure to inorganic arsenical compounds in medications, insecticides, or contaminated well water is frequently identified in patients presenting with this condition. Inorganic arsenic was commonly used to treat psoriasis, asthmatic bronchitis, syphilis, and other conditions in the 1930s and 1940s.

Most lesions are present for many years with no changes occurring; however, they may degenerate into

squamous cell carcinoma. The occasional invasive squamous cell carcinoma may grow rapidly. Histologically, arsenical keratoses show thick hyperkeratosis with a prominent granular layer. Acanthosis is common and may be accompanied by a downward proliferation of the rete ridges. Arsenical carcinoma is almost impossible to distinguish from Bowen's disease. Treatment is usually reserved for painful lesions, which may be softened and mechanically debrided.

BOWEN'S DISEASE

This lesion is frequently described as an intraepidermal carcinoma or as a squamous cell carcinoma in situ, because the basement membrane remains intact. The well-defined, solitary, slightly raised, irregular, red plaque (with or without an adherent scale) may be found anywhere but occurs predominantly on the legs and feet (Fig. 14–5). The lesion appears as a slowly enlarging erythematous macule with a sharp border with slight scaling or superficial crusting. Because the borders are well defined the lesions may be misdiagnosed as psoriasis, seborrheic keratosis, or chronic eczema.

The majority of Bowen's lesions are due to excessive exposure to ultraviolet radiation and are found on sun-exposed areas of the body, but they may also be due to arsenical ingestion. Although potentially malignant, conversion of Bowen's disease to invasive squamous cell carcinoma is infrequent (around 5%) and usually occurs in areas that are continually damaged by irritation or repeated sun exposure.

The histological appearance of Bowen's lesions is squamous cell carcinoma in situ with epidermal thickening by uniformly atypical keratinocytes proliferating at all levels. The lesion is characterized by acanthosis, parakeratosis, and dysplasia. Loss of cellular orientation and maturation, cytoplasmic and nuclear pleomorphism, and increased mitotic activity (both normal and abnormal) occur at different levels within the epidermis.

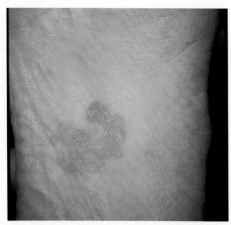

Figure 14–5 Bowen's disease. This intraepidermal carcinoma of the skin of the plantar foot was a well-defined, irregular, slightly raised red plaque with scales and some crust on the surface.

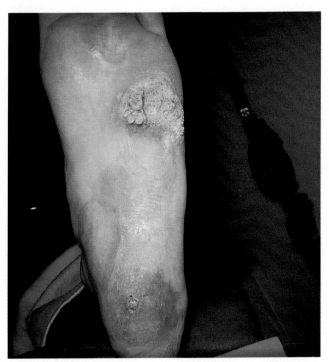

Figure 14–6 **Chronic cicatricial keratosis.** A malignant lesion formed in the center of a chronic scar on the heel of a patient who had undergone multiple surgical treatments to remove recurrent aggressive verrucae on the foot.

Treatment depends on the age and health of the patient and the size and location of the lesion. Excisional biopsy is the treatment of choice, but if the lesion is too large or in an area that makes excision difficult, curet-

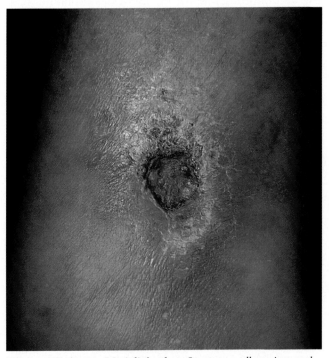

Figure 14–7 **Marjolin's ulcer.** Squamous cell carcinoma developed in a chronic nonhealing leg ulcer after many years.

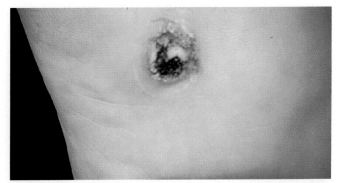

Figure 14–8 **Marjolin's ulcer.** Malignant changes (epithelioma cuniculatum) may occur in areas of chronic draining sinuses as in this case on the foot.

tage and cautery or cryotherapy may be satisfactory alternatives. Extremely large lesions may be treated with 5-fluorouracil cream applied twice a day for 4 to 8 weeks.

CHRONIC CICATRICIAL KERATOSIS

Marjolin's ulcer is the term that refers to malignant changes arising in chronic ulcers, sinuses, scars (especially burn scars), and chronically damaged skin. Carcinomas may develop after many years in areas of chronic cicatricial keratosis (Fig. 14–6), and the majority of these lesions are found on the lower extremities. These include scars from chronic ulcers (Fig. 14–7), puncture wounds or draining sinuses (Fig. 14–8), sites of chronic underlying osteomyelitis (Fig. 14–9), and sites of deep burn scars (Fig. 14–10). Other areas that may show conversion to malignancy include previously frostbitten areas, vaccination scars, chromoblastomycoses, nonheal-

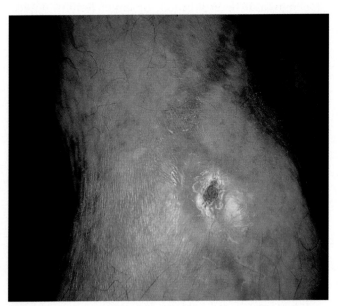

Figure 14–9 **Marjolin's ulcer.** Relatively common malignant changes occurred in a sinus track over the site of chronic osteomyelitis.

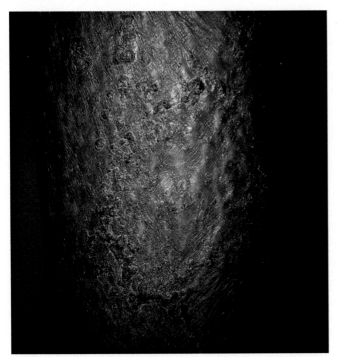

Figure 14–10   Marjolin's ulcer. Classically described location of squamous cell carcinoma formation is around severe deep burn scars on the extremities.

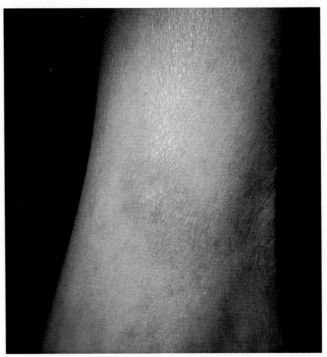

Figure 14–11   Radiation dermatitis. Erythema and hyperpigmentary and hypopigmentary changes may occur after radiation therapy.

ing plantar warts, and hypertrophic lichen planus. A gradual progression from dysplasia to squamous cell carcinoma in situ may occur, but when invasive carcinoma finally develops, it may spread very quickly. This slow progression of dysplasia makes squamous cell carcinomas that occur at sites of chronic skin damage less aggressive than those that develop from actinic keratosis or Bowen's disease. The overall metastatic rate is greater than 40%. Wide local excision is preferred only for very small lesions or grade I lesions that can be radically excised. Grade II or grade III lesions require referral to oncology specialists for prophylactic node irradiation and possible amputation.

RADIATION DERMATITIS

Radiation dermatitis is defined as skin changes that occur after exposure to ionizing radiation. Cutaneous changes include atrophy, scarring, telangiectasia, and pigmentary abnormalities. The early reversible effects include erythema, epilation, and pigmentation that may last from a few months to years. The late nonreversible effects include telangiectasia, dermatitis, and radiation-induced carcinomas. Radiation erythema is characterized by dilatation of the dermal blood vessels and a mild perivascular cellular infiltrate. There is a macular erythematous rash with hyperpigmentary or hypopigmentary changes with considerable thinning of the epidermis (Fig. 14–11).

In chronic radiation dermatitis there is increasing cutaneous atrophy and hyperpigmentation or hypopig-

mentation, and the superficial venules become telangiectatic (Fig. 14–12). The full development of atrophic changes may take many years. The skin becomes thinned, dry, and scaly, and a central ulceration (radioonecrosis) may occur (Fig. 14–13). Chronic radiation dermatitis is permanent and progressive. Squamous cell carcinoma may develop after 7 to 12 years, especially on the hands and feet. The carcinoma always develops

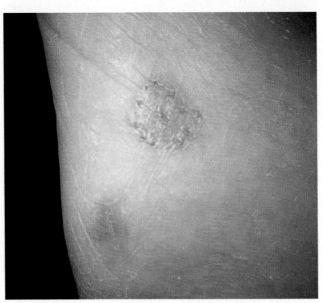

Figure 14–12   Radiation dermatitis. Chronic changes include increased atrophy and telangiectasia with mild xerosis.

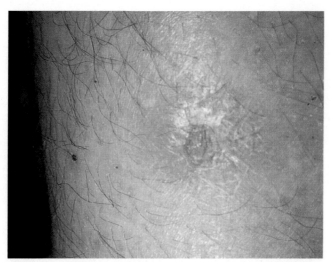

Figure 14–13   Radionecrosis. Ulceration has occurred secondary to inappropriate irradiation of Bowen's disease on the lower leg.

within the area of radiation dermatitis and never in the adjacent normal tissues. The prognoses are poor, recurrences are common, and tumors are often multiple.

VERRUCOUS CARCINOMA

Verrucous carcinoma (epithelioma cuniculatum plantare) is characterized by an indolent tumor of the sole of the foot (Fig. 14–14). This warty-surfaced exophytic

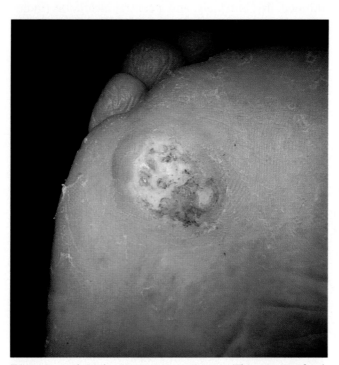

Figure 14–14   Verrucous carcinoma. This warty-surfaced exophytic tumor is found in its characteristic location on the sole of the foot.

tumor may have many sinuses that exude an odoriferous material. This lesion may grow to be a large boggy fungating mass. Many of these lesions have a thick white core with an ulcerated center and an elevated, irregular border. The course of verrucous carcinoma is indolent, ranging from several months' to many years' duration.

This lesion is a low-grade, well-differentiated squamous cell carcinoma that is characterized by papillomatosis, hyperkeratosis, parakeratosis, and acanthosis. It tends to be extremely invasive but never metastatic. Both exophytic and endophytic characteristics are present. Well-differentiated keratinocytes with small nuclei extend into the dermis or subcutis from the epidermis. In some cases, intraepidermal microabscesses are seen.

No cause has been clearly defined, but human papillomavirus has been associated with this lesion and it may be that a plantar wart was present in the early stages of development. Trauma and chronic irritation from treatment may be a contributing factor to the enlargement and proliferation of this condition. The primary treatment is wide and deep surgical excision. The recurrence is minimal if the skin margins are free of tumor after excision.

BASAL CELL CARCINOMA

Basal cell carcinoma is the most common malignant cutaneous neoplasm. Sunlight exposure plays an important role in the cause of this condition, but this lesion may appear in areas not commonly exposed to ultraviolet radiation. The most common location of basal cell carcinoma is on the face, but it may be seen on the lower legs (Fig. 14–15) and the feet (Fig. 14–16). Basal cell carcinoma is a slow-growing destructive lesion that

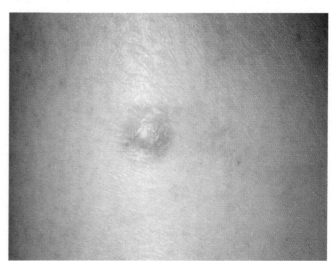

Figure 14–15   Basal cell carcinoma. Nodular basal cell carcinoma on the lower leg was misdiagnosed as a dermatofibroma, which it clearly resembles.

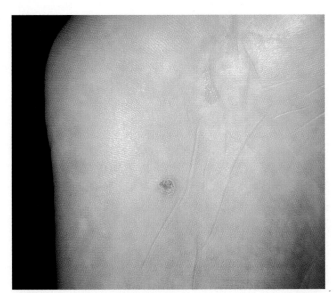

Figure 14–16   Basal cell carcinoma. Superficial form of basal cell carcinoma was found on the plantar sole of the foot. The diagnosis was confirmed by biopsy.

is locally invasive with direct extension but very rarely metastasizes. The cells of a basal cell carcinoma resemble those of the basilar layer of the epidermis. They stain basophilic, have a large nucleus, and form an orderly line around the periphery of tumor nests in the dermis (termed *palisading*). Those lesions with large nests of tumor cells are the least aggressive (nodular form), and those with numerous small nests may be more aggressive (morpheaform). There are several clinical forms of basal cell carcinomas that vary in appearance and malignant potential.

NODULAR BASAL CELL CARCINOMA. This is the most common form of basal cell carcinoma. It begins as a small, white, dome-shaped nodule or papule. Nodular basal cell carcinoma may extend peripherally while remaining flat. As it expands, telangiectatic vessels become more prominent and the tumor may appear erythematous or violaceous (Fig. 14–15). Melanin pigment may be present, giving the tumor a slight brown, black, or blue-black discoloration. The lesion becomes more elevated, forming an oval mass, and it may become multilobular. The center of this lesion may ulcerate and bleed, and then it never seems to heal. Even though the tumor is slow growing, it may extend deeply, destroying the underlying tissues.

CYSTIC BASAL CELL CARCINOMA. A variant of the nodular form appears as a smooth, round, cystic mass that behaves like a nodular basal cell carcinoma. This dome-like tumor may be slightly lobulated, pearl-like in color, with visible telangiectasia. The cystic variant may have a clear fluid if punctured or opened. Unlike the nodular form, this lesion does not break down until much later in its development. Cystic basal cell carcinoma may reach a very large size before medical attention is sought.

PIGMENTED BASAL CELL CARCINOMA. This tumor has similar features of a malignant melanoma with an erosive center and pigmented border. This variant of the nodular lesion may be brown, black, or blue through all or some of the tumor. It still has the characteristic elevated, pearly white, translucent border.

MORPHEIC BASAL CELL CARCINOMA. The name for this variant is derived from its resemblance to a plaque of localized scleroderma (morphea). This form of basal cell carcinoma is frquently misdiagnosed because it does not appear to be a tumor on clinical presentation. Characteristic pearly coloration and telangiectasia are important to the clinical diagnosis. The lesions spread slowly, have subclinical extension beyond the clinically recognized borders, and have a high recurrence rate following treatment.

SUPERFICIAL BASAL CELL CARCINOMA. This is the least aggressive of the basal cell carcinomas characteristically present on the trunk and the most common basal cell carcinoma on the lower extremities and feet (Fig. 14–16). It presents as a red plaque with an adherent scale. The borders are slightly raised, rolled, telangiectatic and pearly white, and the lesion may resemble a plaque of eczema or psoriasis. The round-to-oval, circumscribed tumor spreads by peripheral invasion from a few millimeters to several centimeters.

NEVOID BASAL CELL CARCINOMA SYNDROME (BASAL CELL NEVUS SYNDROME). The nevoid basal cell epithelioma syndrome, also referred to as Gorlin's syndrome, is an autosomal dominant disorder. It occurs with variable penetrance, characterized by multiple basal cell carcinomas that appear at a relatively young age (between puberty and 35 years). Although basal cell carcinoma in this syndrome can cause death due to brain or other vital organ invasion, it rarely leads to metastatic disease. A common feature of this condition (in greater than 60% of the patients) is the presence of palmar and plantar pits (Fig. 14–17). These lesions show the histopathology of basal cell carcinoma, even though basal cell carcinomas are not seen clinically in these areas. Other findings, besides multiple basal cell carcinomas and palmar-plantar pits, include skeletal abnormalities (especially affecting the rib), jaw cysts, and ectopic calcifications of the falx cerebri and other structures. Additional dermatological abnormalities include milia formation, epidermal and sebaceous cysts, lipomas, and fibromas. In addition to these findings, many other associated abnormalities in multiple organ systems may be present.

TREATMENT. In general, treatment of basal cell carcinoma depends on the size, number, location, nature of the lesion, and the physical health of the patient. The most important goals for management are (1) complete removal of the tumor, (2) preservation of as much normal tissue as possible, (3) preservation of function of body parts, and (4) optimal cosmetic results. Obviously, the first goal is the most important. Smaller lesions may be widely excised and primarily closed or repaired by a graft or rotational skin flap. Clinicians not experienced

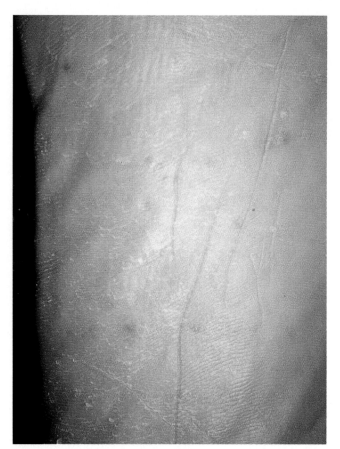

Figure 14–17 **Basal cell nevus syndrome.** Tiny pits on the plantar surface of the soles are characteristic additional features of this condition.

in the treatment of malignant lesions should readily refer patients suspected of having a malignant neoplasm to a specialist.

SQUAMOUS CELL CARCINOMA

Cutaneous squamous cell carcinoma is a primary malignant neoplasm of the keratinizing cells of the epidermis. It is the second most prevalent malignant tumor of the skin. This condition is a potentially dangerous tumor that may infiltrate surrounding tissues and metastasize to lymph nodes and subsequently be fatal. Primary squamous cell carcinoma is most commonly associated with skin damage by solar ultraviolet radiation. As previously discussed, secondary squamous cell carcinoma may result from radiation exposure, carcinogens, chronic skin wounds, scars, genetic disorders, and human papillomaviruses. This tumor may occur as either an ulcer or a nodule. Most squamous cell carcinomas arising in areas of prior sun-damaged skin are less aggressive and less likely to metastasize. On the contrary, squamous cell carcinoma originating in areas of prior chronic ulcers, injury, sinuses, and burn scars are typically more aggressive and have a high frequency of metastases.

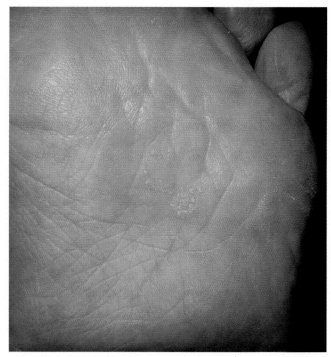

Figure 14–18 **Squamous cell carcinoma.** This early squamous cell carcinoma presented as a verrucous plaque on the sole of the foot.

There is no specific or distinct clinical presentations that establish the diagnosis of squamous cell carcinoma. Typically, squamous cell carcinoma lesions are pink, red, red-brown, to tan. Tumors may appear as light-colored plaques (Fig. 14–18) or as nodules (Fig. 14–19). Early lesions and those in moist areas or with overlying hyperkeratosis may appear white. The pearly trans-

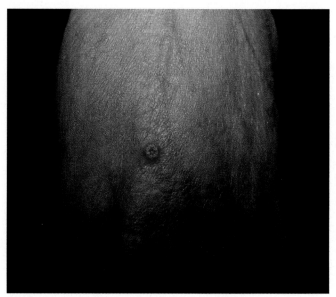

Figure 14–19 **Squamous cell carcinoma.** A small nodular lesion with an erosive center was thought to be molluscum contagiosum. Biopsy confirmed squamous cell carcinoma.

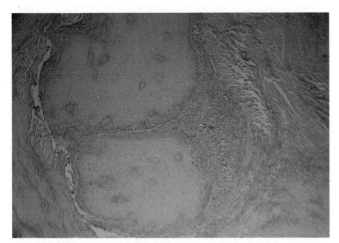

Figure 14–20 Squamous cell carcinoma. Well-differentiated invasive tumor shows dermal infiltration by islands of mature squamous epithelium with obvious keratinization.

lucency and pearl-colored lining of basal cell carcinoma is missing in squamous cell carcinomas. They may have a wide variation in erosion, scaling, crusting, and ulceration. Differentiation is usually difficult, and confirmative diagnosis is based on the findings of the biopsy for histological examination.

The histological appearance of squamous cell carcinoma is variable, as is the disease, and depends on the degree of differentiation (Fig. 14–20). The tumors are classified into well-differentiated, moderately differentiated, minimally differentiated, and poorly differentiated. Differentiation is based on the Broders system. Grade I represents well-differentiated keratinizing neoplasms, and the patient generally has the best prognosis. Grade II represents less keratinization with blurring of the tumor-stroma interface. Grade III demonstrates minimal keratinization with nearly uniform cellular atypia. Grade IV shows a lack of keratinization and evidence of intercellular bridges and may resemble sarcomas. This level represents patients with the worst prognoses.

Squamous cell carcinoma should be managed by the

surgeon, oncologist, and radiotherapist. Surgical excision is the treatment of choice for most lesions (Fig. 14–21), but radiation therapy is effective for some lesions not responsive to surgery. Oncological consultation should take place for every patient with confirmed malignant neoplasm.

KAPOSI'S SARCOMA

Kaposi's sarcoma is an indolent skin tumor usually involving the lower extremities, especially the ankles and feet, of older men of eastern European or Mediterranean origin or Jewish heritage. Kaposi's sarcoma has also been seen in patients with acquired immunodeficiency syndrome (AIDS), particularly homosexual men. In this patient group, the lesions tend to occur on the upper rather than the lower half of the body but appear identical to classic Kaposi's sarcoma.

Clinically, in all groups, the lesions begin as violaceous macules and papules and very slowly progress to form plaques with multiple red-purple nodules (Fig. 14–22). They may be ulcerated or diffusely infiltrative and have many different sizes.

The histopathology of the lesions of Kaposi's sarcoma reveals vascular proliferation (accounting for the violaceous discoloration), hemorrhage, and hemosiderin deposition (Fig. 14–23). Throughout the papillary and reticular dermis there is a proliferation of dilated, thin-walled, irregularly shaped vessels in association with perivascular inflammatory cell infiltrate composed of lymphocytes and plasma cells. Treatment of non–AIDS-associated Kaposi's sarcoma may not be required, but the lesions are responsive to radiation therapy. Several therapeutic protocols are currently available for the treatment of AIDS-related Kaposi's sarcoma.

MALIGNANT MELANOMA

Malignant melanoma is one of the most dangerous cutaneous neoplasms seen on the lower extremities. This malignancy arises from cells of the melanocytic system,

Figure 14–21 Squamous cell carcinoma. *A*, Tumor on anterior shin of leg. *B*, Appearance 1 week after wide excision.

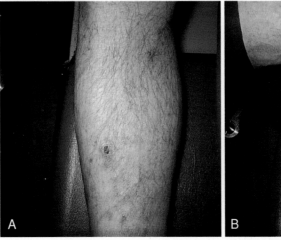
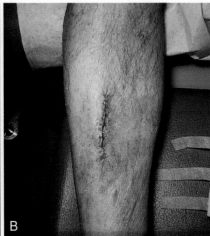

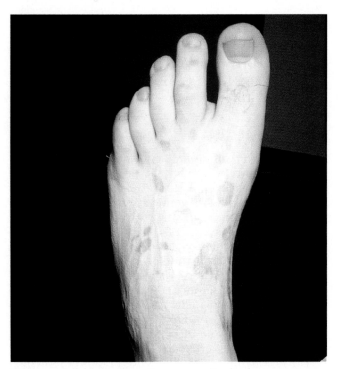

Figure 14–22 **Kaposi's sarcoma.** Purple plaques occur particularly on the dorsa of the feet.

incidence of this condition is greater in patients with fair complexion, red hair, blue eyes, freckles, and poor tanning ability who live in areas where solar exposure is high. Interestingly, the incidence of malignant melanoma is higher in city dwellers than in patients who are outdoor workers. This finding would appear to indicate that acute episodic exposures to sunlight, such as on vacation, cause greater risks than constant occupational sun exposure.

The diagnosis of malignant melanoma is enhanced by recognizing several early findings in lesions that are consistent with this condition. These are the ABCDs of early malignant melanoma recognition. Malignant melanomas have a tendency to have *A*symmetry, *B*order irregularity, *C*olor variegation, and *D*iameter enlargement. As a rule, benign nevi are roughly symmetrical with a regular border and have a uniform tan, brown, or black color. If the nevus could be folded in half, the two sections would match or superimpose on one another (Fig. 14–24). Changes in the appearance, shape, and borders of lesions are important early signs that should always make the physician suspect malignancy. Sudden changes in color or surface characteristics, such as ulceration or bleeding, may also be early indicators of malignant transformation. Because most malignant melanomas develop de novo on skin that

and it has the ability to metastasize to any organ system, including the brain and heart. Metastasis occurs through the lymphatic vessels to the lymph nodes and through the blood vessels to the brain, lungs, heart, bones, and skin. This condition was once considered rare but is now thought to be one of the most common malignant conditions seen by dermatologists and podiatrists. Ultraviolet light, which is increased due to recreational sun exposure and alterations in the protective ozone layer of the upper atmosphere by pollutants, is the most important cause of malignant melanoma. The

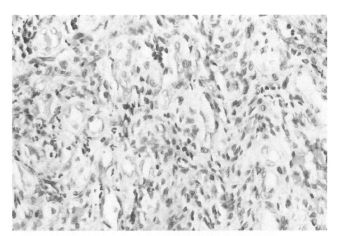

Figure 14–23 **Kaposi's sarcoma.** The early stages of the evolution of Kaposi's sarcoma are characterized by development of irregular cleft-like vascular channels lined by slightly atypical hyperchromatic endothelial cells (hematoxylin and eosin).

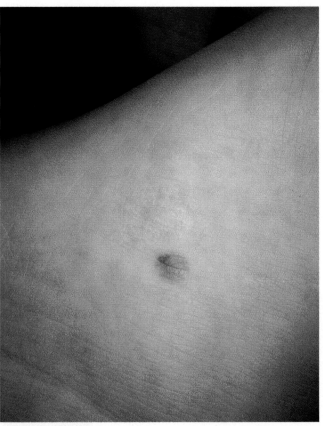

Figure 14–24 **Nevus.** Benign nevus has regular border with symmetrical shape.

was previously normal it is usually easier to notice and see changes. However, about 30% of malignant melanomas develop within or close to previous preexisting junctional nevi. It is usually far more difficult to observe noticeable changes within these lesions.

Clinical classification of malignant melanoma is based on characteristic patterns. The proposed types are superficial spreading melanoma, lentigo maligna melanoma, nodular melanoma, and acral lentiginous melanoma. Those lesions that do not conform to this clinicopathological classification are usually simply labeled as malignant melanoma. These classifications are important in determining the survival rate and potential for metastasis for each lesion. Once a melanocyte becomes neoplastic, it may spread by either radial or vertical growth phases. A radial (horizontal) growth phase in a melanoma is that phase in which the proliferation of well-differentiated malignant melanocytes is confined to the epidermis and there is minimal penetration into the papillary and reticular dermis. This finding provides a slow progression of spread. In the vertical growth phase, more immature groups of cells would be more aggressive and extend and regress at a faster rate. This poorly differentiated cell has no affinity for the epidermis and may grow both horizontally and vertically, penetrating the dermis, producing a mass or palpable nodular lesion.

Superficial spreading melanoma may develop on any portion of the body and at any age with a peak incidence in the late fourth and early fifth decade. It be-

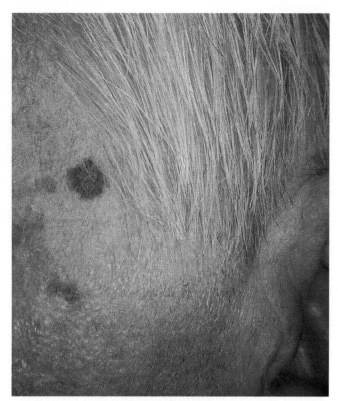

Figure 14–26 Lentigo maligna. This patient had a history of basal cell carcinoma on the cheek in addition to the lentigo. Chronic solar irradiation is one of the causes of this condition.

gins in a nonspecific manner and then changes shape by radial spread and regression (Fig. 14–25). If it is diagnosed early, the prognosis is excellent with a 5-year survival rate of 95%. The lower extremities are involved frequently, and this condition is more common in women. These lesions are raised above the skin surface and have an irregular border with variable and unevenly distributed pigmentation. In the radial growth phase, superficial spreading melanoma displays proliferation of melanocytes that are confined to the epidermis. Ultimately, however, the lesion grows vertically and a nodule develops. It is during this phase that the superficial spreading melanoma may metastasize.

Lentigo maligna melanoma has its predominance on the sun-exposed areas of the body. This lesion begins as a malignant melanoma in situ (lentigo maligna) that grows very slowly; after a number of years, however, it may become invasive (lentigo maligna melanoma). This condition is seen frequently in the elderly, most commonly on the face (Fig. 14–26). The radial growth phase may precede the vertical growth phase by several decades. The vertical growth phase is associated with metastasis in 25% of cases. Clinically, the lesions first appear as a flat pigmented lesion that gradually enlarges. The pigment varies from tan to black, and there may be areas of red, white, blue, or gray. The margin of the lentigo maligna melanoma is irregular, being notched

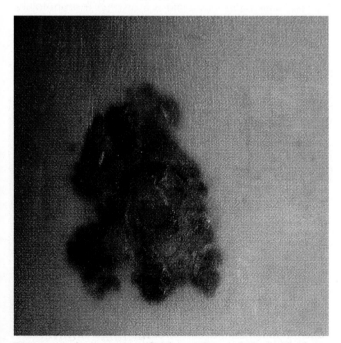

Figure 14–25 Superficial spreading melanoma. The lesion is elevated with irregular borders and is almost totally black except for a reddish brown area in the center. (Courtesy of Dr. Byron Hutchinson.)

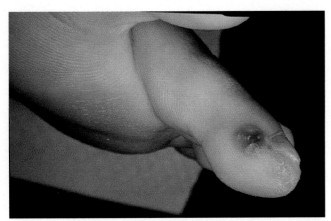

Figure 14–27   Nodular melanoma. This firm nodule on the toe represents the classic presentation. This lesion grows vertically from the beginning, and invasion produces a nodule.

and indented. Ultimately, the lesion becomes nodular and may become quite large.

Nodular melanoma is the most malignant of the four types of melanoma. This lesion is more common in men (2:1 ratio) and occurs most often in the fifth or sixth decade. Nodular melanoma may be found on any body area and occurs as a distinct nodularity with blue, brown, or black pigmentation (Fig. 14–27). It is occasionally amelanotic (flesh colored) and resembles non-pigmented dermal nevi. This lesion is raised, is nodular, and may ulcerate. Nodular melanoma does not appear to have a horizontal growth phase. It grows very quickly and vertically from the beginning. The patient with this type of melanoma has a grave prognosis compared with superficial spreading because of the speed at which it evolves and the depth of penetration that it reaches. Nodular melanoma is the most frequently misdiagnosed form of melanoma because of its rapid onset and the fact that it resembles a blood blister, hemangioma, dermal nevus, or polyp (Fig. 14–28).

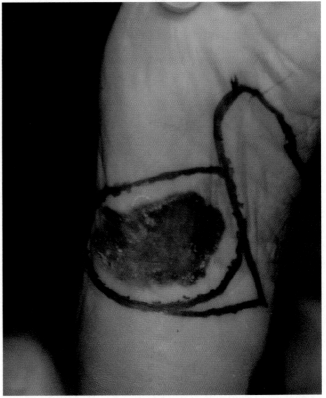

Figure 14–29   Acral lentiginous melanoma. This large lesion on the plantar sole of the foot in an elderly woman began to change in color and shape after many years of remaining quiescent.

Acral lentiginous melanoma is a distinct morphological and biological type of melanoma with a predilection for the palms, soles (Fig. 14–29), and nail beds (Fig. 14–30). It is found frequently in blacks and Asians. The lesions may be similar in appearance and color to lentigo

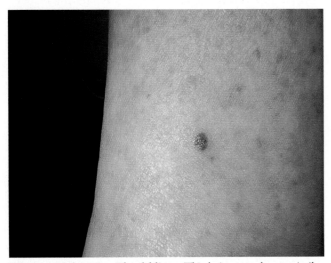

Figure 14–28   Blood blister. This lesion may have a similar appearance to nodular melanoma.

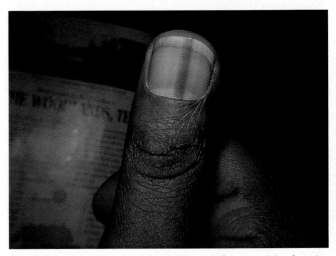

Figure 14–30   Acral lentiginous melanoma. Macular pigmentation suddenly appearing in a band originating from the proximal nail fold (Hutchinson's sign) may be suggestive of acral lentiginous melanoma.

maligna melanoma. They have a tendency to be flat due to an extended horizontal growth phase and may remain latent for many years. The peak incidence is during the sixth or seventh decade.

The majority of acral lentiginous melanomas are found on the plantar skin, especially in the weight-bearing areas. In subungual lesions, 92% are on the thumb or hallux. Small areas of elevation and increased color may be associated with vertical growth (deep invasion). In this case, the tumor may become very aggressive and metastasize. The sudden appearance of a subungual pigmented band originating at the proximal nail fold (Hutchinson's sign) is extremely suggestive. The presence of a vascular nodule in association with discoloration or erosion of the nail plate is indicative of an invasive growth phase (Fig. 14–31). Histological examination shows that cells of the vertical growth phase display a high degree of cytological pleomorphism, abundant mitotic activity, and minimal pigment in the cytoplasm. This lesion, when seen on the toes, may be misdiagnosed as pyogenic granuloma. There can be partial or decreased pigmentation, which leads to further problems with attempts at visual diagnosis. Clinically, other acral malignant melanomas may be difficult to identify. Advanced malignant melanoma of the sole or

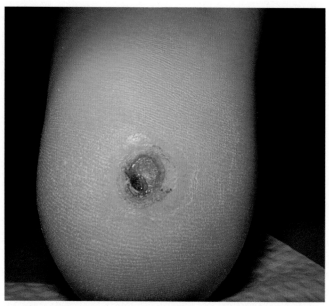

Figure 14–32 Advanced malignant melanoma. The lesion on the weight-bearing heel is partially amelanotic and is ulcerated, making the clinical diagnosis very difficult.

heel of the foot may be partially or totally amelanotic and may show ulceration (Fig. 14–32). Patients with ulcers more than 3 mm in breadth have been associated with a poor prognosis.

All lesions suspected of being malignant melanomas should be sampled, or the patient should be referred to a dermatologist or an oncologist. Histological evaluation is essential to the correct diagnosis and to determination of the thickness, level of invasion, and type and mitotic activity of the lesion. A properly performed biopsy will obviate unnecessary radical surgery or amputation should the lesion be found benign.

Decisions concerning the type and extent of surgery depend on the type, level, and thickness of the lesion. The American Joint Committee on Cancer has adopted a staging system for malignant melanomas based on the primary tumor thickness, the presence of node metastasis, and the presence of distant metastasis.[1] This system utilizes the combined level of invasion (Clark's System of Microstaging) and the measurement of thickness (Breslow's System of Microstaging). The categories and stage groupings are summarized in Table 14–1. Based on this classification, the 5- and 10-year survival rates by stage are, respectively, 97% and 95% for stage I, 77% and 68% for stage II, 48% and 40% for stage III, and 0% and 0% for stage IV. The four-stage system delineates distinct prognostic groups of patients that are more evenly divided than in any other staging system. This grouping also aids the physician in choosing the most effective treatment program. Patients with malignant melanoma should be examined regularly for local recurrence, metastasis, and new malignancy, and they should be monitored for the rest of their lives.

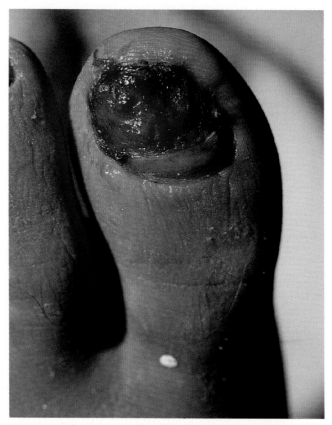

Figure 14–31 Acral lentiginous melanoma. There is complete loss of the distal nail plate and bed. Distally, there is a large vascular nodule (which is amelanotic) representing the vertical growth phase. This lesion was misdiagnosed as a pyogenic granuloma.

TABLE 14–1 Melanoma Staging System (American Joint Committee on Cancer)

Stage	Description
Primary Tumor (pT)	
pTX	Primary tumor cannot be assessed.
pT0	No evidence of primary tumor
pTis	Melanoma in situ (atypical melanotic hyperplasia, severe melantoic dysplasia), not an invasive lesion (Clark's level I)
pT1	Tumor 0.75 mm or less in thickness and invades the papillary dermis (Clark's level II)
pT2	Tumor more than 0.75 but not more than 1.5 mm in thickness and/or invades to papillary-reticular dermal interface (Clark's level III)
pT3	Tumor more than 1.5 mm but not more than 4 mm in thickness and/or invades the reticular dermis (Clark's level IV)
pT3a	Tumor more than 1.5 mm but not more than 3 mm in thickness
pT3b	Tumor more than 3 mm but not more than 4 mm in thickness
pT4	Tumor more than 4 mm in thickness and/or invades the subcutaneous tissue (Clark's level IV) and/or satellite(s) within 2 cm of the primary tumor
pT4a	Tumor more than 4 mm in thickness and/or invades the subcutaneous tissue.
pT4b	Satellite(s) with 2 cm of primary tumor
Lymph Node (N)	
NX	Regional lymph nodes cannot be assessed.
N0	No regional lymph node metastasis
N1	Metastasis 3 cm or less in greatest dimension in any regional lymph node(s)
N2	Metastasis more than 3 cm in greatest dimension in any regional lymph node(s) and/or in-transit metastasis
N2a	Metastasis more than 3 cm in greatest dimension in any regional lymph node(s)
N2b	In-transit metastasis
N2c	Both (N2a and N2b)
Distant Metastasis (M)	
MX	Presence of distant metastasis cannot be assessed.
M0	No distant metastasis
M1	Distant metastasis
M1a	Metastasis in skin or subcutaneous tissue or lymph node(s)
M1b	Visceral metastasis
Stage Grouping	
Stage Ia	pT1, N0, M0 (localized melanoma < 0.75 mm or level II)
Stage Ib	pT2, N0, M0 (localized melanoma 0.76 to 1.5 mm or level III)
Stage II	pT3, N0, M0 (localized melanoma 1.5 mm to 4 mm or level IV)
Stage IIIa	pT4, N0, M0 (localized melanoma > 4.1 mm or level V)
Stage IIIb	Any pT, N1, N2, M0 (limited nodal metastases involving only one regional lymph node basin or <5 in-transit metastases, but without nodal metastases)
Stage IV	Any pT, any N, M1, M2 (advanced regional metastases or any patient with distant metastases)

REFERENCE

American Joint Committee on Cancer: Manual for Cancer Staging, 3rd ed, pp 143–144, 1988.

BIBLIOGRAPHY

Berlin SJ, Clancy JT, Giordano ML: Kaposi's sarcoma of the foot: A review and report of 156 cases. J Am Podiatr Med Assoc 79:311–317, 1989.

Bowen JT: Precancerous dermatoses: A study of two cases of chronic atypical epithelial proliferation. J Cutan Dis 30:241–243, 1912.

Breslow A: Thickness, cross-sectional area and depth of invasion in the prognosis of cutaneous melanoma. Ann Surg 172:902–905, 1970.

Breslow A: Prognostic factors in the treatment of cutaneous malignant melanoma. J Cutan Pathol 6:208–210, 1979.

Broders AC: Squamous cell epithelioma of the skin. Ann Surg 73:141–146, 1921.

Brownstein MH, Shapiro L: Verrucous carcinoma of skin: Epithelioma cuniculatum plantare. Cancer 38:1710–1712, 1976.

Clark WH Jr: The histogenesis and biologic behavior of primary human malignant melanoma of the skin. Cancer Res 29:705–711, 1969.

Clark WH Jr, Mihm MC: Lentigo maligna and lentigo maligna melanoma. Am J Pathol 55:39–67, 1969.

Frankel AH, Warren AM: Verrucous squamous cell carcinoma. J Foot Surg 25:307–310, 1986.

Friedman HI, Cooper PH, Wanebo HJ: Prognostic and therapeutic use of microstaging of cutaneous squamous cell carcinoma of the trunk and extremities. Cancer 56:1099–1105, 1985.

Gorlin RJ: Nevoid basal-cell carcinoma syndrome. Medicine 66:98–113, 1987.

Graham JH, Helwig EB: Bowen's disease and its relationship to systemic cancer. Arch Dermatol 80:133–136, 1959.

Green JG, Ferrara JA, Haber JA: Epithelioma cuniculatum plantare. J Foot Surg 26:78–83, 1987.

Guadara J, Segi A, Labruna V, Welch M, Gazivoda PL: Transformation of plantar verruca into squamous cell carcinoma. J Foot Surg 31:611–614, 1992.

Hale D, Dockery GL: Giant keratoacanthoma of the plantar foot: A report of two cases. J Foot Surg 32:75–84, 1993.

Hilton L, Simpson RR, Simpson RR: Differential diagnosis of plantar palmar keratoderma. J Am Podiatr Assoc 68:578–584, 1978.

Horn L, Sage R: Verrucous squamous cell carcinoma of the foot. J Am Podiatr Med Assoc 78:227–232, 1988.

Hutchinson BL: Malignant melanoma in the lower extremity: A comprehensive overview. Clin Podiatr Med Surg 3:533–550, 1986.

Jones RR, Spaull J, Spry C, Jones EW: Histogenesis of Kaposi's sarcoma in patients with and without acquired immune deficiency syndrome. J Clin Pathol 39:742–748, 1986.

Kallibjian AE, Choos JN: Keratoacanthoma or verrucous carcinoma? A case report. J Foot Ankle Surg 32:584–590, 1993.

Kaplan RP: Cancer complicating chronic ulcerative and scarring mucocutaneous disorders. Adv Dermatol 2:19–23, 1987.

Leis SB, Bayne O, Karlin JM, Scurran BL, Reiner M: Squamous cell carcinoma: An unusual early complication of postoperative osteomyelitis. J Foot Ankle Surg 33:21–27, 1994.

Levi MJ, Boykoff TJ, Levy SE: Acral lentiginous malignant melanoma. J Am Podiatr Med Assoc 79:519–520, 1989

Lewis J, Mendicino RW: Squamous cell carcinoma of the great toe. J Foot Ankle Surg 33:482–485, 1994.

Lifeso RM, Bull CA: Squamous cell carcinoma of the extremities. Cancer 55:2862–2867, 1985.

Marczak L: Epidermal inclusion cyst of the heel. J Am Podiatr Med Assoc 80:660–661, 1990.

McCarthy DJ: Helomata and tylomata. In McCarthy DJ, Montgomery R (eds): Podiatric Dermatology, pp 53–73. Baltimore, Williams & Wilkins, 1986.

McCarthy DJ: Cutaneous malignancies of the human foot. In McCarthy DJ, Montgomery R (eds): Podiatric Dermatology, pp 235–254. Baltimore, Williams & Wilkins, 1986.

Menn JJ, Boberg J: Fibroepithelial polyps: An unusual case report. J Am Podiatr Med Assoc 80:496–498, 1990.

Muehlman C, Rahimi F: Aging integumentary system: Podiatric review. J Am Podiatr Med Assoc 80:577–582, 1990.

Norton JR, Kaspar GD: Bowen's disease: A case report. J Foot Surg 17:120–123, 1978.

Novicki M: Burn scar carcinoma: A review and analysis of 46 cases. J Trauma 17:808–817, 1977.

Rabinowitz AD: Skin tumors. Clin Dermatol 1:54–66, 1983.

Schiraldi FG, Korostoff SB, McElgun T: Acral lentiginous melanoma. J Am Podiatr Med Assoc 77:554–556, 1989.

Simmonds WL: Management of actinic keratosis with topical 5-fluorouracil. Cutis 18:298–300, 1976.

Smith PJ, Hylinski JH, Axe S: Verrucous carcinoma: Epithelioma cuniculatum plantare. J Foot Surg 31:324–328, 1992.

Techner LM, Eannace RJ: Squamous cell carcinoma in situ (Bowen's disease). J Am Podiatr Med Assoc 77:662–664, 1989.

Vance CE, Levy L: Recognizing arsenical keratosis. J Am Podiatr Assoc 66:91–94, 1976.

Wallace GF, Peters S: Verrucous carcinoma with a dorsal sinus tract. J Am Podiatr Med Assoc 85:271–273, 1995.

Wolf WB, Cohen LS: Intraepidermal squamous cell carcinoma (Bowen's disease of the dorsum of the foot). J Am Podiatr Assoc 68:688–690, 1978.

Zivot ML, Kanat IO: Malignant melanoma: A clinical and surgical review: I. Introduction and general discussion. J Am Podiatr Med Assoc 79:367–374, 1989.

Zivot ML, Kanat IO: Malignant melanoma: A clinical and surgical review: II. Diagnosis and treatment. J Am Podiatr Med Assoc 79:421–431, 1989.

MECHANICAL INJURIES

INTRODUCTION

Superficial trauma to the cutaneous and soft tissue layers secondary to mechanical pressure, irritation, and injury is often an overlooked and neglected area of dermatology. Many physicians consider these lesions to be unimportant or inconsequential, and they can relegate treatment to home care by the patient or delegate a staff technician to do minor treatment. In reality, many of these mechanical injuries are very uncomfortable for the patient and proper diagnosis and treatment may be very beneficial. Conditions range from simple blister formation to deep scars from puncture wounds. Other associated conditions include callus formation, hyperkeratoses, ulcerations, bruises, scratches, and foreign-body injuries.

BLACK HEEL SYNDROME

Black heel syndrome is an asymptomatic irregular hemorrhage caused by sudden shear forces that fracture or tear small superficial blood vessels. This relatively common entity is a traumatic lesion that has been termed *calcaneal petechiae* and *talon noir.* However, the definition of post-traumatic punctate hemorrhage of the skin is probably more accurate. This is commonly seen in patients involved in competitive sports such as basketball and running. The lesions usually appear as punctate, discrete, dark brown to black macules on the sole of the foot or edge of the heel (Fig. 15–1). Because this lesion is often confused with melanoma, it is important that it be quickly differentiated. This condition is usually asymptomatic, and thus it may be disregarded as far as treatment is concerned. If the condition persists or becomes bothersome, lining the heel of the shoe with felt helps.

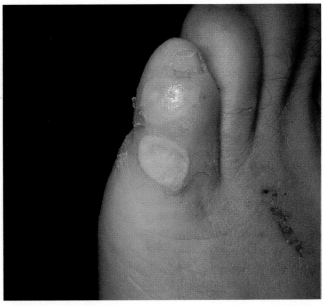

Figure 15–2   Friction blister. Common location of friction blisters is on the tops of the toes.

BLISTERS

Blisters are usually secondary to friction and shearing forces on the skin of the lower extremities. The most common areas of involvement are the ends and tops of the toes (Fig. 15–2), the ball of the foot (Fig. 15–3), and the posterior heel (Fig. 15–4). Blisters are characterized by their generalized appearance of an oval or a circum-

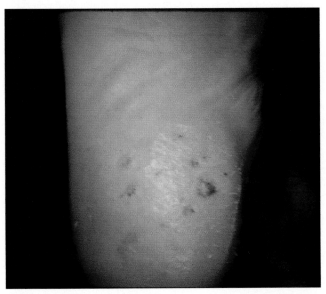

Figure 15–1   Black heel. Multiple punctate intradermal hemorrhages on the plantar heel of an athlete are due to shearing forces.

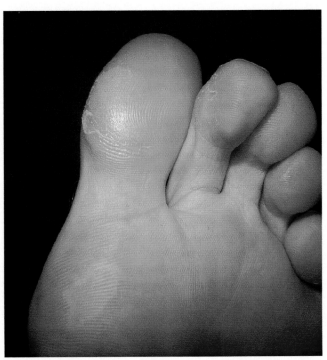

Figure 15–3   Friction blister. Plantar weight-bearing ball of the foot shows simple friction blisters.

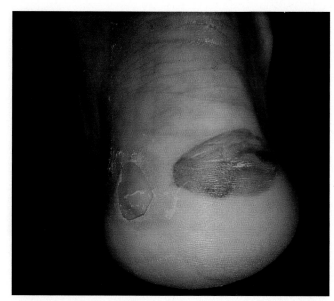

Figure 15-4 Friction blister. On posterior heel region smaller fluid blister has been deroofed and larger blister has a hemorrhagic component indicating continued pressure after blister formation.

scribed elevation of the skin containing clear fluid between the layers of the epidermis. In some cases, there may be a hemorrhagic component if the pressure or friction continues to an area of blister formation. The elevated portion of the blister is termed the *roof* and the remaining layers are the *floor* or *base* of the blister. Preventative measures include using talc to reduce the friction, wearing two pairs of socks (one lighter pair covered by regular absorbent socks), and wearing properly fitted shoes with cushion insoles that reduce shearing forces on the plantar foot. Patients should be instructed to apply an adhesive bandage or a moleskin felt pad to blister-prone areas and to prevent getting the shoes or socks wet. Extremes of dryness and wetness decrease friction, whereas intermediate moisture tends to increase friction. Skin that is warm or hot will form blisters more easily than will cool or cold skin.

Treatment of blisters begins with draining the blister, applying an antiseptic, and covering the area with a dry sterile protective dressing. Deroofing blisters causes increased irritation and inflammation, leading to greater discomfort and increased risk of secondary infection (Fig. 15–5). The blister roof should be preserved with fluid drainage performed by multiple aspirations during the first 24 hours or a single aspiration at some time between 24 and 36 hours. This technique appears to allow the blister roof to adhere to the floor of the blister, resulting in decreased discomfort and much earlier healing.

BRUISES

When blood extravasates into the intracutaneous or subcutaneous layers the condition is termed *purpura*.

Purpura does not blanch on pressure and is classified as either petechiae or ecchymoses. Small macular areas of purpura are called petechiae, and when the lesions are larger and of variable shape and color, they are called ecchymoses, or common bruises. There are several causes of purpura, and the differential diagnosis should be completed to rule out platelet abnormalities, coagulopathies, and other like disorders. In this section, the condition being reviewed is directly or indirectly related to nonpathological hemorrhagic bruising.

Bruising may be due to direct local trauma or injury (see Fig. 9–48), which is termed a *contusion,* and is usually a local hemorrhage with soft tissue injury. When there is considerable bleeding there may be blistering (Fig. 15–6). Purpuric bruises may also occur at distal areas from trauma or surgery (Fig. 15–7). The hemorrhage that occurs at a superior portion of the body may seek an area of less pressure or simply relocate, owing to gravity, to a more distal region of the body. This finding is very common on the lower leg and ankle when injury or surgery is performed and bruising is noted in the heel or toes several days later. This condition is usually asymptomatic, but in some cases the pressure of the hemorrhagic fluid causes discomfort. Moist, warm compression will speed the resolution of this condition and allow early healing.

BURSITIS

A bursa is a closed, flat, synovial-lined sac that is present in areas subject to excessive friction or pressure. These

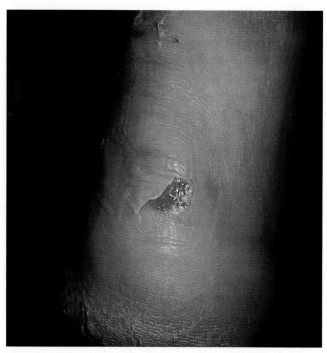

Figure 15-5 Friction blister. Posterior heel blister has been partially deroofed, causing increased pain and inflammation.

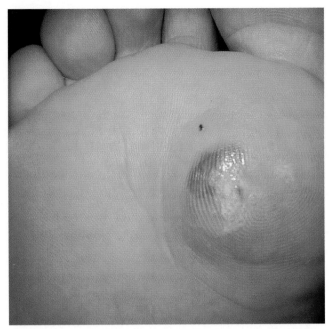

Figure 15–6   Bruise. Trauma-induced hemorrhage with blister formation is evident on the ball of the foot.

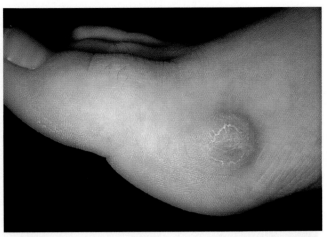

Figure 15–8   Adventitious bursa. Common bursitis occurred over the dorsomedial aspect of the first metatarsophalangeal joint.

sacs are located near joints or where skin, muscle, and tendon move over bony prominences. Bursae may be either adventitious (acquired) or anatomical. Pathological bursae may represent either of these types, which have become thick-walled and distended from chronic irritation, inflammation, infection, or pressure. These inflamed bursae are smooth to palpation, unilobular, distended, and usually tender. Symptoms of pain and inflammation may be associated with adventitious bur-

sae located at the dorsomedial first metatarsophalangeal joint (Fig. 15–8), at the superficial Achilles tendon (Fig. 15–9), around digits, and at the dorsolateral fifth metatarsophalangeal joint (Fig. 15–10). Inflammatory bursitis may be seen in cases of gout (Fig. 15–11) and rheumatoid arthritis (Fig. 15–12).

Treatment involves relief of pressure and irritation and reduction of inflammation with rest, padding and strapping, local and systemic anti-inflammatory drugs, physical therapy, intralesional injections of cortisone, and, if necessary, surgical intervention. Care must be

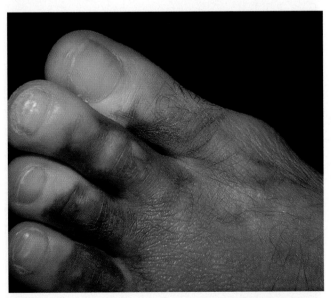

Figure 15–7   Bruise. This purpuric bruising is seen in the toes in a patient who had ankle surgery. The blood extravasated from the superior area and collected in the distal digits.

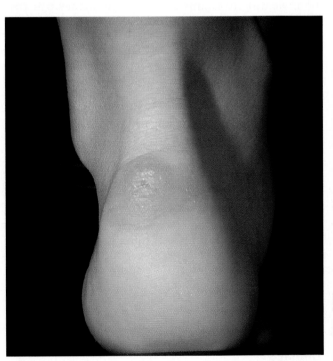

Figure 15–9   Adventitious bursa. Superficial Achilles bursitis occurred at the posterior heel area.

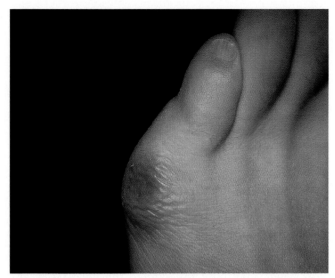

Figure 15–10   Adventitious bursa. Typical irritated bursa are located over the dorsolateral aspect of the fifth metatarsophalangeal joint.

taken with intralesional injections of corticosteroid because of the potential for atrophy and discoloration (Fig. 15–13).

DECUBITUS AND NEUROTROPIC ULCERS

The decubitus ulcer (pressure ulcer) is most often due to prolonged pressure on a body part resulting in a breakdown of the tissue leading to ulceration of the skin. The increased pressure for extended times causes compression of the capillary circulation leading to ischemia. Onset of a pressure ulcer is usually preceded by intense erythema over a body prominence that, when untreated, rapidly progresses to a necrotic tissue ulcer (Fig. 15–14). This type of ulceration spreads widely with peripheral undermining. Its depth may extend through the skin, subcutaneous tissue, and muscle exposing the underlying bone. The sacral areas, trochanter and ischial tuberosity, and the heels are the

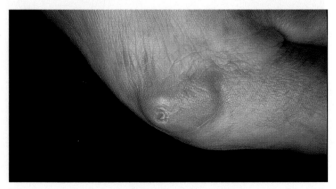

Figure 15–11   Inflammatory bursa. Large area of bursitis over the first metatarsophalangeal joint is secondary to gout.

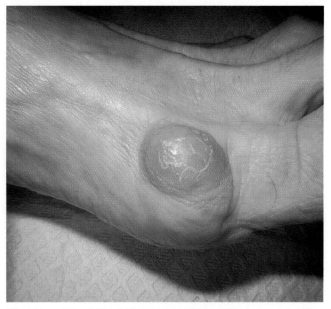

Figure 15–12   Inflammatory bursa. Bursa over the first metatarsophalangeal joint is seen in rheumatoid arthritis.

most common areas for decubitus ulcers. The common denominator of all pressure ulcers is ischemia of the tissues from shearing forces and external pressure. Shearing forces produced by repeated sliding of a patient up in bed may produce an area of thick necrosis referred to as a neuropathic eschar (Fig. 15–15). This tissue is

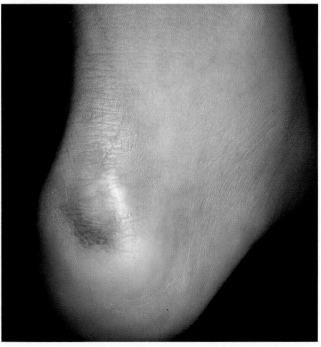

Figure 15–13   Corticosteroid complication. Atrophy and discoloration are noted at the posterior heel after several cortisone injections of the superficial heel bursa.

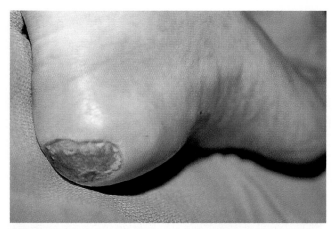

Figure 15–14   Decubitus ulcer. Left heel of a bedridden patient.

very difficult to remove, and the underlying ulcer is slow to heal.

The best treatment of decubitus ulcers is prevention. Careful examination of pressure points on the body reveals areas of early erythema. Frequent rotation and moving of bedridden or wheelchair-bound patients prevents long-term pressure from occurring in one area. Protective clothing, bed sheets, lambs' wool padding, rubber or air cushions, elevation of the heels off the bed, heel protectors, and skin lubricants offer additional relief of pressure from prominent areas. Once an ulcer forms, treatment consists of local wound care to clear any tissue necrotic borders and the ulcer base. In the early stages, occlusive dressings and antibiotics may be recommended. If there is an adjacent dermatitis, the ulcer is treated with a hydrogel until the surrounding skin

heals. The ulcer is then treated as a clean ulcer with hydrocolloid dressings and occlusion. A multidisciplinary approach by internal medicine, podiatric, nursing, and rehabilitation staff is usually required to heal this type of ulcer.

Neuropathic or neurotropic ulcers of the lower extremities are also common in bedridden and elderly patients. They are essentially due to insensitivity and increased pressure combined to allow tissue breakdown. The neurotropic ulcer is typically a punched-out or sharply demarcated ulcer surrounded by a thick peripheral border of callus (Fig. 15–16). The skin around the ulcer is usually anhidrotic, and the tissue is warm. Repetitive mechanical pressure or cyclical biomechanical trauma under areas of weight bearing or bony prominence may cause ulceration. These ulcers are generally referred to as *mal perforans* (Fig. 15–17). Long-standing ulcers may lead to additional problems because the deep scar layers may bind the skin to the deep fascia and bone, placing the skin under increased mechanical stress. The underlying collagen network is replaced with fibrous scar tissue, which does not have the capacity to adapt and dissipate stress forces. This condition causes further tissue breakdown and prevents adequate healing. When this type of ulcer is carefully debrided, it is apparent that the entire periphery of the lesion is firmly adhered to the underlying fascia or bone (Fig. 15–18). A *black eschar* may develop within deep adherent ulcers (Fig. 15–19).

Neurotropic ulcers may be classified by the Wagner six-grade method of categorizing ulcers:

Grade 0: Skin intact, possible osseous deformity may place foot at risk

Grade 1: Localized, superficial ulceration

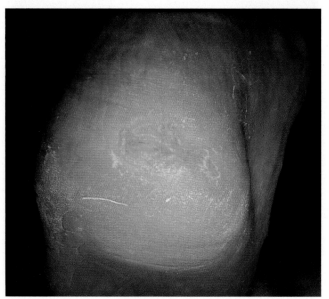

Figure 15–15   Neuropathic eschar. Repeated shearing forces and external pressures over the heel result in a thickened area of necrosis.

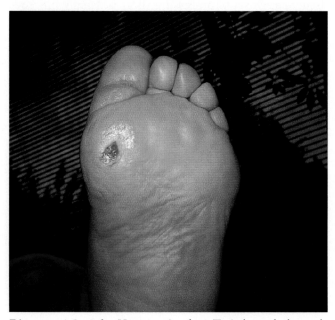

Figure 15–16   Neurotropic ulcer. Typical punched-out ulceration on a weight-bearing area of the sole of the foot.

Grade 2: Deep ulcer with extension to tendon, ligament, bone, or joint
Grade 3: Deep abscess with osteomyelitis
Grade 4: Gangrene of toes or forefoot
Grade 5: Gangrene of the whole foot.

Treatment of this type of ulcer is similar to the management of other ulcerations of the lower extremities. Protection of the area is crucial. Local wound care with debridement and antibiotics follows the standard guidelines. In this condition, additional surgical management may be warranted with osseous correction by either exostectomy or osteotomy of the underlying pathology to reduce pressure areas as needed. Excision of the ulcer with primary closure or skin grafting may be necessary in some cases. Occasionally, some ulcers lend themselves to repair by rotational skin flaps. The advantages of covering the ulcer site with a rotation skin flap or other skin plasty procedure are more rapid healing, a more pliable scar that may better withstand pressure, and a quicker return to activity. A covered ulcer decreases additional risks of infection and a continued need for constant wound care. A black eschar that is attached to bone is left untreated until it starts to spontaneously separate. If the black eschar is separating from the borders of the ulcer, there is underlying softness, or the surrounding skin is erythematous, tender, or appears infected, it is surgically removed. The necrotic tissue is removed, and the ulcer is then managed as either a clean or dirty ulcer.

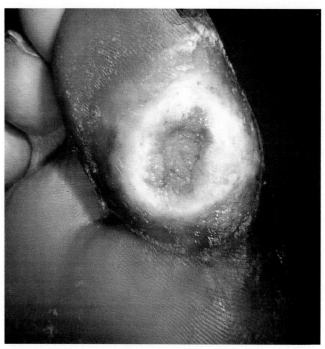

Figure 15–18   Neurotropic ulcer. Debridement of the callus border shows that the lesion is firmly attached to the underlying fascia and bone and does not move with manipulation.

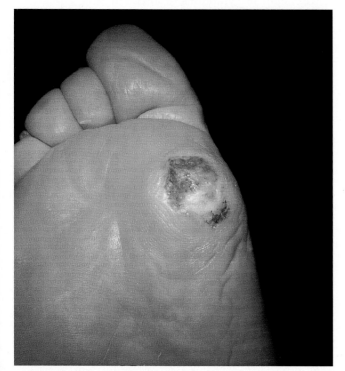

Figure 15–17   Neurotropic ulcer. Mal perforans with thick callus rim that is very difficult to heal unless all pressure can be relieved from the weight-bearing areas.

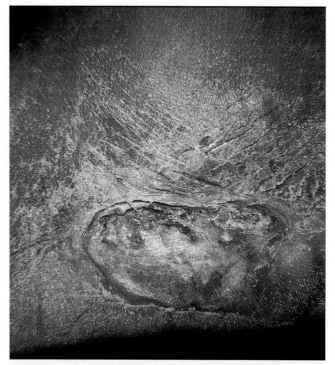

Figure 15–19   Black eschar. A large neurotropic ulcer on the foot has a firmly attached black eschar that is starting to separate at the margins.

FISSURES

Skin fissures are discussed elsewhere in this book but are mentioned here in connection with external trauma. Fissures on the skin of the foot represent a continuum of skin response patterns to various types of mechanical trauma. Acute friction and shearing forces usually cause blister formation; pressure applied for extended periods of time produces ulcerations; and repetitive friction and pressure eventually lead to callus formation or increased thickening of the stratum corneum. Once orthokeratotic hyperkeratosis develops over the thin epidermis it may be damaged by stretch or torque of the skin. Fissures are cracks or rents within the thickened stratum corneum, and they may be seen on any area of the body. This condition is common on the heel and may be represented by transverse fissures (Fig. 15–20) due to stretching of the skin or by vertical fissures (Fig. 15–21) secondary to twisting or torquing of the skin. Treatment involves debridement of the overlying hyperkeratotic tissue, hydration of the stratum corneum, and softening of the skin with emollients. If there is any secondary bacterial infection, it should be addressed at the same time. Protective socks, shoes, and bedding are required to complete the treatment program.

FOREIGN BODIES AND PUNCTURE WOUNDS

Puncture wounds are responsible for many different clinical presentations on the lower extremities. Many of these injuries are simple punctures of the skin with no foreign body implanted, secondary scarring, infection, or other complication. However, complications af-

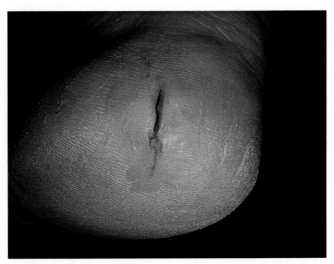

Figure 15–21   Heel fissure. These vertical cracks are secondary to dry, thick skin that is placed under torque and compression during running.

ter puncture wounds to the foot are numerous and include abscess formation, infection, cellulitis, inclusion cyst, joint sepsis, and osteomyelitis. With the use of the Resnick and Fallot classification system four categories of puncture wounds can be listed according to the depth and level of severity of injury.

Type I: Superficial cutaneous penetration
Type II: Subcutaneous or articular joint involvement with signs or symptoms of infection
Type IIIA: Established soft tissue infection including pyarthrosis and retained foreign body
Type IIIB: Foreign-body penetration into bone
Type IV: Osteomyelitis secondary to puncture wound injury.

In some cases, the foreign body that caused the injury is retained within the skin. Distinctive patterns may be seen as a result of various unabsorbable substances that penetrate the skin. A variety of histological reactions are noted in association with these foreign-body agents, such as nonspecific inflammation, granulomatous reaction, and nonreactive implantation.

Nonspecific inflammation usually results when the reaction to the penetrating foreign body is relatively mild, painless, and nonpruritic and quickly festers, ulcerates, and heals over with no scarring. Treatment is usually not necessary in most cases of mild nonspecific inflammation.

The *granulomatous reaction* is a hypersensitivity reaction with focal accumulations of mononuclear cells of varying degrees of differentiation. Cells range from undifferentiated proliferative monocytes to phagocytic macrophages, mixed macrophages, and purely secretory or vesicular epithelioid cells. Giant cells are commonly seen as well. Three types of granulomatous reactions are presented based on the tissue changes noted. A *benign foreign-body granuloma* is characterized by a

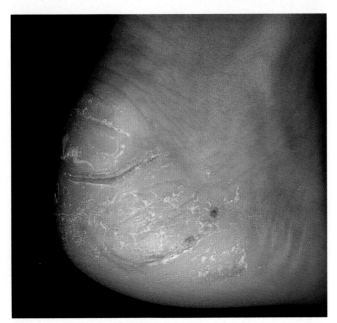

Figure 15–20   Heel fissure. The cracked skin on the posterior aspect of the heel occurred with excessive dorsiflexion of the foot causing stretch to this area.

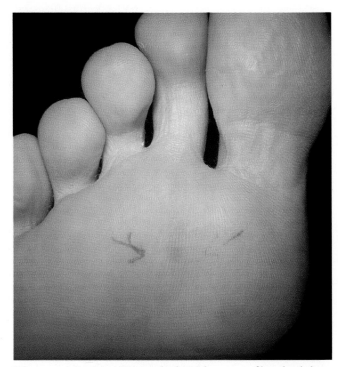

Figure 15–22   Foreign body. Nylon carpet fiber shards have penetrated the skin on the sole of the foot causing an inflammatory reaction.

simple macrophage response to a penetrating foreign body into the dermis. Typically, the foreign body cannot be broken down or rejected and is eventually surrounded by foreign-body giant cells and walled off. This creates a solid granuloma that has to be surgically removed. A *cytotoxic foreign-body granuloma* results when there is both an acute and a chronic inflammatory response, as well as a granulomatous reaction to the foreign body. This condition results when keratin material is penetrated into the dermis layer along with the foreign body. This same reaction is seen when cactus or other plant spines penetrate the skin. The final form is *hypersensitivity foreign-body granuloma,* which is much more complex and is composed of activated macrophages that differentiate into epithelioid cells. Histologically, these epithelioid cells appear as enlarged mononuclear cells with an oval nucleus with chromatin distributed throughout the nucleoplasm and a prominent nucleolus.

The *nonreactive penetration* foreign body is simply one that is implanted within the skin and no secondary foreign-body reaction or granulomatous reaction occurs. The material is retained indefinitely with no secondary problems noted. This benign form of foreign-body penetration is the basis of tattoos.

Various substances may be embedded in the skin and underlying tissues with different responses noted by the examining physician. Acrylic or nylon fibers may be accidentally embedded into the skin of the feet, especially by walking on a new carpet (Fig. 15–22). Careful evaluation of each individual lesion

shows a characteristic dome with the central area surrounded by a white rim and an external peripheral erythematous ring (Fig. 15–23). Histologically, macrophages and foreign-body giant cells surround and phagocytize the nylon fibers.

Foreign-body reactions to particles of wood and wood-fiber products that have been inoculated into the skin may also be seen in the foot (Figs. 15–24 and 15–25). Clinically, these lesions typically appear as elevated dome-like nodules with a white or yellow center and a pink or red border. Intracellular wood fiber material is identified within vacuoles of foreign-body giant cells as fasciculated inclusion bodies. Excision or deep curettage of the lesions is usually curative.

Particles or slivers of glass may also be embedded into the skin of the foot (Fig. 15–26). This usually occurs when a glass or bottle was broken at home and subsequently the patient stepped on pieces left after the clean-up process. Reactions may range from benign inert to reactive granulomatous. In most cases, surgical removal of the glass is necessary to stop the reaction.

Metal, stones, and sharp objects such as needles and pins may also penetrate the skin and become lodged underneath, creating a deeply buried foreign-body reaction (Fig. 15–27). Radiographs of the foot in cases of suspected foreign-body penetration may be successful in identifying the objects (Fig. 15–28). Once foreign objects have been identified they may be removed surgically, if indicated. Triangulation techniques and computed tomography may greatly enhance the ability to locate deeply buried objects.

Foreign-body reactions to human and animal hair

Figure 15–23   Foreign body. A close-up of a nylon carpet fiber foreign-body reaction shows a characteristic elevated central area surrounded by a white rim and peripheral erythema.

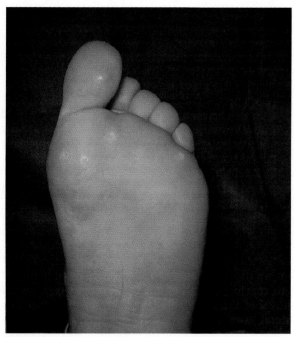

Figure 15–24　Foreign body. Multiple areas of foreign-body reactions are present on the sole of foot secondary to running on a cedar woodchip track.

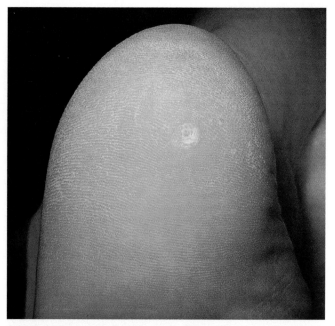

Figure 15–26　Foreign body. This patient remembered stepping on a piece of glass many months earlier.

(Figs. 15-29 and 15–30) may be seen in barbers, beauticians, pet groomers, and pet owners, who may develop interdigital sinuses of the fingers or toes or well-developed and discrete lesions on the soles of the feet. Careful excision or curettage of the lesions frequently reveals the hair (Fig. 15–31).

Additional foreign-body lesions include silicate cutaneous granulomas from the bristly spines of the sea ur-

chin (Fig. 15–32) and coral heads (Fig. 15–33), inclusion cysts from puncture wounds (Fig. 15–34), and sterile suture foreign-body reactions (Fig. 15–35). The spines of many of the ocean's sea urchins are brittle and are broken easily and retained within the skin of the foot when stepped on. Foreign-body reactions may occur weeks or months after the original injury. Once the foreign-body granuloma forms it may persist indefi-

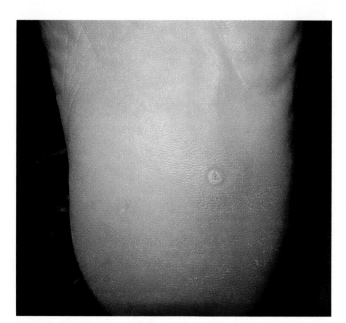

Figure 15–25　Foreign body. This patient stepped on a wooden toothpick that broke-off in his heel. A typical foreign-body reaction occurred.

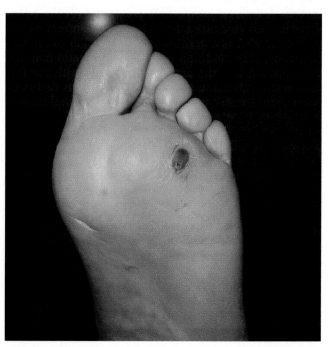

Figure 15–27　Foreign body. A hematoma located on the plantar foot should alert the physician to consider a penetrating foreign body.

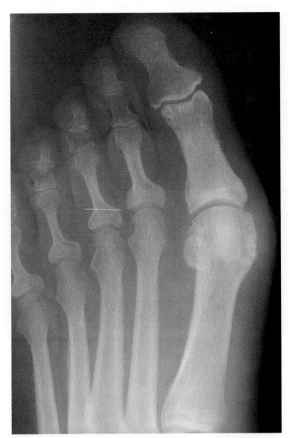

Figure 15-28 Foreign body. A radiograph of the foot showed a broken needle buried within the tissue below the third toe.

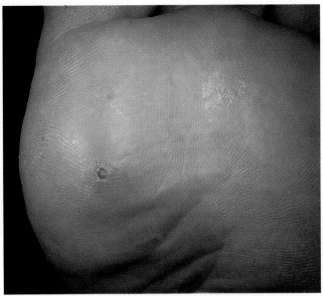

Figure 15-30 Foreign body. An acutely reactive lesion on the foot is secondary to penetration of the plantar skin by an animal hair.

nitely or spontaneously resolve. Intralesional injection of corticosteroid may be necessary, and surgical excision may be performed if the lesion continues to be symptomatic. The silica-tipped darts of the cnidoblast cells of the hard coral heads may enter a traumatic laceration or enter undamaged skin on the feet when the swimmer rubs up against or steps on the coral. The darts release a toxin that produces an acute inflammatory reaction and cellulitis. Eventually, many of these injuries become secondarily infected with bacteria. (See Chap-

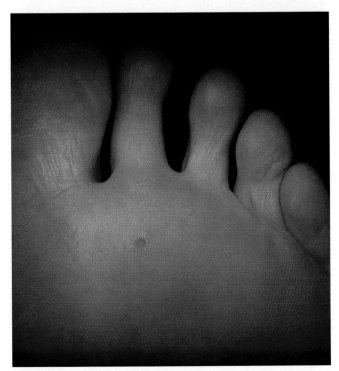

Figure 15-29 Foreign body. Removal of this well-defined lesion from the plantar foot of this beautician revealed a curled human hair.

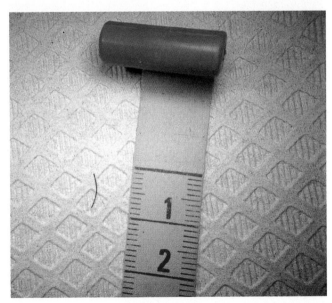

Figure 15-31 Foreign body. A short, black dog hair was removed from the plantar lesion of this pet owner (same patient as in Figure 15-30).

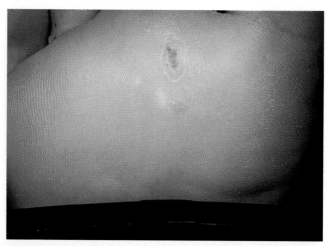

Figure 15–32   Foreign body. A sea urchin spine granuloma was noted several months after injury was sustained while snorkeling in the ocean.

ter 8 for additional discussion on treatment of sea urchin spines and coral injuries.)

Epidermal inclusion cysts occur when fragments of epithelium are implanted deep within the wound during lacerations or puncture wounds. Sterile suture abscesses and foreign-body reactions sometimes occur when the body does not completely dissolve absorbable suture materials. These granulomatous reactions are usually self-limiting; however, early removal will speed healing and decrease scar formation.

Lesions caused by nonreactive foreign bodies such as tattoos and pencil lead (Fig. 15–36) are usually asymptomatic and do not need to be treated in any way. Many of these lesions will become reactive after sev-

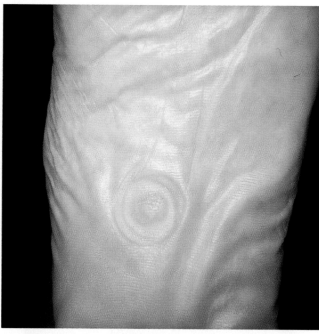

Figure 15–34   Foreign body. Epidermal inclusion cyst was noted after puncture of the plantar foot with a nail.

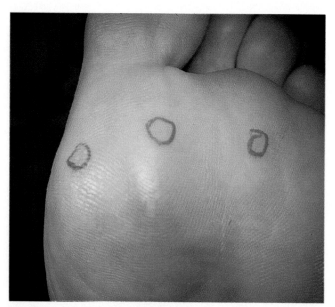

Figure 15–33   Foreign body. Silica-headed darts of the cnidoblast cells of coral heads may enter traumatic lacerations of the skin and create erythematous foreign-body reactions.

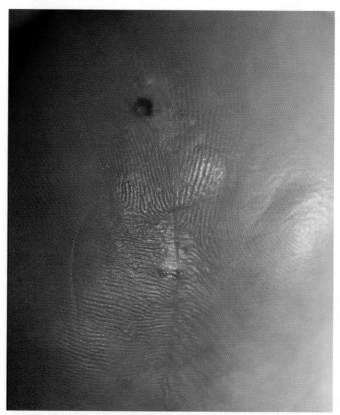

Figure 15–35   Foreign body. A sterile suture abscess reaction is noted at the central and superior border of this surgical incision.

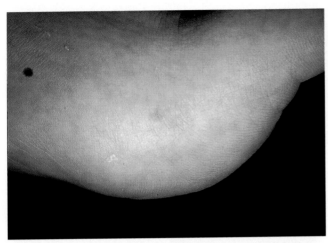

Figure 15–36   Foreign body. A nonreactive pencil lead "tattoo" resulted from implantation of a pencil tip into the skin of the foot many years earlier.

eral years of dormancy. These latent or delayed granulomatous lesions resemble histopathologically the most chronic foreign-body granulomas, and it is difficult to ascertain why these lesions persisted for so long without reactivity.

In all cases of puncture wounds, the following questions must be considered:

Is a foreign body still present?
Has the patient received up-to-date tetanus prophylaxis?
Is any infection present?
Is there injury to underlying vital structures?
Is there any concurrent disease processes going on that might prolong or delay treatment?
What are the long-term risks or complications of treatment or the provision of no treatment?

Attending to all of these issues will provide the patient with a higher chance of obtaining a good result and decrease many of the complications seen with puncture wounds and foreign-body injuries.

HYPERKERATOSES AND TYLOMAS

Abnormalities in keratinization may represent thickenings referred to as corns, calluses, tylomas, or hyperkeratoses. The normal basket-weave pattern seen in the stratum corneum is referred to as orthokeratotic scale. When the stratum corneum is increased in thickness, the term *hyperorthokeratotic,* or simply *hyperkeratotic,* is used. In general, hyperkeratosis indicates an increased keratinocyte activity, as seen in the corn or callus, in which the hyperkeratosis is due to stimulation of the epidermis by intermittent or increased pressure. Hyperkeratoses may be diffuse and generalized and are frequently referred to as calluses or tylomas. If the hyperkeratoses are more distinct and

isolated, they are usually referred to as corns or helomas. Several unrelated lesions mimic or have similar appearances to corns and calluses. These conditions include arsenical keratosis, eccrine poroma, keratodermas, knuckle pads, plantar verrucae, and porokeratosis plantaris discreta.

Diffuse hyperkeratotic tissue is generally found on the weight-bearing surface of the sole of the foot and is usually asymptomatic (Fig. 15–37). This form is seen more often in patients who regularly go barefoot. Occasionally, this form may become dry and fissured at the edges of the callus. The more isolated varieties of hyperkeratosis are frequently painful, and patients commonly complain of burning pain in these lesions. Close evaluation of these lesions may show a central conical core of keratin at the point of greatest pressure. Discrete isolated lesions may be similar to cutaneous horns, but careful debridement will lift this keratin plug off completely, leaving visible skin lines underneath (Fig. 15–38). Other distinct areas of hyperkeratosis formation include the medial aspect of the great toe, called a *hallux pinch callus* (Fig. 15–39); the proximal plantar aspect of the great toe, which is often secondary to an interphalangeal joint sesamoid (Fig. 15–40), and the distal plantar hallux, which is frequently associated with a hallux limitus condition (Fig. 15–41). Calluses formed under the metatarsal heads on the ball of the foot that are resistant to regular conservative treatments of debridement and protective padding are often referred to as *intractable plantar keratosis.* These lesions may be seen

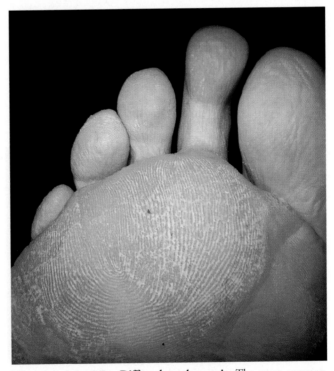

Figure 15–37   Diffuse hyperkeratosis. The most common form of hyperkeratotic skin is the asymptomatic generalized version found on the weight-bearing aspect of the foot.

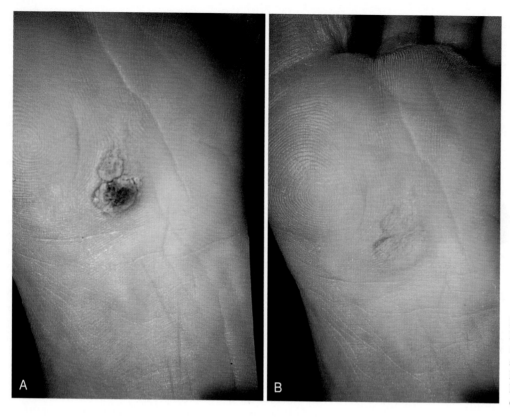

Figure 15–38 Isolated hyperkeratosis. *A,* This lesion may be skin-colored or pigmented and look similar to the cutaneous horn (see Fig. 13–8). *B,* When the keratotic plug is removed, the underlying skin lines may be seen.

under the first metatarsal head (Fig. 15–42), the fifth metatarsal head (Fig. 15–43), or below any or all of the lesser metatarsal heads of the foot (Fig. 15–44).

Treatment of the diffuse type of hyperkeratotic tissue build-up is relatively simple with protective insoles and regular treatment of the area with a pumice stone or callus abrader. Having the patient refrain from walking barefoot may also be beneficial. The more isolated forms of hyperkeratosis are generally more difficult to resolve. Treatments may be as simple as controlling the abnormal pressures and biomechanical forces on the foot

with cushioned inserts, special shoes, or prescription custom-made functional orthotic devices. Local tissue debridement and protective padding reduce much of the pain associated with these lesions (Fig. 15–45). Surgical removal of underlying bone pathology or realignment of the metatarsal bones may also be required (Fig. 15–46). Isolated hyperkeratotic tissue may also be found on the heels, arches, ankles, or any other area of

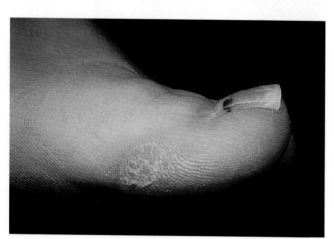

Figure 15–39   Isolated hyperkeratosis. The medial hallux pinch callus is seen in patients with excessive pronation and may occur as a burning discomfort or numbness.

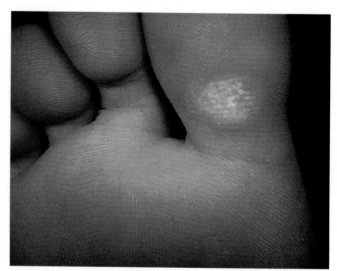

Figure 15–40   Isolated hyperkeratosis. The proximal plantar hallux callus is usually associated with an interphalangeal joint sesamoid.

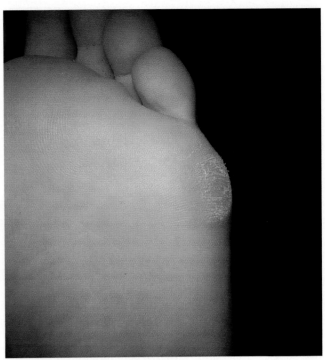

Figure 15–41   Isolated hyperkeratosis. The distal plantar hallux callus is frequently associated with a hallux limitus condition.

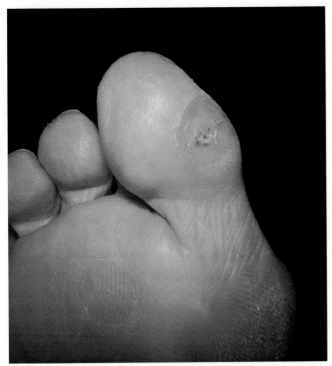

Figure 15–43   Isolated hyperkeratosis. Located below the fifth metatarsal head and associated with a tailor's bunionette, this lesion resolved with bunionette surgery.

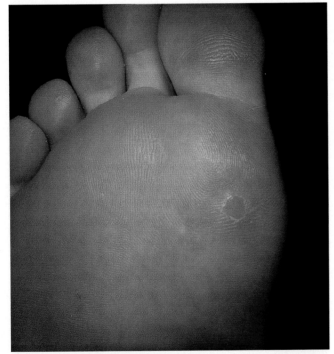

Figure 15–42   Isolated hyperkeratosis. The intractable plantar keratosis under the first metatarsal head sesamoid was very resistant to conservative care.

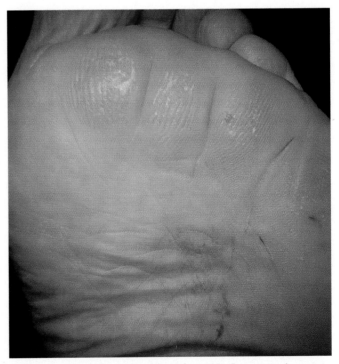

Figure 15–44   Isolated hyperkeratosis. In some patients, especially those with rheumatoid arthritis, intractable lesions may form below the lesser metatarsals.

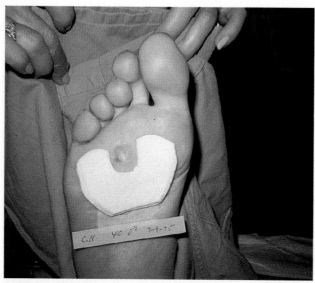

Figure 15–45   Isolated hyperkeratosis. The lesions may be debrided sharply to remove most of the dead tissue and then be protected by felt padding. (Courtesy of Dr. Steven LeBaron.)

the body where intermittent or increased pressures have allowed thickening of the skin.

The discrete helomas, also called corns, may be found in several different forms, including *heloma durum* (hard corn), *heloma milliare* (seed corn), *heloma mollé* (soft corn), *heloma neurofibrosum* (neurovascular corn), and *heloma vasculare* (vascular corn). Heloma durum is a col-

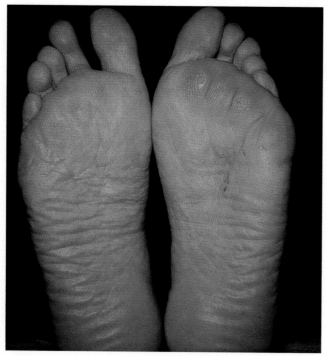

Figure 15–46   Isolated hyperkeratosis. The right foot shows resolution of long-standing intractable lesions after metatarsal surgery to relieve the pressure on the ball of the foot. (Same patient as Figure 15–44.)

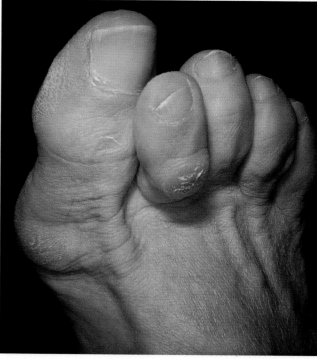

Figure 15–47   Heloma durum. A hard corn will frequently form over prominent areas, such as on the dorsal surface of the second toe.

lection of dense compacted tissue that is frequently located over the pressure areas of the toes (Fig. 15–47), especially the dorsal lateral aspect of the fifth toe (Fig. 15–48) and the plantar distal aspect of the middle lesser toes (Fig. 15–49). Treatment ranges from simple debridement and padding to topical keratolytics to sur-

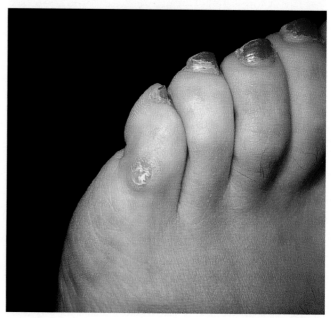

Figure 15–48   Heloma durum. The most common location for this hard corn is over the dorsolateral aspect of the fifth toe.

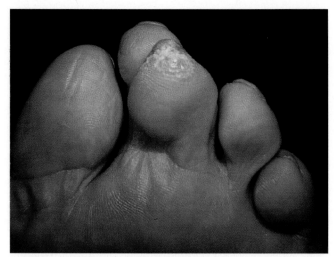

Figure 15–49 Heloma durum. A hard corn may be found on the distal plantar aspect of plantar flexed or rigid toes.

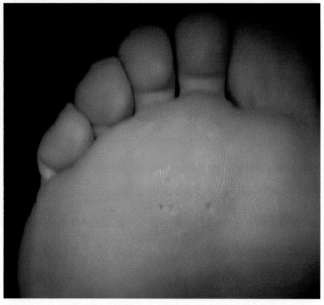

Figure 15–51 Heloma milliare. Small pinpoint seed corns may be found on the plantar ball of the foot and are usually asymptomatic.

gical removal of the underlying osseous pathologic process.

Heloma milliare is frequently found on the sole of the foot in non–weight-bearing areas (Fig. 15–50). It may be located on any skin surface, such as the heel, arch, and ball of the foot (Fig. 15–51). Each small, circumscribed lesion ranges from less than 1 to 3 mm in diameter and is usually asymptomatic. Seed corns may be single or multiple. Anhidrosis or excessive dryness of the skin is frequently present with adjacent fissuring. Treatment involves rehydration of the skin, topical emollients, treatment of secondary fungal infections, and simple removal of the larger lesions with curettage or sharp dissection followed by the application of silver nitrate.

Heloma mollé is a soft corn that is found between the toes in the deep web space (Fig. 15–52) or on the inner sides of the toes (Fig. 15–53). It is usually soft because it has absorbed moisture that causes maceration. However, this painful lesion is not always soft and moist and may be firm and dry if it is located more distally on the toes. This soft corn results from increased friction and pressure from adjacent bony prominences or nail edges rubbing against normal tissue. Treatment includes drying of the digital interspace area, debridement of the heloma, and padding or surgical removal of the offending digital bone or nail condition causing the lesion.

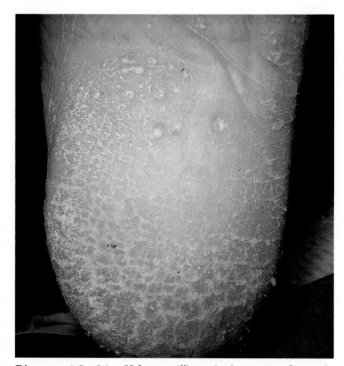

Figure 15–50 Heloma milliare. Seed corns are frequently found on the plantar sole of the foot in non–weight-bearing areas.

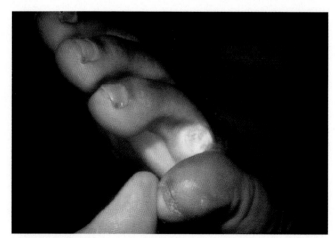

Figure 15–52 Heloma mollé. The soft corn is usually located on the deep web-space area between the toes.

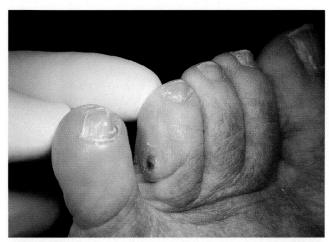

Figure 15–53   Heloma mollé. The soft corn may be located at any level along the inner aspect of two adjacent toes that are rubbing together.

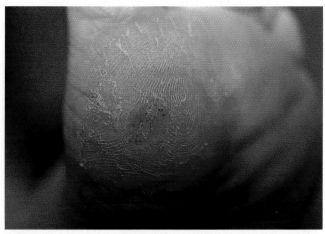

Figure 15–55   Heloma vasculaire. The vascular corn is very thin, and the superficial vessels bleed easily. This lesion is frequently symptomatic, even after treatment.

Heloma neurofibrosum is a painful lesion that is referred to as a neurovascular corn because it contains a plexus of vascular and nerve elements. This lesion may have visible blood vessels and is often confused with a plantar wart. A neurovascular corn is usually located at a point of increased pressure or pinching of the skin such as around the medial hallux, first metatarsophalangeal joint, medial heel, or fifth metatarsophalangeal joint (Fig. 15–54). Protection and padding of the area is usually beneficial. Application of silver nitrate after debridement may be curative. Alcohol sclerosing injections are the treatment of choice and are very useful in reducing the size and symptoms of this lesion.

Heloma vasculare is a very thin symptomatic lesion that is characterized by several superficial capillary loops within the central region (Fig. 15–55). This lesion is more common on plantar weight-bearing or pressure points such as under the plantar first and fifth metatarsal heads. Attempts at debridement of the lesion are unsuccessful, and it will bleed easily and heal slowly. The use of silver nitrate to cauterize the area is helpful. Judicial utilization of alcohol sclerosing injections may

also eliminate the vascular corn. Care must be taken to prevent ulceration within the central core of the lesion.

UNRELATED LESIONS

Unrelated lesions that may be visually similar to corns and calluses must be identified to obtain the most beneficial results from treatment.

Arsenical keratoses (see Fig. 14–4) are discrete hyperkeratotic lesions found on the palms and soles secondary to arsenic exposure, either from environmental causes or in medications. These lesions may mimic heloma milliare (seed corns) or discrete intractable keratoses.

Eccrine poromas (Fig. 15–56) are slow-growing, painless, superficial, smooth-surfaced, partially flattened le-

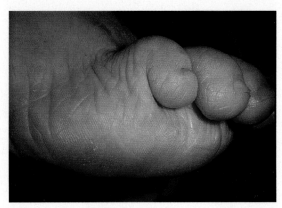

Figure 15–54   Heloma neurofibrosum. Small neurovascular plexus may be seen within the lesion located on the plantar lateral aspect of the fifth metatarsophalangeal joint.

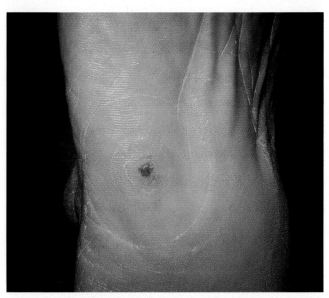

Figure 15–56   Eccrine poroma. This painless, superficial, slow-growing lesion is more common on the digits. It often resembles a pyogenic granuloma.

sions that resemble pyogenic granulomas, dermatofibromas, or amelanotic melanomas. The lesions are generally rubbery to firm and can expand up to 3 cm in maximum diameter. Some tumors may become infected or ulcerate. They may occur on any surface but are more common on the toes (especially interdigitally), palms, or soles. Most eccrine poromas are found in women during the fourth decade. Histologically, eccrine poromas show sheet-like downgrowths of epithelium (Fig. 15–57). The squamoid cells of these downgrowths are polyhedral but smaller than midepidermal keratinocytes. Their cytoplasm is pale due to increased glycogen content. Treatment is usually surgical excision of the entire unit and underlying tissue with direct suture closure.

Keratodermas, especially localized forms (Fig. 15–58) and regional forms (Fig. 15–59), may be similar to diffuse generalized or isolated forms of hyperkeratosis. These forms of keratodermas may be associated with systemic manifestations. Most types are inherited as autosomal dominant traits. Diffuse hyperkeratosis of the palmar and plantar skin may become so thick that it tends to crack. The punctate form of palmoplantar keratoderma (Fig. 15–60) looks very similar to arsenical keratoses with the exception that a central translucent center is commonly present in each lesion. These keratodermatous conditions are all persistent and difficult to treat. Treatment consists of debridement of the hyperkeratotic lesions with keratolytics such as salicylic acid paste (25% to 40%) or sharp debridement with scalpel blades (Fig. 15–61). Topical vitamin A and emollients may also be helpful. Cushioned or shock-absorbing insoles may reduce some of the pressures that accelerate the formation of the keratoderma.

Knuckles pads may be either congenital (Fig. 15–62) or acquired (Fig. 15–63) and are characterized by well-defined, plaque-like fibrous thickenings. The congenital form is commonly seen in dark-skinned individuals and is often dominantly inherited. They consist of thick-

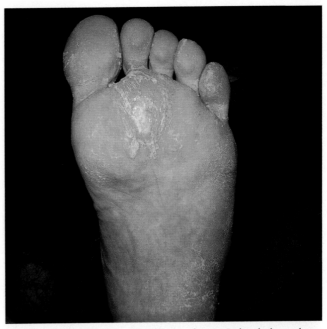

Figure 15–58   Localized keratoderma. Isolated plantar keratoderma of the weight-bearing ball of the foot may be yellow or orange and may involve the hands.

ened skin overlying the interphalangeal joints and knuckles of the hands and feet. Dupuytren's contractures or plantar fibromatosis may be associated. The lesions may resemble helomas, but usually very little hyperkeratotic tissue is present. The knuckle pads are usually hypopigmented with a slightly hyperpigmented

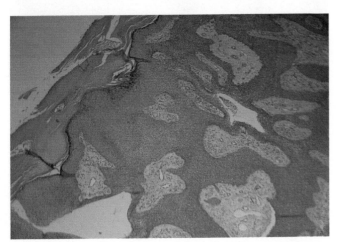

Figure 15–57   Eccrine poroma. Scanning magnification shows sheet-like downgrowths of epithelium cells that are polyhedral but smaller than normal keratinocytes. Their cytoplasm is pale due to increased glycogen content.

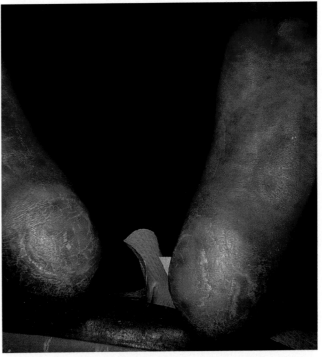

Figure 15–59   Palmoplantar keratoderma. Regional keratoderma may involve most of the weight-bearing surfaces of the foot.

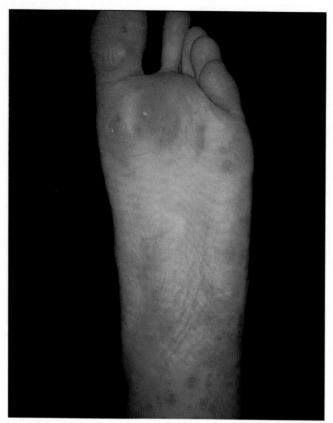

Figure 15–60   Punctate palmoplantar keratoderma. These lesions are difficult to differentiate from arsenical keratoses and heloma milliare.

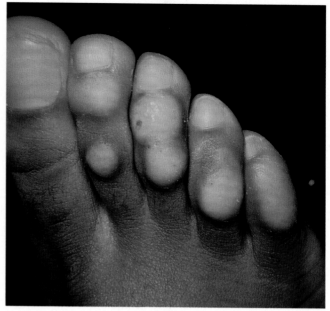

Figure 15–62   Congenital knuckle pads. These are usually seen in dark-skinned individuals over the interphalangeal joints of the hands and feet.

thickening of the dermal collagen fibers. The acquired form of knuckle pads is usually seen in dancers, especially ballet dancers. The condition results from chronic irritation, pressure, and friction; however, there is typically little or no hyperkeratotic tissue build-up. Simple protection and padding of the toes is all that is neces-

border. The skin lines are frequently lost, and the pads may be shiny. The pads appear during adolescence and are usually permanent. There is no successful treatment for this condition, but intralesional injections of cortisone may improve the appearance of the lesions. Histologically, the specimens may show hyperkeratosis and

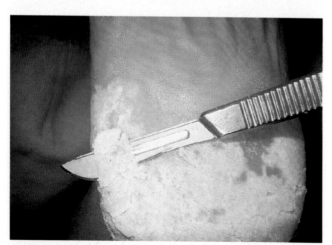

Figure 15–61   Keratoderma. Treatment may involve sharp debridement of the lesions following topical emollients or keratolytics applied to soften the tissue. (Courtesy of Dr. Steven LeBaron.)

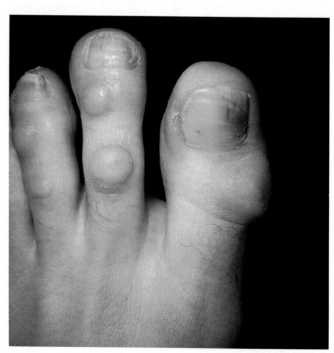

Figure 15–63   Acquired knuckle pads. Typically seen in the extensor surfaces of the toes of ballet dancers, these lesions resolve when dancing is discontinued.

sary, and the lesions usually dissipate once dancing is discontinued.

Porokeratosis plantaris discreta is represented by 1- to 3-mm diameter punctate lesions found on the weight-bearing aspect of the sole of the foot (Fig. 15–64). The lesion is probably developed by direct pressure on the plantar surface of the skin. There is some debate as to whether the underlying ducts of sweat glands are involved. The lesion is characterized by hyperkeratosis of the epidermal sweat duct with the formation of a cornoid lamella superficially. These distinct lesions appear as white or yellow-white lesions that are most tender with side-to-side pressure. They do not have vascular elements and do not show pinpoint bleeding when debrided. This lesion may penetrate to a depth of up to 1.5 cm. Histologically, the features of porokeratoses resemble those of the tylomas and helomas, showing a central horny plug containing areas of parakeratosis. Sweat ducts below the plug of keratin may be dilated, but this is not the likely cause of this condition. Treatment includes topical keratolytics, debridement, padding, intralesional injections of alcohol sclerosing solution, enucleation of the plug with desiccation of the base, or surgical excision of the lesion.

Plantar verrucae (Fig. 15–65) may be seen as a punctate single lesion or multiple seed warts (see Fig. 7–11) on the weight-bearing areas of the foot and may easily be mistaken for solitary hyperkeratotic lesions or heloma milliare.

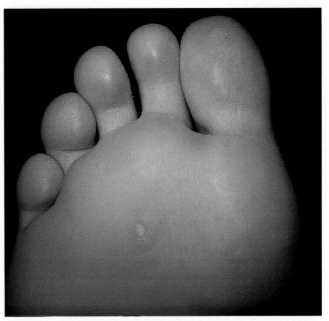

Figure 15–65 **Plantar verruca.** Individual endophytic plantar warts may be mistaken for nucleated hyperkeratotic lesions. Debridement usually shows small pinpoint capillary bleeding.

SCRATCHES, ABRASIONS, AND BURNS

Scratches are linear injuries to the skin secondary to sharp objects breaking the intact barrier of the epidermis. These lesions may be caused deliberately by the patient (see Chapter 17) or may be induced accidentally. They may be superficial scratches (Fig. 15–66), which tend to heal quickly and without scarring in the noncompromised patient, or they may be deep scratches

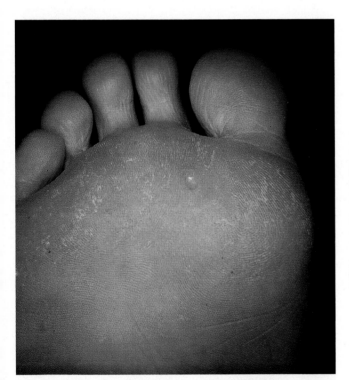

Figure 15–64 **Porokeratosis plantaris discreta.** A discrete, white or yellow-white punctate lesion is most painful when palpated from side to side. There are no vascular elements within the lesion.

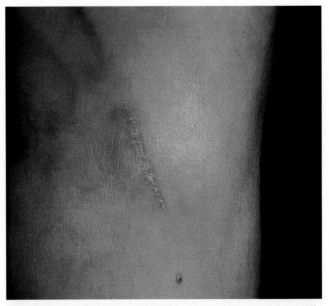

Figure 15–66 **Superficial scratch.** These wounds usually heal very quickly and without complications in the noncompromised patient.

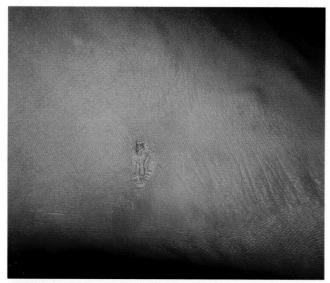

Figure 15–67 Deep scratch. This injury has a higher chance of complications with infection and scarring.

(Fig. 15–67), which may penetrate the upper dermis or all layers of the skin. In this latter case, many would consider this a laceration rather than a scratch. The deep scratch may result in a scar formation after healing. Treatment is usually not necessary in the superficial injury, but in the deeper scratch it is necessary to prevent secondary infections and superficial protective bandaging is helpful during the early stages of healing.

Abrasions result with the superficial removal of the epidermal layers of the skin. This injury occurs with traumatic rubbing or scraping combined with pressure. Abrasions may result from a large variety of injuries or conditions, including new shoes (Fig. 15–68), stubbing

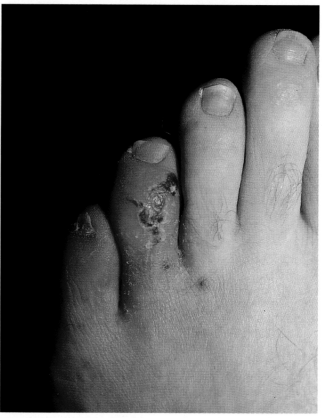

Figure 15–69 Abrasion. Injury to the dorsal toe was sustained secondary to stubbing the toes on the bottom of a door.

injuries to the toes (Fig. 15–69), aggressive shaving of the lower legs (Fig. 15–70), and accidents (Fig. 15–71). Characteristically, abrasive injuries result in bleeding, secondary weeping, pain, and loss of superficial skin layers. In abrasions secondary to accidents such as

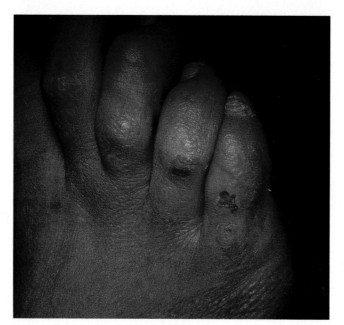

Figure 15–68 Superficial abrasion. The patient had worn a new pair of shoes that caused abrasions on the lateral toes.

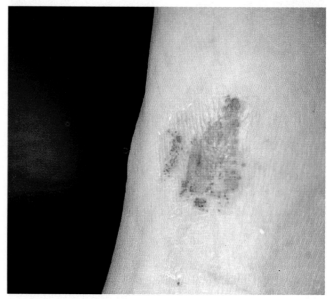

Figure 15–70 Abrasion. Wide and superficial abrasion injury is due to shaving leg without a safety razor.

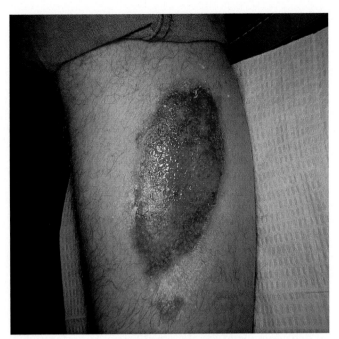

Figure 15–71   Abrasion. Large area of injury to lateral calf with embedded debris occurred after a motorcycle accident.

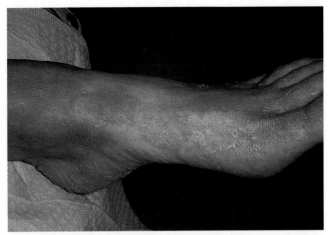

Figure 15–73   Superficial second-degree burn. This superficial burn with blister formation to the dorsum of the foot was caused by a hot grease spill.

falling off skateboards, bicycles, or swings or being involved in motorcycle or automobile accidents, there may be a large amount of embedded debris in the wound. These larger wounds are similar to burns, and secondary infections may occur. Treatment of the smaller superficial abrasions is simply cleansing the wound and allowing it to heal. More involved and larger abrasions need more thorough cleansing to remove all embedded debris. Protective dressings and antiseptics will usually prevent infection.

Burns are very common injuries to the feet and legs and may result from a variety of external causes such as sun exposure, open flames, hot liquids (boiling water or grease), hot pipes, motor vehicle exhausts, hot-water bottles, and heating pads. Plaster of Paris casts may also cause thermal burns owing to the exothermic reaction when the plaster dries too fast, which forms an insulating layer that does not allow equal distribution of heat to transfer out of the bandage (Fig. 15–72).

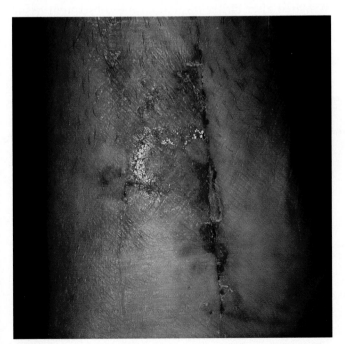

Figure 15–72   Plaster of Paris burn. The patient received a thermal burn to the anterior ankle from the cast that was applied after surgery.

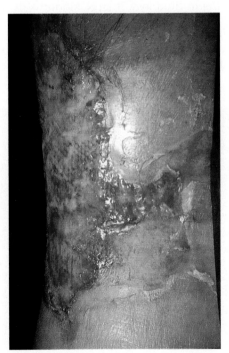

Figure 15–74   Deep second-degree burn. There is loss of the upper protective skin layers with characteristic mottled appearance due to a boiling water injury.

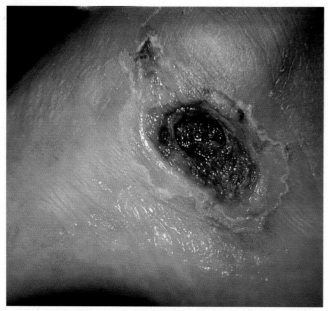

Figure 15–75   Third-degree burn. The full-thickness burn at the medial aspect of the foot resulted from contact with a hot motorcycle exhaust pipe.

Initially, with exposure to heat or flames, the skin becomes hyperemic and vasodilatation occurs within the skin capillaries. As the heat continues or intensifies there is an increase in the capillary permeability and, consequently, coagulation, thrombosis, and stasis occur. Coagulation necrosis follows with loss of water, protein, and sodium from the skin surface. Once the outer layer of protective skin is lost the tissue will begin to dehydrate owing to fluid loss. If large amounts of tissue are lost the patient will rapidly become dehydrated. In severe burns and widespread injuries, acidosis and shock may follow. The depth of burns depends on the thickness of the skin at the area of damage, the intensity of

heat, and the length of time the burning agent is applied to the skin.

Burns are classified as partial thickness or full thickness and as first, second, or third degree. First-degree burns show erythema with no blistering. The most common form of first-degree burn is with sunburn to the skin from overexposure to ultraviolet rays. Second-degree burns may be either superficial or deep. Superficial second-degree burns show erythema with blister formation (Fig. 15–73). These burns are usually very painful for several days. Deep second-degree burns frequently show more extensive loss of the epidermis due to blistering, but blisters are not always present. The skin may be dry and anesthetic or wet and painful and may appear mottled (Fig. 15–74). Third-degree burns show destruction to the full thickness of the skin as well as to all of its appendages (hair, sweat glands, and sebaceous glands). These burns are usually anesthetic, leathery, and discolored, and they may have thrombosed blood vessels present at the periphery or deep layers (Fig. 15–75). This injury is usually the most difficult to accurately estimate the amount of damage until debridement of the damaged tissues is performed.

The initial treatment of burns begins with an immediate assessment of the patient and the circulatory status of the extremity. Initially, the burn area may be covered with towels soaked in cool water or saline until the patient's general status is evaluated. Ice should *not* be applied to the burn area because a cold thermal injury may be added to the hot thermal injury. Blisters should not be broken. However, blisters that are already broken should be debrided and covered with a topical antibiotic cream, such as silver sulfadiazine.

When a significant amount of protective layer skin is sloughed after blister formation, the subsequent tissue necrosis, wound dehydration, and wound pain can be decreased by applying sterile porcine xenografts (Fig. 15–76). Porcine xenografts should be placed dermal

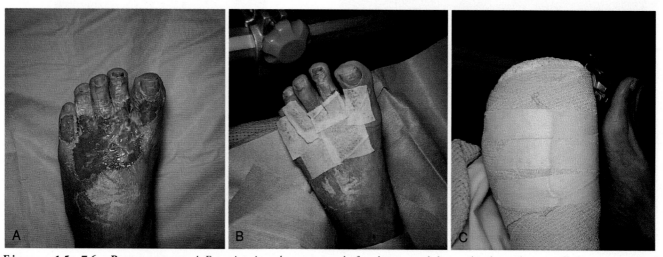

Figure 15–76   Burn treatment. *A*, Extensive tissue loss was noted after deep second-degree skin burn due to spilled grease. *B*, Initial porcine xenografts were applied to promote vascular granular bed and decrease fluid loss and pain. *C*, Mildly compressive sterile bandaging promotes additional protection of the burn site.

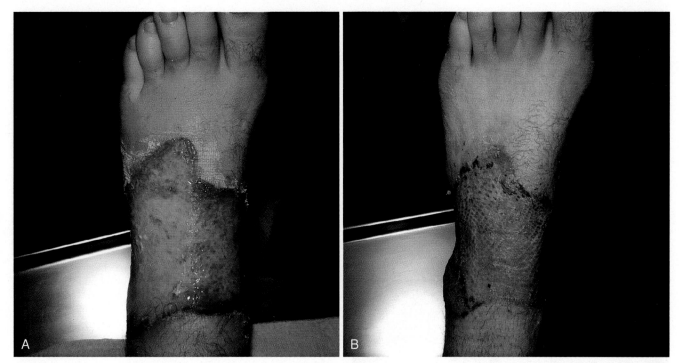

Figure 15-77   Skin grafting. *A,* Deep second-degree burn after almost 3 weeks of wound care. *B,* After meshed split-thickness skin grafting to burn site.

side against the wound. Healing by reepithelialization proceeds faster and with potentially fewer complications than under artificial dressings or scab formation. In infected burn wounds the xenograft is changed daily with local wound care debridement. In noninfected burn wounds the graft is changed on a weekly basis. When the xenograft lifts easily off the wound, it is replaced. If it is adherent to the wound base it is left alone and simply redressed. In many cases, the first porcine xenograft applied seems to "take" and becomes firmly attached to the wound. After a few weeks of being adhered the xenograft is firm and dry and eventually lifts off easily in the dressings. At this point significant wound healing should be noted. If the lesion is still present, a new xenograft or split-thickness skin graft may be applied. Covering the grafts with sterile bandages with mild compression also decreases the patient's pain by reducing air exposure and motion in the area. The mild compression also has the benefit of preventing additional contractures during healing. Second-degree burns should be healed within 3 weeks. When there is failure to heal within this time the wound should be debrided and grafted with split-thickness skin grafts (Fig. 15–77). External compression is continued on the healed skin graft for several months (up to 1 year) to prevent hypertrophic scar formation and scar contracture.

SUBUNGUAL HEMATOMA

Subungual hematoma may be caused by a variety of conditions that cause trauma to the nail plate, which causes bleeding under the nail and immediate pain. Hemorrhage beneath the nail plate allows blood to fill the small space between the plate and the nail bed (Fig. 15–78). This hemorrhage below the nail plate causes increased pressure, which is characterized as throbbing pain. The quantity of blood may be sufficient to cause separation and loss of the nail plate. Initially, the subungual hematoma appears red to bluish red, and later it may appear dark brown to blue-black (Fig. 15–79). This condition may be due to direct trauma (see Fig. 15–78) or may be indirect, such as is seen in runners (Fig. 15–80), tennis players, or golfers and in patients with

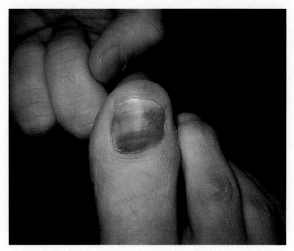

Figure 15-78   Subungual hematoma. Characteristic appearance of subungual hemorrhage after direct trauma to the hallux toenail.

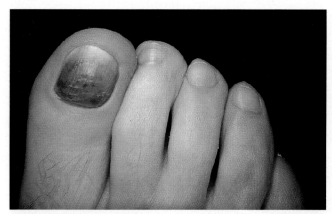

Figure 15–79 Subungual hematoma. Later stages of hematoma may appear darker brown or blue-black.

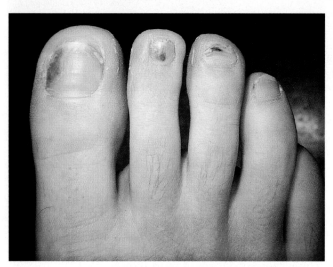

Figure 15–80 Subungual hematoma. Typical hemorrhage is noted under the toenails in runners.

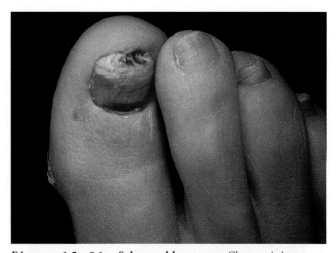

Figure 15–81 Subungual hematoma. Characteristic appearance of hemorrhage below a thick toenail was caused by pressure from shoes.

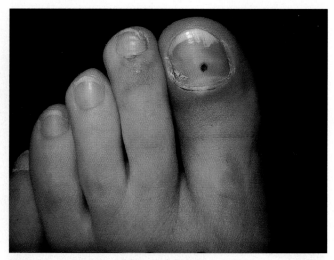

Figure 15–82 Subungual hematoma. Placing a small hole in the nail plate will allow drainage of the blood underneath in the acute stages. Once the blood has coagulated and dried it will not be possible to drain it.

thick toenails who wear close-toed shoes (Fig. 15–81). When the subungual hematoma is due to direct injury to the toe it is important to take radiographs of the toe to rule out a distal phalanx fracture.

Treatment of subungual hematoma is by drainage of the trapped blood beneath the nail plate. In many instances a small hole may be place in the nail with a fine-point drill, heated paper clip, or hand cautery unit (Fig. 15–82). Once the blood has been drained the toe may be placed in a mildly compressive bandage for protection. This will also compress additional fluids out from beneath the nail. In more severe cases of injury, or in later stages of hematoma formation, the entire nail plate should be avulsed to relieve the underlying pressure and to inspect the nail bed for lacerations. These lacerations should be cleansed and repaired for the best long-term results.

BIBLIOGRAPHY

Attinger C: Use of skin grafting in the foot. J Am Podiatr Med Assoc 85:49–56, 1995.

Bodman MA: Pedal nail and skin problems. In Robbins JM (ed): Primary Podiatric Medicine, pp 283–317. Philadelphia, WB Saunders, 1994.

Cortese TA, Fukuyama K, Epstein W: Treatment of friction blisters: An experiment model. Arch Dermatol 97:717–721, 1968.

Crissy JT, Peachey JC: Calcaneal petechiae. Arch Dermatol 83:501–502, 1961.

Dockery GL: Skin Grafting Techniques. In Jay RM (ed): Current Therapy in Podiatric Surgery, pp 14–17. Philadelphia, BC Decker, 1989.

Dockery GL: Nails. In McGlamry ED, Banks AS, Downey MS (eds): Comprehensive Textbook of Foot Surgery, 2nd ed, pp 277–303. Baltimore, Williams & Wilkins, 1992.

Dockery GL, Nilson RZ: Intralesional injections. Clin Podiatr Med Surg 3:473–485, 1986.

Farrington GH: Subungual hematoma: An evaluation of treatment. BMJ 21:742–744, 1964.

Friedman SL: Palliative care. In Robbins JM (ed): Primary Podiatric Medicine, pp 167–182. Philadelphia, WB Saunders, 1994.

Goldenberg RA, Goldenberg EM, Estersohn HS: Needle localization of foreign bodies using computed tomography. J Am Podiatr Med Assoc 78:629–631, 1988.

Graziano TA, Baratta JB, Menditto L, Ramirez L: A surgical alternative in the management of chronic neurotrophic ulcerations of the foot. J Foot Surg 32:295–298, 1993.

Hernandez PA, Hernandez WA, Hernandez A: Clinical aspects of bursae and tendon sheaths of the foot. J Am Podiatr Med Assoc 81:366–372, 1991.

Herring KM, Richie DH: Friction blisters and sock fiber composition: A double-blind study. J Am Podiatr Med Assoc 80:63–71, 1990.

Hetherington VJ, Hash G: Evaluation of lower extremity ulcerations. J Foot Surg 31:599–602, 1992.

Hyman AB, Brownstein MH: Eccrine poroma: An analysis of forty-five new cases. Dermatologica 138:29–38, 1969.

Krell B, Sink CA, Kwiecinski MG: Burns of the lower extremity: Surgical and nonsurgical considerations and treatment. J Foot Surg 28:42–50, 1989.

Lavalette R, Pope M, Dickstein B: Setting temperatures of plaster casts. J Bone Joint Surg [Am] 64:907–911, 1982.

Mahan KT, Marks JA: Puncture wounds. In McGlamry ED, Banks AS, Downey MS (eds): Comprehensive Textbook of Foot Surgery, 2nd ed, pp 1430–1439. Baltimore, Williams & Wilkins, 1992

Malay DS: Injuries to the nail bed and associated structures. In Scurran BL (ed): Foot and Ankle Trauma, pp 107–118. New York, Churchill Livingstone, 1989.

Marcinko DE, Tursi FJ: Pedal burn contractures. J Am Podiatr Med Assoc 78:396–398, 1988.

McCarthy DJ: Helomata and tylomata. In McCarthy DJ, Montgomery R (eds): Podiatric Dermatology, pp 53–73. Baltimore, Williams & Wilkins, 1986.

Michota RS, Peridiue RL, Mason WH: A clinical report of 60 cases of porokeratosis plantaris discreta. Curr Podiatr 26:6–12, 1977.

Milione V, Kanat I: Burns: A review of pathophysiology, treatment, and complications of thermal injury. J Foot Surg 24:373–381, 1985.

Pien FD, Kistner RL, Partsch B, et al: Retrospective study of hospitalized patients with chronic leg ulcers in Hawaii. J Foot Surg 33:546–550, 1994.

Rabinowitz AD: Skin tumors. Clin Dermatol 1:54–66, 1983.

Resnick CD, Fallat LM: Puncture wounds: Therapeutic considerations and a new classification. J Foot Surg 29:147–153, 1990.

Ritz G, Kushner D, Friedman S: A successful technique for the treatment of diabetic neurotrophic ulcers. J Am Podiatr Med Assoc 82:479–481, 1992.

Samitz MH: Occupational dermatoses. Clin Dermatol 1:25–34, 1983.

Shilling JJ: Glass fragments retained in the foot. J Am Podiatr Med Assoc 84:89–90, 1994.

Stein RA, Clarke S: Foreign bodies in the foot. J Podiatr Med Assoc 83:284–287, 1993.

Tuerk D: Burns and frostbite. In Scurran BL (ed): Foot and Ankle Trauma, pp 153–165. New York, Churchill Livingstone, 1989.

Wagner FW: A classification and treatment program for diabetic, neuropathic, and dysvascular foot problems. AAOS Instr Course Lect 27:143–165, 1979.

Weisfeld M: Understanding porokeratosis plantaris discreta. J Am Podiatr Assoc 63:138–144, 1973.

Yale JF: Dermatologic and toenail disorders. In Yale's Podiatric Medicine, pp 131–246. Baltimore, Williams & Wilkins, 1987.

Young G, Johnson JD: An algorithmic approach to the diagnosis and management of lower extremity ulcerations. Lower Extremity 1:29–36, 1994.

16

PEDIATRIC DERMATOLOGY

INTRODUCTION

Pediatric dermatology overlaps considerably with adult dermatology, and most of the conditions in this chapter are discussed in more detail elsewhere under general topics for each disease. Because several conditions are seen primarily in children and are less common in adults, these conditions are emphasized and the others are covered to a lesser extent.

ALLERGIC CONTACT DERMATITIS

The frequency of this condition is less in children than in adults. It is quite unusual to see allergic contact dermatitis in children younger than 3 years of age. This type of dermatitis occurs after a variable number of contacts with a sensitizer. The rash occurs locally at the site of contact with the allergen but may also spread to adjacent areas. The most common sensitizers causing allergic contact dermatitis are the *Rhus* plants (poison ivy and poison oak), paraphenylenediamines (shoe dyes), nickel compounds, rubber products, ethylenediamines, and the chromates. In children, the foot is frequently in shoes for extended periods of time and the increased heat and perspiration can exacerbate allergic contact dermatitis to shoe materials (Fig. 16–1). The process of increased heat, perspiration, and allergic dermatitis may allow spread of the vesicular papules by increased vascularity, and the clinical presentation may lead to a misdiagnosis of tinea pedis. In many instances the proper diagnosis is delayed due to extended treatment of the condition with topical antifungal creams.

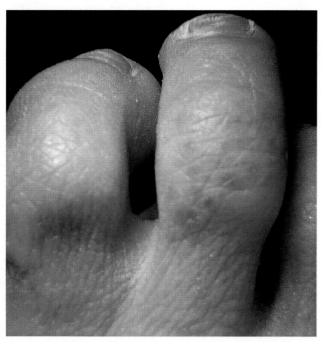

Figure 16–1   Allergic contact dermatitis. This condition was secondary to exposure to shoe material and involved the dorsa of the toes of both feet.

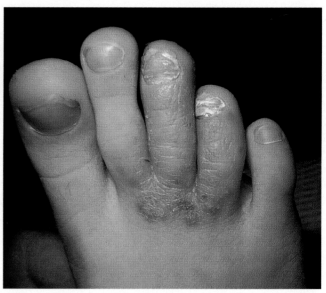

Figure 16–2   Atopic dermatitis. Characteristic lesions on the toes of a 7-year-old girl with toenail involvement were misdiagnosed as a fungal infection.

It is difficult to differentiate irritant contact dermatitis from allergic contact dermatitis. Generally, irritant contact dermatitis is localized and looks more like a burn with blisters, edema, and erythema. Allergic contact dermatitis, in contrast, appears more polymorphic, with erythema, vesiculation, pruritic papules, and edema.

Treatment is directed toward detection of the allergen by patch testing and avoidance of the offending agent. Local treatment includes soothing foot soaks, short courses of topical corticosteroids, and control of excessive perspiration (see Chapter 10 for additional treatments).

ATOPIC DERMATITIS

Atopic dermatitis is extremely common in children and is known as atopic eczema and allergic eczema. This condition is typically referred to as "atopy" and is considered a chronic disorder that lasts for many years, even decades, causing long-term problems of recurrent dermatitis. There is frequently a family history of atopic dermatitis or eczema, allergic rhinitis, and asthma. The characteristic lesions of atopic dermatitis consist of erythema, papulovesiculation, and scaling (Fig. 16–2). The chronic lesions are frequently lichenified. In widespread cases, the flexor surfaces of the antecubital and popliteal fossae are involved. There may be lesions around the head and neck, especially around the eyes, mouth, and behind the ears. The feet are frequently involved, and the skin may show thickening, accentuated skin lines with xerosis, and dystrophic toenails (Fig. 16–3). The hands typically show generalized lichenification with accentuated skin lines but without nail involvement (Fig. 16–4). General principles of treatment in

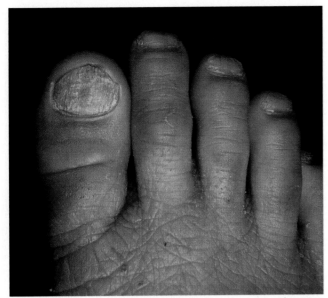

Figure 16–3 **Atopic dermatitis.** Chronic atopy with xerosis and nail dystrophy occurred in a 12-year-old boy with severe asthma.

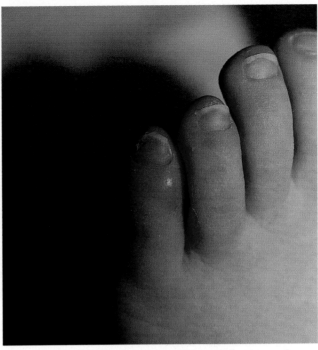

Figure 16–5 **Blister.** Friction blisters may be seen on the toes after the child has been wearing a new pair of shoes.

clude elimination of inflammation and infection, hydration of the skin, and control of all factors that cause exacerbations of the dermatitis. Specific therapy is found in Chapter 10.

BLISTERS

Blisters are common in children and are usually caused by friction and pressure. A new pair of shoes may cause

a toe blister (Fig. 16–5). Another area in which a common blister may be found in children who have just received a new pair of shoes is the heel (Fig. 16–6). A hemorrhagic blister may be seen in pre-walkers or very young children who have been fitted with their first pair of firm leather shoes or new shoes that are too small (Fig. 16–7). Blisters should not be deroofed but drained. A topical antiseptic and protective dressing are all that is usually necessary. If the area becomes red or swollen, a topical antibiotic may be applied. Protection from additional friction and pressure is necessary to prevent recurrence.

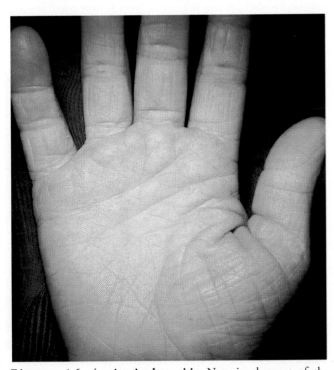

Figure 16–4 **Atopic dermatitis.** Note involvement of the hands with lichenification and accentuation of the skin lines.

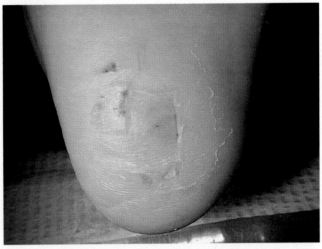

Figure 16–6 **Blister.** This common blister has been deroofed and is often found on the heel in a child starting school with new shoes.

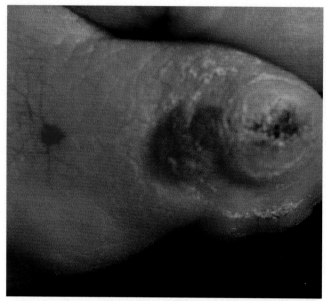

Figure 16–7   Hemorrhagic blister. This painful blood blister is seen in toddlers and very young children who have been wearing firm leather shoes that may be too small.

CANDIDIASIS

Cutaneous candidiasis is usually caused by the yeast-like fungus *Candida albicans.* Local occlusion resulting in heat, moisture, and maceration, cutaneous trauma, and preexisting ulcerations or fissures may all be factors that predispose a child to candidiasis. The clinical manifestations of cutaneous candidiasis include intertrigo (Fig. 16–8), which may be seen at a very early age; toenail involvement (Fig. 16–9); and generalized skin infection (Fig. 16–10). Inguinal and interdigital candidiasis may be seen in neonates after infection contracted in pas-

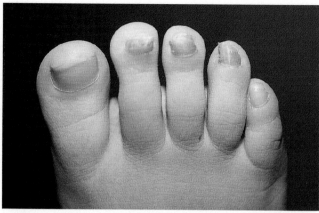

Figure 16–9   Candidal nail infection. Candidiasis involving the nails may lead to severe deformity that appears intractable unless the proper diagnosis can be made.

sage through the vagina. This infection is usually seen after 2 weeks or more and usually produces surprise in the parents and physician. In the very young child the interdigital infection from *C. albicans* is characterized by desquamation, erythematous fissuring, maceration, and peripheral erythema.

Candidiasis of the toenails is common in children and is characterized by marked destruction and onychauxis of the nails. They may thicken considerably and become discolored. Localized cutaneous candidiasis is more common on the plantar skin of the foot, and in chronic stages shows a considerable amount of desquamation with peeling and cigarette paper–like scaling of the skin. Many cases will have a characteristic fissuring. Treatment is based on the proper diagnosis and involves application of a topical imidazole group of drugs, such as clotrimazole, or nystatin cream. In more advanced cases

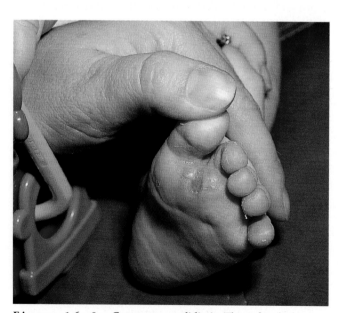

Figure 16–8   Cutaneous candidiasis. This infant had a candidal infection at the interdigital space of the foot.

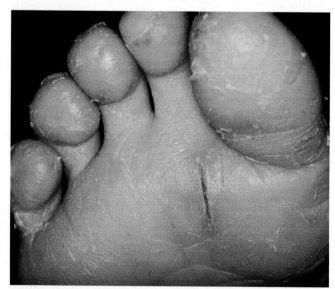

Figure 16–10   Chronic cutaneous candidiasis. In long-standing candidiasis of the feet in children there may be extensive exfoliative scaling of the skin with prominent fissures.

with oral thrush, skin involvement, and nail infections, oral ketoconazole may be very useful.

CUTANEOUS LARVA MIGRANS

Larva migrans is a characteristic cutaneous eruption, referred to as "creeping eruption," caused by larvae of various nematode parasites (see Fig. 8–31). The most common species in the United States is the cat or dog hookworm, *Ancyclostoma braziliense*. The adult nematodes are found in the intestines of cats and dogs, where they deposit ova that are secreted in the animal's feces. The ova hatch into larvae in the soil or sand where they are deposited. The larvae then penetrate human skin that comes into contact with them. Children are more susceptible than adults to cutaneous larva migrans because they tend to spend more time sitting, standing, lying, and playing in the sand or soil of contaminated beaches and playgrounds. Penetration usually occurs on the hands, feet, legs, or buttocks. After the larvae have entered the skin they begin to migrate, causing an inflammatory reaction that forms a bizarre and irregular pattern (see Fig. 8–30). Once the inflammatory reaction becomes visible the patient may experience moderate to intense pruritus. The larva are located deep in the epidermis and stay directly ahead of the advancing tip of the visible inflamed tunnel. Because the larva are not in the actual lesion but are ahead of it by several millimeters (up to 1 cm), biopsy specimen findings are frequently negative.

Treatment begins with an explanation to the patient and the parents of the condition. Light freezing of the advancing border tip of the larva tract with ethyl chloride spray will usually stop the forward progression. Topical thiabendazole 10% aqueous solution may be helpful in early and mild infections during the beginning stages. Oral thiabendazole, 25 mg/kg of body weight, given twice daily after meals for 2 days, is usually sufficient in resolving this condition. If necessary, an additional 2 days of treatment may be warranted.

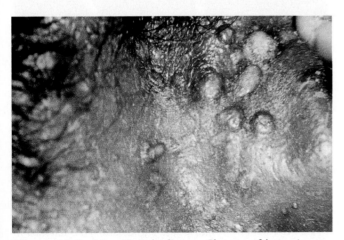

Figure 16–11   Darier's disease. Close-up of keratotic papules shows that some are associated with hair follicles whereas others are not.

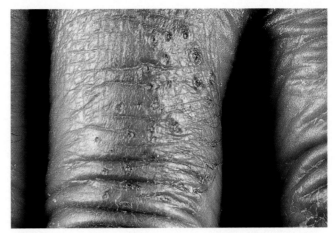

Figure 16–12   Darier's disease. Small symmetrical, dark, red-brown, wart-like papules are seen on the dorsal aspect of the fingers. Similar lesions may be seen on the toes.

DARIER'S DISEASE

Darier's disease (keratosis follicularis) is an uncommon, autosomal dominantly inherited disorder of keratinization that begins in early youth (end of first decade to beginning of second decade) and is caused by imperfect development of the tonofilament-desmosome complex. These cellular structures are responsible for the attachment of one epidermal cell to another and to the basement membrane. Cells separate from one another (acantholysis) and show signs of premature keratinization (dyskeratosis). This papulosquamous disease is characterized by symmetrical eruptions of small, firm red-brown papules that may involve the chest, back, forehead, scalp, hands, and feet. The lesions first appear as skin-colored papules that are covered with a yellow to tan, rough-textured, scaly crust (Fig. 16–11). The lesions may coalesce to form large plaques. Small flat-topped, dark, wart-like papules may be seen on the dorsum of the foot or hand (Fig. 16–12). Well-defined, small, white to yellow, punctate keratoses, either raised or with a central pit, may be seen on the palms or soles of the foot (Fig. 16–13). The fingernails and toenails may also be affected, with thinness, fragility, splintering, and longitudinal ridges and notches at the distal margins (Fig. 16–14). Mucous membrane lesions may occur and appear as white, depressed papules of the cheeks, palate, and gums. Histologically, this disease demonstrates zones of hyperorthokeratosis associated with focal acantholytic dyskeratosis, a reaction pattern consisting of suprabasal acantholysis and dyskeratosis of the sloughed acantholytic keratinocytes (Fig. 16–15).

There is no known cure for Darier's disease. The patients should be instructed to minimize sunlight exposure, heat, and high humidity conditions, which may exacerbate the symptoms of Darier's disease. Symptomatic treatment includes vitamin A cream under occlusion. The synthetic retinoid isotretinoin may also be effective in reducing the lesions, especially when combined with oral vitamin E, 1200 IU daily. Topical sali-

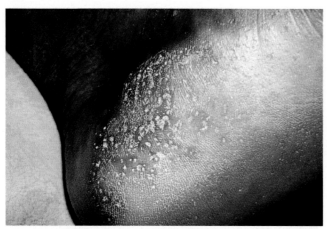

Figure 16–13   Darier's disease. Multiple small, punctate, white-to-yellow keratoses are found on the sole of the foot.

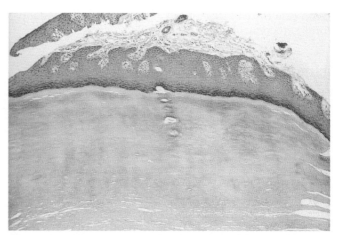

Figure 16–15   Darier's disease. Photomicrograph of lesion demonstrates small foci of suprabasal acantholysis, epidermal hyperplasia, and hyperkeratosis.

cylic acid, sulfur compounds, tar, and calamine lotion may be helpful to reduce the hyperkeratosis and inflammation in large crusts. Topical or systemic corticosteroids provide excellent short-term resolution of the condition, but the lesions usually return and the long-term use of these medications is not recommended.

DERMATOPHYTE INFECTIONS

Dermatophyte infections are common in older children and adolescents, and it appears that they occur in males more frequently than in females. They are caused by a number of anthropophilic fungi, especially *Trichophyton rubrum, Epidermophyton floccosum,* and *Trichophyton mentagrophytes.* The eruption is of the web spaces of the toes and is characterized by maceration with peeling, scal-

ing, and erythema (Fig. 16–16). The condition is usually pruritic and may be painful if there is much fissuring of the tissues. The infection is frequently asymmetrical with one foot more involved than the other. This infection may spread from the interdigital spaces onto the plantar or lateral aspects of the foot and occurs as a pruritic, vesicular, and scaling usually unilateral eruption (Fig. 16–17). Although once thought to be rare, tinea pedis does occur in infants and young children (see Fig. 6–3). If tinea pedis is untreated or mistreated with topical corticosteroids, it may spread onto the dorsum of the digits and tends to have an increase in erythema (Fig. 16–18). When the infection is caused by *T. rubrum* there is usually no vesicular response and the changes on the skin may be very subtle (Fig. 16–19). Most all fungal infections on the feet in children

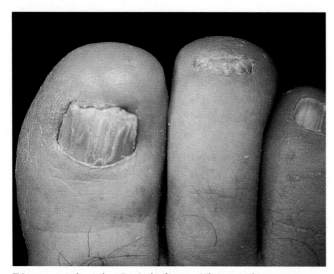

Figure 16–14   Darier's disease. There are characteristic toenail changes with longitudinal ridges, subungual thickening, and notching at the distal margins.

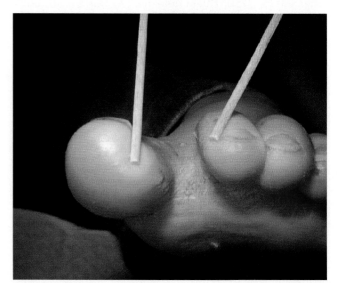

Figure 16–16   Tinea pedis. This dermatophyte infection of the toe web spaces starts as maceration and continues with peeling, fissuring, and erythema.

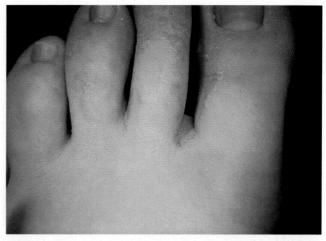

Figure 16–19   Tinea pedis. When the causative agent is *Trichophyton rubrum* there may be dry, powdery scales with peeling of the skin.

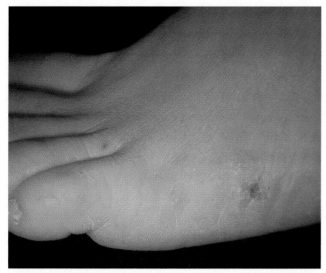

Figure 16–17   Tinea pedis. The infection may spread to the sides and plantar aspect of the sole.

will resolve within 2 to 3 weeks with twice-a-day applications of topical antifungal creams.

EPIDERMOLYSIS BULLOSA SIMPLEX

Epidermolysis bullosa is the general term for a group of inherited dominant and recessive conditions that feature the formation of blisters after minor irritation or trivial trauma. The pathogenesis is unknown, and these diseases are classified as scarring or nonscarring and histologically by the level of blister formation. The clinical classification is based on the presence of scarring and dystrophic changes of the skin. The intraepidermal forms (epidermolysis bullosa simplex) do not have dystrophic changes or scarring. The junctional forms (junctional epidermolysis bullosa) have dystrophic atrophy. Dermal forms (dystrophic epidermolysis) result in both atrophy and scarring. Classification by level of blister formation shows that the intraepidermal types demonstrate a split through the epidermal basal cells: the junctional types split through the basement membrane area, and the dermal forms split through the upper dermis.

The most common condition involving the lower extremities is the condition called epidermolysis bullosa simplex (Weber-Cockayne disease), which is also referred to as recurrent bullous eruption of the hands and feet. Clinically, this condition is characterized by the onset of blisters to the hands and feet early in childhood or adolescence; however, in a few cases the disease may not manifest until adulthood. Hyperhidrosis is a frequently associated condition. The feet are more severely affected than the hands in most patients. Hot weather, increased humidity, walking, or exercise aggravates the condition. The blisters have a characteristic appearance with thick walls that heal slowly. Normal-appearing clear blisters and hemorrhagic-appearing blisters may occur in the same area. Blisters are usually localized to the palm of the hand (Fig. 16–20) and the sole of the foot (Fig. 16–21). The nails and buccal mucosa are spared in this condition, and there is no gum involvement. Genetic counseling is advised to avoid the more dystrophic forms of epidermolysis bullosa.

Treatment for this blistering disorder is one of prevention or control of friction, trauma, tight clothing, heat, and humidity. Patients are advised to avoid injury, seek cooler climates, wear soft leather well-fitting shoes that are well vented, soak their feet in cool water with Epsom salts to decrease hyperhidrosis, and apply topical antiseptics to any blisters that form. Blisters should not be deroofed but left intact. Once the blisters break, they should be protected from additional irritation or

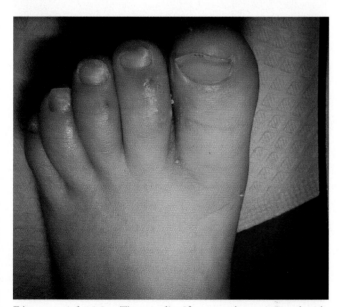

Figure 16–18   Tinea pedis. If untreated or mistreated with corticosteroids, the eruption may spread to the dorsa of the toes and show an increase in erythema.

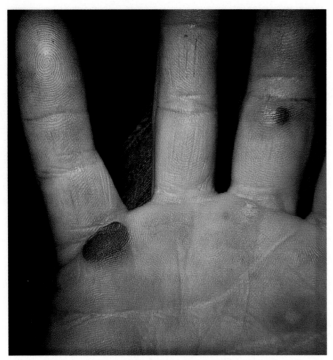

Figure 16–20 Epidermolysis bullosa simplex. This young patient had recurrent blistering on both hands that healed without scarring.

friction. If the blisters become infected, appropriate topical antibiotics are applied. The application of protective cushioned insoles or ones with activated charcoal is also helpful. Patients should also wear protective gloves for sports and play to decrease blister formation on the hands.

ERYTHEMA NODOSUM

Erythema nodosum is an acute reaction that occurs as red, elevated, painful nodules on the lower extremities. The nodules are usually distributed symmetrically on the front of the shins (see Fig. 10–34) or on the dorsum of the foot (see Fig. 10–35). The individual lesions last for 7 to 10 days, and the entire process is over within 1 month. Each nodule may reach 4 cm in diameter but are usually smaller. They are usually bright red initially but gradually turn to yellow-green, blue, or purple, just like a bruise. This condition might be a type of vasculitis of the same general type as anaphylactic purpura and erythema multiforme and secondary to a provoking antigenic stimulus. Streptococcal or viral infections may also be the precipitating cause. In many cases, the patient may feel unwell and have a fever, malaise, arthralgia, or sore throat during the eruptions. Drugs are responsible for most cases identified in children, including barbiturates, sulfonamides, and antibiotics. In female patients older than 13 years of age, the drugs most often associated with erythema nodosum are 13-*cis*-retinoid acid and oral contraceptives.

Erythema nodosum may also be seen in very young women during the early stages of their first pregnancy. Because the condition is self-limited, treatment is symptomatic with cool compresses to the inflamed nodules and bed rest. In painful conditions, oral anti-inflammatory medications may reduce the redness and swelling. Aspirin is not recommended in children with fevers.

ERYTHEMA MULTIFORME

This condition, like erythema nodosum, is not a true disease in its own right, but the characteristic presentation of its skin lesions is distinct and readily recognizable. This acute skin reaction is a self-limited syndrome, thought to be secondary to drug reactions, *Mycoplasma* infections, or viral infections (especially post-herpetic reactions). Patients present with distinctive skin lesions with or without mucosal lesions. Erythema multiforme is common in children but is rarely seen before 3 years of age. Over 50% of reported cases occur in persons younger than the age of 20 with a slightly increased ratio in males. The condition may last 3 or 4 weeks before complete recovery occurs, and it may range from mild symptoms to potentially fatal reactions. Erythema multiforme usually runs its course within 2 to 3 weeks. This is typical for cases triggered by herpes simplex. Those cases due to *Mycoplasma* infections or drugs tend to last longer and be more severe. Recurrences are common if linked to repeated herpetic infections, whereas drug-induced reactions are more episodic.

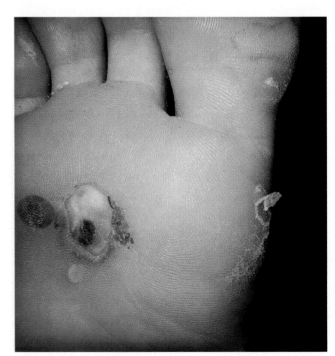

Figure 16–21 Epidermolysis bullosa simplex. Characteristic blisters, both clear and hemorrhagic, are seen on the pressure areas of the plantar foot.

Three types of erythema multiforme are classified based on the degree of skin damage done to the skin or mucous membranes. In general, these types are considered separate from one another, but there may be considerable overlap between them.

The *iris type* is the most common form of erythema multiforme and the simplest to recognize clinically. The lesions are characterized by symmetrical, round, and pink, red, or purple "target" lesions occurring on the extremities. Typically, lesions are seen on the backs of the hands and forearms, palms, soles, lower legs, and feet (Fig. 16–22). These annular lesions resemble a target in that the central area is more involved than the periphery. Typical iris type erythema multiforme is a relatively benign illness with no significant complications.

The *vesiculobullous type* shows a greater degree of vascular damage than the simple iris form. There may be vesicles or bullae in the central region of the target lesion. The adjacent and surrounding involved skin may show less damage. Unlike the simple form, this condition may be much more widespread with a greater area of the body involved. Painful, denuded areas result when the blisters break. There is usually mucosal involvement.

The most severe form of erythema multiforme is the *Stevens-Johnson type,* which may be fatal. There is significant involvement of the skin and mucous membranes. The joints, kidneys, gastrointestinal tract, and lungs are often involved, resulting in a high fever with systemic disturbances.

The diagnosis of erythema multiforme in general is based on clinical presentation. Management begins with treatment or removal of the offending agent if possible. Additional treatment depends on the severity of the condition. In the simple iris type of erythema multiforme the treatment is symptomatic, with cooling soaks or lotions and mouthwashes. The vesiculobullous and severe types of erythema multiforme may require systemic corticosteroids. Hospitalization and referral for medical management may also be necessary in the more severe cases.

EXANTHEMS

The word *exanthem* is defined as any eruptive disease or eruptive fever, and it generally refers to a condition that "bursts forth or blooms." Exanthematous conditions are characterized by symmetrical, widespread, erythematous macules or papules (maculopapular lesions). Disorders that begin with exanthems may be initiated by bacteria, viruses, or drugs. Some are accompanied by mucosal or oral lesions referred to as *enanthems.* Exanthems were classically categorized by a consecutive numbering system according to their historical appearance and general description: first disease, measles; second disease, scarlet fever; third disease, rubella; fourth disease, coxsackievirus or echovirus; fifth disease, erythema infectiosum; and sixth disease, roseola infantum. Of these conditions the most common and the most likely to be seen by physicians treating the foot and leg are the viral exanthems (see Chapter 7) and the drug-induced exanthems (see Chapter 10).

ECHOVIRUS AND COXSACKIEVIRUS EXANTHEMS. The most common exanthematous eruptions are caused by the enteroviruses echovirus and coxsackievirus. Many of these viruses begin with an eruptive rash, which is more common in children than in adults. The patients may also have systemic features of fever, nausea and vomiting, sore throat, lymphadenopathy, and diarrhea. The rash may appear at any time during the infection and is usually generalized. Lesions appear as erythematous maculopapules with areas of confluence (Fig. 16–23). There may also be adjacent vesicles, petechiae, or urticaria. The rash usually heals without scaling, pigmentation, or scarring. Treatment is symptomatic.

Another viral exanthem common to children is hand-foot-and-mouth disease, which is a very distinctive complex caused by coxsackievirus A16 virus. This viral infection is seen frequently in the late summer and early fall in children younger than 15 years of age. Most children with this infection have symptoms of sore throat, fever, malaise, or abdominal pain before the visible rash that forms on the hands, feet, and mouth (see Figs. 7–32 and 7–33). Treatment of this condition is also symptomatic and supportive.

DRUG EXANTHEMS. Cutaneous drug reactions are common side effects of drugs. The most common form of exanthematous rash secondary to drugs is called a mor-

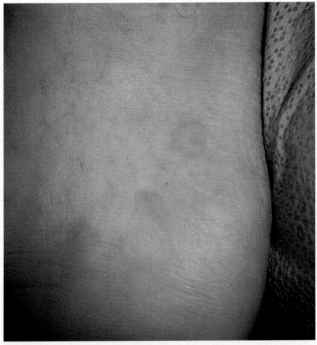

Figure 16–22 Erythema multiforme. Typical target-like configuration of the skin lesions on the foot is noted. (Courtesy of Dr. Jeffrey C. Page.)

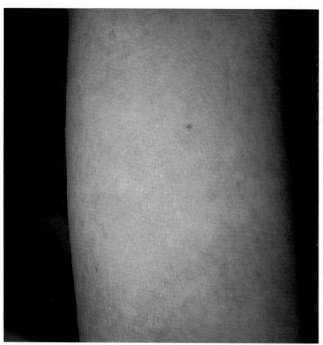

Figure 16–23 Viral exanthem. Typical symmetrical erythematous maculopapular rash involves the trunk and extremities.

billiform eruption. These lesions are macular and papular rashes that may become confluent. The pattern is usually one of general distribution that often spares the face, palms, and soles. Often lesions are present on the glabrous areas of the body and on the tops of the hands and feet (Fig. 16–24). Drug exanthems may be indistinguishable from viral exanthems, but there may be more pruritus and slightly more scaling with drug reactions than are seen with viral exanthems. Additionally, if there is intense pruritus the child may scratch or excoriate the area, making visual identification slightly more difficult (Fig. 16–25).

The clinical presentation of the rash is usually 7 to 10 days after the onset of starting the medication, but it may not be visible until after the drug has been stopped. In some cases, the patient has taken this drug before or has been taking it for an extended time with no problems, but once sensitization occurs, a reaction may follow within a short amount of time. Once a drug exanthem is present it will usually last for up to 2 weeks, and then it will fade—in many cases even if the medication is continued. Treatment of the maculopapular rash is not necessary unless there is intense pruritus. Oral antihistamines will decrease much of the itch and, in some cases, topical soothing lotions (e.g., calamine) may be beneficial.

FIXED DRUG REACTIONS

The fixed drug reaction is a unique expression of a drug allergy that occurs at the same site on the body each

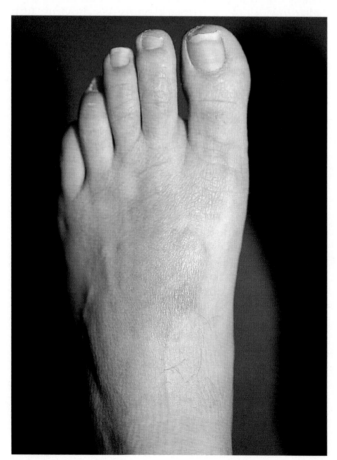

Figure 16–24 Drug exanthem. Characteristic asymmetrical, confluent maculopapular rash on top of the foot occurred after a reaction to ampicillin.

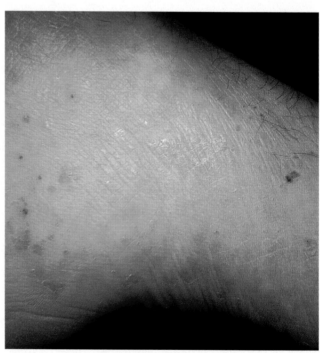

Figure 16–25 Drug exanthem. In some cases, the intense pruritus causes the patient to scratch and excoriate the lesions, making clinical recognition more difficult.

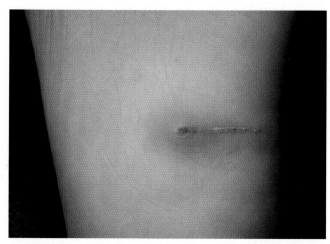

Figure 16–26   Foreign body. This 2-year-old boy stepped on a broken clam shell on the beach, which precipitated an infection.

time the drug is given to the patient (see Figs. 10–38 through 10–40). The characteristic lesions are single or multiple, round-to-oval, dusky red plaques that appear shortly after ingestion of the drug and reappear each time the same drug is taken. Mild to intense pruritus may be present. Blistering may occur with desquamation and crusting, followed by increased pigmentary changes. Lesions are common on the back, legs, and feet but may occur on any body area. Many different drugs have been implicated in fixed drug reactions, including antibiotics, anti-inflammatory agents, aspirin, barbiturates, phenolphthalein, sulfonamides, and tetra-

cycline. Treatment is usually not necessary except to control excessive pruritus.

FOREIGN BODIES AND PUNCTURE WOUNDS

Puncture wound injuries and foreign-body penetrations are very common in young children who tend to play barefoot or in thin-soled shoes. Many different agents have been implicated in these injuries (see Chapter 15). Young children are more susceptible to secondary contamination or infection after puncture wounds, especially if foreign material is left imbedded in the wound (Fig. 16–26). In these cases, it is advisable to open the wound, remove all foreign debris, flush the deep layers, and close the skin with nonreactive sutures (Fig. 16–27). Appropriate tetanus prophylaxis should be considered. Treatment with antibiotics is usually not necessary because the removal of the foreign body is almost always curative.

In some cases there may be spreading cellulitis present from the puncture wound site (Fig. 16–28). In this instance, the wound is debrided of all foreign-body material and the cellulitis decreases immediately (Fig. 16–29). Appropriate foot soaks and antibiotics are then started, if necessary.

If the foreign body is not obvious, as in the case shown in Figure 16–30 of a young boy who presented with a puncture wound on the bottom of his foot, then radiographs should be taken to help identify any visible items. The boy reported that he had tried to "smash" a wooden drawing pencil with his foot and the pencil had penetrated through the shoe and into his

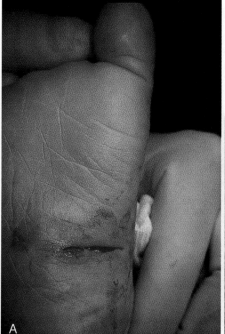

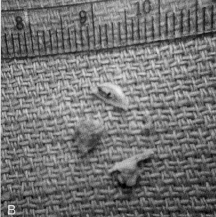

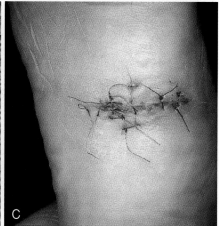

Figure 16–27   Foreign-body treatment. *A,* Incision of the puncture site with removal of external damaged skin. *B,* Excision of deep fragments of clam shell and debris. *C,* Suture repair of incision with nonreactive suture.

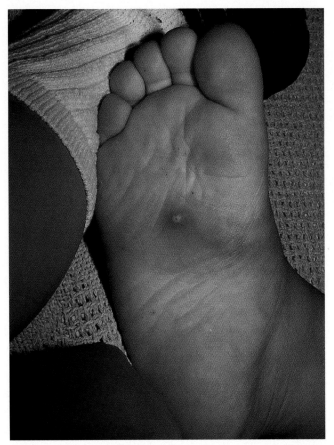

Figure 16–28   Foreign body. In this young child a splinter was demonstrated by bright-red spreading cellulitis to above the ankle.

foot. A close examination of the shoe showed the remaining broken portion of the pencil (Fig. 16–31). At that point, radiographs were taken of the foot and the deep fragments of the pencil and pencil lead could be clearly seen (Fig. 16–32). This finding necessitated opening of the wound with careful debridement and power-flush irrigation of the surgical site (Fig. 16–33).

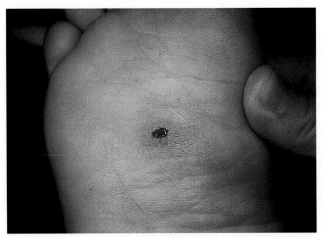

Figure 16–29   Foreign body. After simple debridement of the foreign body the cellulitis quickly dissipated.

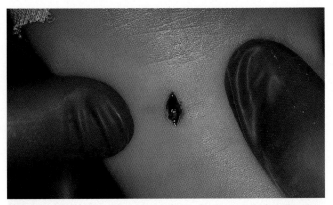

Figure 16–30   Foreign body. A puncture wound to the plantar foot occurred, but no obvious foreign material was visible.

In all cases of puncture wounds, the following questions should be asked:

1. Is foreign body material still present in the wound?
2. Has the patient received up-to-date tetanus prophylaxis?
3. Are there any signs or symptoms of infection?
4. Are there other injuries to underlying vital structures (e.g., tendons, nerves, blood vessels)?
5. Is there any concurrent disease process that might delay or prolong the treatment?
6. What are the long-term risks or complications of treatment or the provision of no treatment?

Answering all of these questions will provide the patient with a higher chance of obtaining a good endresult after puncture wound or foreign-body injuries.

GRANULOMA ANNULARE

Granuloma annulare is a benign inflammatory, selflimiting granulomatous process with a variable clinical presentation of unknown cause. Although this disorder may occur at any age, it is predominantly a disease of

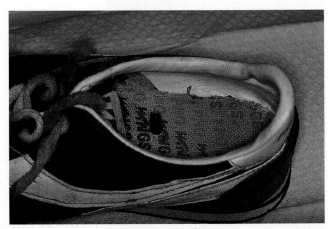

Figure 16–31   Foreign body. Examination of the shoe identified a portion of a broken drawing pencil through the insole.

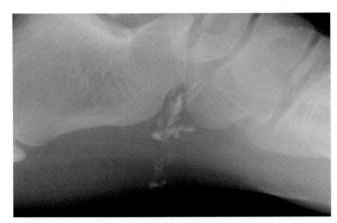

Figure 16–32 Foreign body. Radiographic evaluation showed numerous foreign objects consistent with pencil and lead buried deep within the foot.

children and young adults. Granuloma annulare is very common in young females (female-to-male ratio, 2:1) with 70% of patients younger than 30 years of age and more than 40% younger than 15 years of age. Hand involvement is found in 60% of patients and foot involvement is found in more than 70% of all patients with granuloma annulare. The cause is unknown, but it has been reported to follow insect bites, sun exposure, viral infection, and certain medications, such as antibiotics, anti-inflammatory agents, and oral contraceptives. The lesions may spontaneously resolve in 3 months to many years, with the average remission occurring in 2 years from onset. Recurrences are com-

mon, but the newer lesions tend to spontaneously resolve sooner than the original lesions. The condition has several variants, including the classic type, subcutaneous type, papular type, nodular type, perforating type, and disseminated type.

The *classic type* is the most common type, and it occurs in both children and young adults. This type is characterized by a skin-colored or violaceous, well-defined, lesion arranged in a complete or half-circle configuration measuring from 1 to 5 cm in diameter. The lesions are most common on the dorsa of the hands and feet (Fig. 16–34). The center of the lesion may be erythematous and slightly depressed. These typical-appearing lesions may be solitary or multiple, with over 50% of patients presenting with a single lesion.

The *subcutaneous type* consists of multiple, asymptomatic, skin-colored to slightly erythematous, subcutaneous lesions measuring 1 to 5 mm in diameter. They commonly occur on the dorsa of the hands and feet (Fig. 16–35), but they may also occur on the palms, legs, buttocks, fingers, or scalp.

The *papular type* is an atypical form that occurs with individual papules from 1 to 3 mm in diameter. The lesions are slightly infiltrated, erythematous, and discrete (Fig. 16–36). Individual papules may have a tendency to coalesce. The papules may be umbilicated and may be associated with insect bites in children. This type is also more common in patients with diabetes mellitus.

The *nodular type* is characterized by the presence of one or more superficial or deep nodules. When the nodules are deep, they tend to be solitary and may be confused with juxta-articular rheumatic nodules in chil-

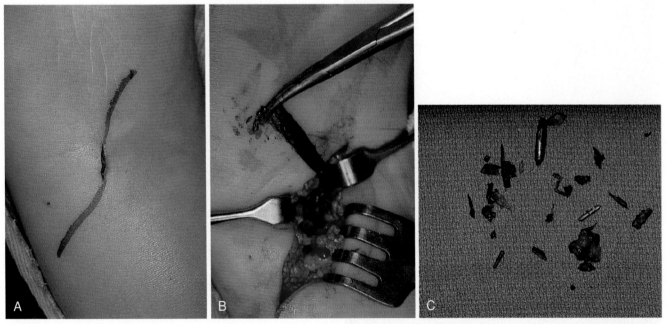

Figure 16–33 Foreign body. *A,* Incision was placed on the plantar foot to minimize weight-bearing scarring but achieve maximum exposure. *B,* All visible and palpable foreign-body items were excised and removed. *C,* Multiple pieces of the pencil and soft lead fragments were removed from within the foot.

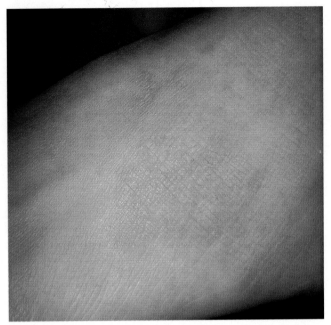

Figure 16–34   Granuloma annulare. A classic solitary annular lesion occurred on the top of the foot in a young girl.

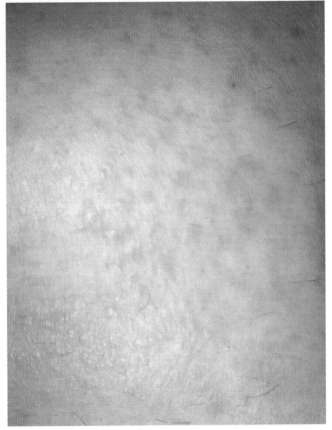

Figure 16–36   Granuloma annulare. Papular type has multiple generalized papules that are erythematous, raised, and discrete.

dren (Fig. 16–37). In some cases, both subcutaneous and nodular forms may be seen together (Fig. 16–38).

The *perforating type* is characterized by superficial, small, papular lesions that develop central umbilication and perforation. In some cases, several small perforations occur in each lesion and small central plugs or

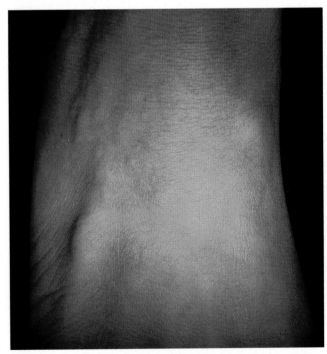

Figure 16–35   Granuloma annulare. Subcutaneous type has multiple small deep dermal or subcutaneous lesions on the dorsum of the foot.

crusts may form (Fig. 16–39). Frank ulceration with discharge of creamy fluid may occur in this type of lesion but is considered very rare.

The *disseminated type* is characterized by numerous, widespread, skin-colored, pink, or yellow-tan papules or nodules located on the trunk and all extremities (Fig. 16–40). In this type it is common for the patient to have multiple lesions that are pruritic and may become circinate or reticular. The patients are usually younger than age 10 or older than age 40. Biopsy is required for a confirmed diagnosis of granuloma annulare (Fig. 16–41), but it is not necessary because the clinical presentation is relatively consistent. An interesting finding, in many cases, is that the lesion frequently heals spontaneously after a sectional biopsy. It is not uncommon for the lesion to be gone by the time the pathology report has been received on the biopsy specimen.

The histological appearance of granuloma annulare shows that there is a superficial perivascular lymphocytic infiltrate. Mononuclear cells are present among collagen bundles in association with variable mucin deposition. In well-developed lesions there are zones of mucinous necrobiosis of collagen surrounded by mononuclear cells. Multinucleated giant cells may also be present. Treatment is not necessary in many cases because the condition is self-limiting and usually asymp-

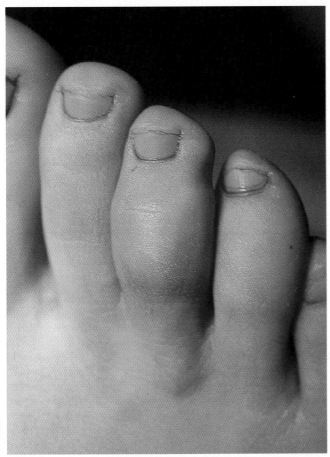

Figure 16–37   Granuloma annulare. Nodular type at third digit may be confused with juxta-articular rheumatoid nodule in children.

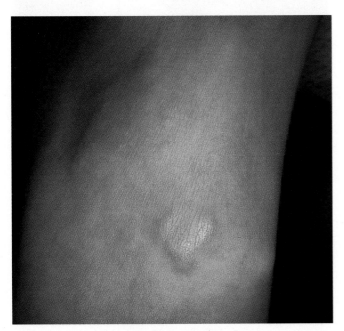

Figure 16–38   Granuloma annulare. In some cases more than one type of lesion may be identified, as in this case with subcutaneous and nodular forms adjacent to one another.

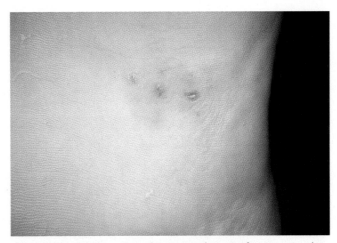

Figure 16–39   Granuloma annulare. Perforating type has three central perforations on lesion located on the foot.

tomatic. In those cases that occur with pruritus or spreading, treatment may be performed with intralesional injections of dexamethasone or betamethasone sodium phosphate. In larger or nodular lesions, triamcinolone injections may be more effective but may also cause more dermal atrophy or pigmentary changes.

HYPERHIDROSIS

Hyperhidrosis can be defined as an increase in sweat production above normal. Eccrine hyperhidrosis has many causes or associations but, for the purposes of this chapter, the discussion is limited to the local increase in sweat production involving the palms and soles (volar hyperhidrosis).

Excessive emotional sweating of the palms and soles may be seen in all races of both sexes. This condition frequently becomes a clinical problem in childhood and can persist into adulthood. This form of hyperhidrosis is not in response to heat and is noted by patients or their parents to be increased under conditions of stress.

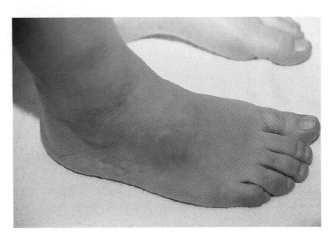

Figure 16–40   Granuloma annulare. Disseminated type has circinate and reticular lesions located on all extremities and on the trunk.

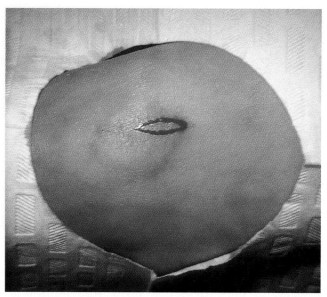

Figure 16–41   Granuloma annulare. A sectional biopsy of a typical lesion is performed for accurate diagnosis of the condition.

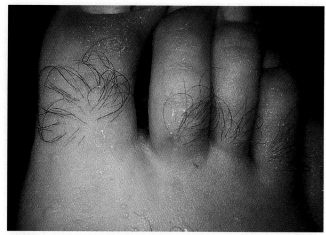

Figure 16–42   Hyperhidrosis. Excessive sweating may be prominent on the hands and feet during an examination.

The patients may exhibit normal sweating patterns when they are totally inactive or in a relaxed state but immediately become hyperhidrotic in active or stressful states. No morphological abnormalities of the sweat glands have been reported.

The primary complaint of most patients with this disorder is the problem of social embarrassment from the excessive wetness of their hands and feet and from the odor that is commonly found with excessive foot perspiration. There may be itching, burning, and blistering of the feet from the increased moisture. There is also an increased incidence and severity of dermatophyte, bacterial, and viral infections. This can lead to tinea pedis, pitted keratolysis, and verrucae. Because this condition may also be associated with excessive axillary sweating, there may be complaints of soiling of clothing. Excessive sweating may be an accessory factor in causing contact dermatitis by leaching out sensitizing agents from shoes or insoles (see Fig. 10–17). Excessive sweating with intense pruritus may be a prodrome for dyshidrotic eczema (see Fig. 10–53). Clinically, the hands and feet may show such a high level of sweating that it may actually bead up with small droplets in a moccasin–like distribution (Fig. 16–42) that may drip off the part during the examination. Patients with hyperhidrosis may also present with plantar skin on the sole that is erythematous, shiny, and very uncomfortable (Fig. 16–43), or they may present with plantar skin that is pale, thick, and boggy from absorption of excessive sweat (Fig. 16–44). The latter type is usually associated with bromhidrosis as well.

The chronic course of volar hyperhidrosis does not usually vary without some form of treatment. The management of very mild disorders begins with personal hygiene habits developed by the patient. The patient should avoid occlusive shoes and synthetic or wool socks. Leather and fabric shoes are encouraged as well as the use of cotton socks to wick moisture away from the skin. Socks should be changed midday if necessary. Absorbant foot powders may also help in relieving mild conditions. The treatment of mild to moderately severe cases consists of regular soaking of the feet in a solution of warm water and magnesium subsulfate (Epsom salts). The patients are instructed to mix 2 tablespoons per quart of warm water and soak the feet for approximately 20 minutes each day. The combined effect of

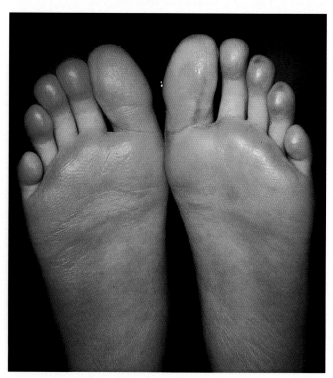

Figure 16–43   Hyperhidrosis. The soles are red, shiny, and very uncomfortable.

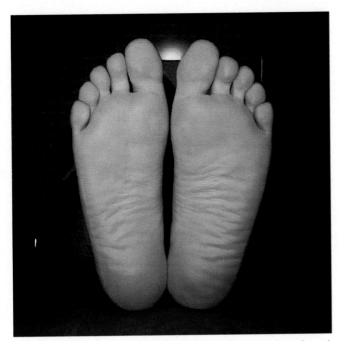

Figure 16–44   Hyperhidrosis. The soles are pale, soft, and boggy due to excessive moisture absorption.

soaking with an astringent is to reduce the skin surface of bacteria and to reduce the hyperhidrosis. Normal saline (0.9% sodium chloride) may also be used for the drying effect, which results after soaking for approximately 20 minutes and then allowing the solution to evaporate from the skin while air drying the lower extremity. This solution may be approximated by adding 1 tablespoon of table salt to 480 mL of water. If used on a routine basis, astringent salts may cause excessive drying of the skin, which can be countered by the use of topical emollients or skin creams.

Aluminum compounds are frequently provided for antiperspirant and astringent effects. These astringents precipitate protein and decrease perspiration. Aluminum acetates (Burow's solution) contain approximately 5% of aluminum acetate and are diluted 1:10 to 1:40 for use as a wet dressing for the feet. This may be one of the most commonly used astringents for wet dressings, which, unlike the aldehydes, does not stain the skin and allows drying and soothing of hyperhidrotic tissue. Aluminum chloride hexahydrate may provide a much better type of wet compress dressing. Aluminum sulfate and calcium acetate combinations are dispensed in powder or tablet form and quickly dissolve in warm water to create an aluminum diacetate combination. The liquid form of aluminum chloride hexahydrate may be applied directly to the skin as an antiperspirant solution. The agents are effective astringents and may also be antibacterial. Patients should be instructed to discontinue soaking or applying medication if excessive dryness occurs. It is probably sufficient to soak the feet once or twice a week once the hyperhidrosis is improved.

For severe cases of hyperhidrosis the addition of stronger agents may be necessary. Aldehydes induce a decrease in perspiration by blockage within the stratum corneum. Formaldehyde is a potent wide-spectrum antiseptic and germicide that has been used as a solution in water to decrease perspiration. The main disadvantage of this particular agent is that it is very irritating to the skin at concentrations required to achieve the desired response. Consequently, it is seldom recommended for its anhidrotic action of the soles.

Glutaraldehyde solution is also a potent dialdehyde with a wide range of germicidal activity that is also rapidly sporicidal and actively decreases hyperhidrosis with regular use. Glutaraldehyde solution is generally applied three times per week for 1 to 2 weeks until the excessive perspiration is under control. Initially, a 10% solution is recommended for soaking of the feet and may cause a temporary brown discoloration. A 2% solution will not cause the discoloration and may be used for regular application; however, this concentration may not reduce excessive sweating. This glutaryl 2% solution has a pH of 7.5 and is available as a nonprescription product for general use. It may cause some irritation to the skin with chronic application.

Methenamine in gel form, which releases formaldehyde and ammonium chloride locally, may be used topically. Methenamine in a 5% gel applicator or in a 10% solution may be used to control moderate hyperhidrosis of the soles. It is very effective and usually does not induce contact sensitization.

Biofeedback techniques may also be very effective in decreasing excessive palmoplantar hyperhidrosis and the chronic symptoms of plantar sole sweating. These relaxation techniques may be added to the other antiperspirant and astringent topical agents for more effective and long-lasting results in the treatment of a sometimes embarrassing and problematic condition of severe hyperhidrosis.

Iontophoresis using tap water or combinations of anticholinergic drugs such as glycopyrrolate may effectively reduce hyperhidrosis of the soles for many weeks. The use of iontophoresis with tap water only is a very safe and effective way of inducing hypohidrosis.

In many cases, severe hyperhidrosis that is nonresponsive to standard methods of treatment may respond to psychotherapy and by the judicious use of tranquilizing agents.

ICHTHYOSIS VULGARIS

The primary ichthyosiform dermatoses include a variety of disorders that are characterized by generalized scaling of the skin. They are congenital disorders and are frequently due to an error of lipid metabolism. The most common form is an autosomal dominant ichthyosis, ichthyosis vulgaris. Ichthyosis vulgaris is rarely present at birth but begins in early childhood. It usu-

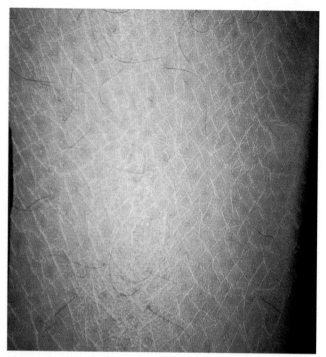

Figure 16–45   **Ichthyosis vulgaris.** Scaling is usually more severe on the lower legs and may resemble lamellar ichthyosis.

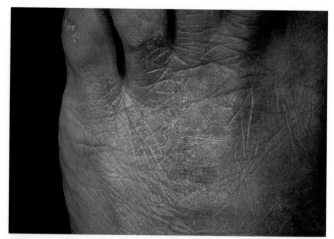

Figure 16–46   **Ichthyosis vulgaris.** Atopic eczema of the feet may also be associated with other clinical symptoms of ichthyosis, such as scaling, fissuring, and keratosis pilaris.

ally improves during the summer and worsens in the winter and during cold, dry weather.

Clinically, this form of ichthyosis presents as small scales outlined with white fissures located primarily on the trunk and extensor surfaces of the extremities (Fig. 16–45). The margins of the scales may be turned up, which give the skin a very rough feeling. The scaling is most prominent on the lower extremities and may be severe enough to resemble the lamellar form of ichthyosis. Keratosis pilaris of the arms and legs may be present, as is atopy in the form of hay fever, asthma, or eczema of the hands or feet (Fig. 16–46). Even in milder forms, there may be a significant accentuation of the skin lines (dermatoglyphics) on the palms (see Fig. 16–4) and feet (Fig. 16–47). This condition is usually lifelong but may improve with time. Histologically, ichthyosis is characterized by mild to moderate hyperkeratosis and reduced or absent keratohyalin granules. Treatment is with daily applications of emollients, alpha-hydroxy acids, or 40% to 60% propylene glycol in water applied under occlusion two or three times a week. Moving to humid, warm climates may be curative.

JUVENILE PLANTAR DERMATOSIS

A generalized scaly plantar dermatitis seen in children is known as chronic pediatric plantar dermatitis, pediatric winter itch, plantar atopic dermatitis, or juvenile plantar dermatosis. This condition is commonly misdiagnosed as tinea pedis or contact dermatitis. Clinically,

it occurs as an erythematous dermatitis with slight scaling and increased plantar skin creases and fissuring over the plantar surface of the forefoot (Fig. 16–48). The digits and the dorsum of the foot may also be involved. There is absence of toe web space involvement, negative fungal test results, and negative patch test results for shoe product sensitivities. There may be a positive family history of atopic dermatitis.

This condition is often described as being much worse during the winter months with some improvement or clearing during the warmer summer months. There may be a relationship between frictional dermatitis caused by shoes in children prone to atopic dermatitis. Treatment includes the wearing of properly fitting shoes or open-toed shoes, control of associated hyperhidrosis, application of emollient creams after warm water foot soaks, wearing of cotton socks, application of mild corticosteroid cream, and, if infection is present, systemic antibiotics.

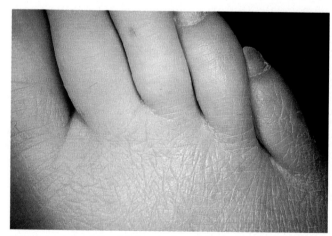

Figure 16–47   **Ichthyosis.** In milder forms, there may be accentuation of the skin lines over the dorsum of the foot and toes.

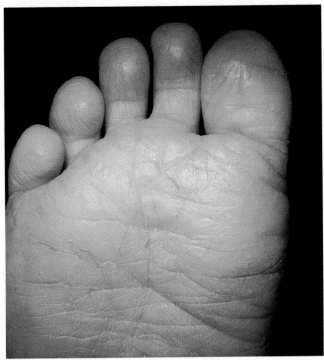

Figure 16–48 Juvenile plantar dermatosis. Increased skin markings and fissures are seen with generalized scaling dermatitis on the plantar forefoot area.

JUVENILE RHEUMATOID ARTHRITIS

Juvenile rheumatoid arthritis is a common pediatric connective tissue disease that has no known cause. Girls are affected twice as often as boys. This condition usually occurs before 16 years of age with peak onsets between 1 and 3 and 8 and 12 years of age. Polyarthritis is usually present in one or more joints and is characterized by effusion (swelling) with clinically increased heat, pain, and limitation of motion (Fig. 16–49). The

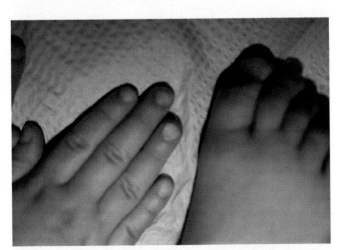

Figure 16–49 Juvenile rheumatoid arthritis. Polyarthritis involves the fingers and toes with joint swelling, increased heat, pain, and limited motion.

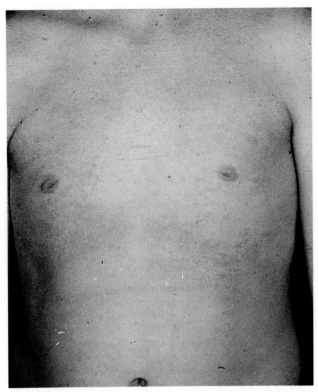

Figure 16–50 Juvenile rheumatoid rash. This erythematous dermatitis is macular and papular and distributed primarily over the trunk, neck, and extremities. It may be transient and most prominent during episodes of fever.

rheumatoid rash appears in over 90% of all patients with juvenile rheumatoid arthritis (Fig. 16–50). This rash is more common in patients with polyarthritis and less common in oligoarthritis. Clinically, the rash has an erythematous to pink color and consists of macules and papules involving the trunk, neck, extremities, palms, and soles. The Koebner or isomorphic response may be activated by rubbing or scratching the lesions during the urticarial or pruritic phase. Patients should be referred to a rheumatologist for management.

JUVENILE RHEUMATIC FEVER

Rheumatic fever is an inflammatory disease principally of the heart, joints, central nervous system, skin, and subcutaneous tissue. This condition is secondary to a delayed sequela to pharyngeal infection with group A streptococci. The skin manifestations of rheumatic fever are of considerable diagnostic value. The three cutaneous lesions that may be associated with rheumatic fever are subcutaneous nodules, erythema papulatum, and erythema marginatum.

Subcutaneous nodules usually appear late in the disease and are more common in adults. These nodules are firm, free moving, and painless and occur over joints, over bony prominences, and commonly around the extensor tendons, particularly of the hands and feet (Fig.

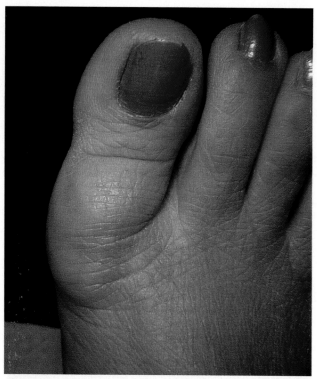

Figure 16–51   Rheumatic subcutaneous nodule. These nodules present along the extensor tendons on the feet in a young girl with a history of rheumatic fever.

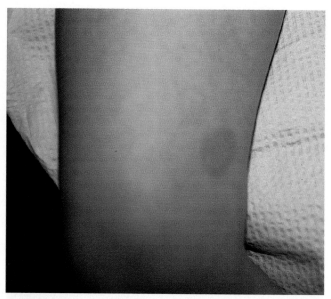

Figure 16–52   Erythema marginatum. A characteristic lesion on the inner thigh in a 12-year-old girl with rheumatic fever was evanescent.

16–51). Erythema papulatum, which is rare in rheumatic fever, consists of asymptomatic papular lesions that appear on the extremities and buttocks and may persist for hours to days. Erythema marginatum is a relatively specific rash of rheumatic fever. Clinically, this condition is characterized by an oval, elevated, pink to salmon-red rash that may be present on the face, trunk, extremities, hands, and legs. These annular-appearing lesions may persist from 2 hours to several days and show rapid peripheral spreading. They may develop smooth polycyclic or festooned outlines or develop into irregular geographic-like patterns. In a few cases, a well-developed, raised, oval lesion appears on the trunk or extremity as a solitary lesion (Fig. 16–52). These lesions are usually present during the active disease process and are frequently associated with carditis, but they may appear without it. These patients should be referred to a rheumatologist for treatment consisting of bed rest, primary and secondary antibiotic prophylaxis, and antirheumatic therapy.

OSTEOCHONDROMA

Although not a dermal lesion, the solitary osteochondroma is frequently seen in patients between 10 to 20 years of age and is frequently misdiagnosed as a skin tumor or subungual exostosis. Subungual exostoses are not true osteochondromas but they may have similar features. Osteochondroma is characterized by a cartilaginous capped osseous protrusion, most often located at the metaphysis area of long tubular bones or at the subungual area of the distal phalanges (Fig. 16–53). This lesion is primarily composed of bone and is produced by progressive endochondral ossification of the growing cartilage cap. As the bone tumor enlarges, the

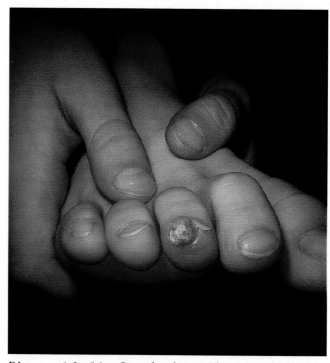

Figure 16–53   Osteochondroma. This 9-year-old boy presented with a painful lesion on the third toe that had been previously misdiagnosed as a subungual wart.

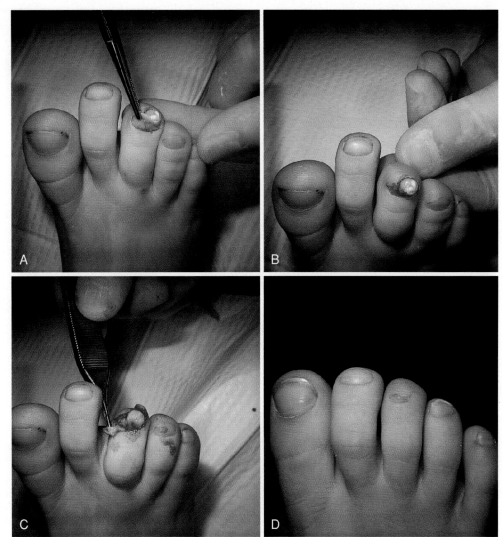

Figure 16–54 Osteo-chondroma. *A,* The toenail is avulsed to obtain clear exposure to the underlying lesion. *B,* Total exposure clearly shows the cartilage cap of the lesion. *C,* The lesion is surgically dissected to the underlying bone and completely resected. *D,* Follow-up at 6 weeks shows the toenail is regrowing without deformity.

pressure on the nail plate or on adjacent neurovascular bundles may elicit pain. In symptomatic cases, the treatment of choice is surgical excision. Subungual lesions usually require nail avulsion and surgical excision of the entire tumor (Fig. 16–54).

PITTED KERATOLYSIS

This common condition in children and adolescents is caused by several different bacterial organisms (see Chapter 5). The characteristic lesions are many small circular punched-out pits found in the stratum corneum (Fig. 16–55) or irregular shaped superficial erosions that may form bizarre patterns on the skin (Fig. 16–56). This disorder is frequently associated with hyperhidrosis and bromhidrosis and is seen more often in boys than girls. Treatment starts with removing shoes and socks that do not air or breathe well. Controlling the hyperhidrosis with astringent foot soaks is helpful. Topical treatment of the involved areas with 2% erythromycin or 1% clindamycin solution daily for 2 weeks

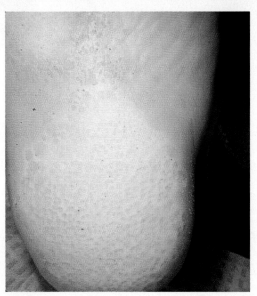

Figure 16–55 Pitted keratolysis. Characteristic punched-out pits formed on the weight-bearing heel in a teenager with secondary hyperhidrosis.

is usually curative. In severe cases, oral erythromycin, 1 g daily for 2 weeks, may be necessary.

PRURIGO NODULARIS

Nodular prurigo is a variant of lichen simplex chronicus and is characterized by a discrete hyperkeratotic nodule that occurs mainly on the lower extremities as multiple lesions or as a single lesion (Fig. 16–57). This condition may be seen on the arms in younger patients. As the name implies, pruritus is the main symptom. Many patients report that the area started as a scratch, insect bite, or small puncture wound. The principal lesion is created by repeated scratching and picking at this isolated area. The lesions are typically erythematous or brown, dome-shaped, and lichenified, with a smooth, crusted, or warty central surface, often with a halo of postinflammatory pigmentation. This lesion is frequently misdiagnosed as a plantar wart in children. Treatment consists of protection of the area from repeated rubbing and scratching. Cryosurgery or intralesional cortisone injections may reduce the size of the lesion as well as the pruritus. In chronic or recurrent cases, surgical excision of the lesion may be warranted.

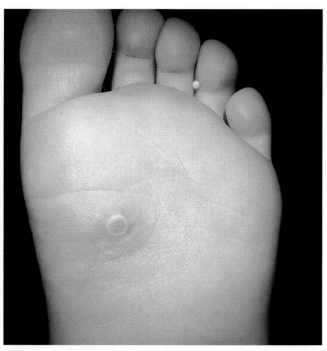

Figure 16-57 Prurigo nodularis. A single discrete lesion on the sole of a young child is characterized by a firm, pink, dome-shaped nodule with an excoriated summit and a surrounding halo of postinflammatory pigmentation.

BIBLIOGRAPHY

Abahussein AA, Al-Zayir AA, Mostafa WZ, Okoro AN: Inherited epidermolysis bullosa. Int J Dermatol 32:561–568, 1993.

Baden HP: Darier-White disease (keratosis follicularis) and miscellaneous hyperkeratotic disorders. In Fitzpatrick TB, Eisen AZ, Wolff K, Freedberg IM, Austen KF: Dermatology in General Medicine, 3rd ed, pp 520–525. New York, McGraw-Hill, 1987.

Baruch K: Pediatric dermatology. Clin Podiatr Med Surg 3:399–411, 1986.

Brady M: Hands and feet that blister and peel: Dyshidrosis. J Pediatr Health Care 7:37–38, 1993.

Cockayne EA: Recurrent bullous eruption of feet. Br J Dermatol 50:358–360, 1938.

Cooper KD: Atopic dermatitis: Recent trends in pathogenesis and therapy. J Invest Dermatol 102:128–137, 1994.

Cullen SI: Topical methenamine therapy for hyperhidrosis. Arch Dermatol 111:1158–1160, 1975.

Dockery GL: Podiatric dermatologic therapeutics. In McCarthy DJ, Montgomery R (eds): Podiatric Dermatology, pp 311–335. Baltimore, Williams & Wilkins, 1986.

Duller P, Gentry WD: Use of biofeedback in treating chronic hyperhidrosis: A preliminary report. Br J Dermatol 103:143–145, 1980.

Gessner R, McCarthy DJ: Podiatric implications of Darier's disease. J Am Podiatr Med Assoc 78:563–571, 1988.

Greger G, Cantanzariti AR: Osteochondroma: Review of the literature and case report. J Foot Surg 31:298–300, 1992.

Hanifin JM: Atopic dermatitis in infants and children. Pediatr Dermatol 38:763–789, 1991.

Hood AF, Mihm MC: Hand-foot-and-mouth disease. In Fitzpatrick TB, Eisen AZ, Wolff K, Freedberg IM, Austen KF (eds): Dermatology in General Medicine, 3rd ed, pp 2297–2300. New York, McGraw-Hill, 1987.

Howland HW, Golitz LE, Weston WL, Huff JC: Erythema multiforme: Clinical, histopathologic, and immunologic study. J Am Acad Dermatol 10:438–446, 1984.

Huff JC, Weston WL, Tonnesen MG: Erythema multiforme: A critical review of characteristics, diagnostic criteria, and causes. J Am Acad Dermatol 8:763–775, 1983.

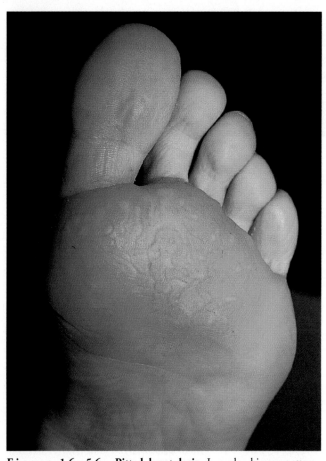

Figure 16-56 Pitted keratolysis. Irregular bizarre patterns may form on the skin as superficial erosions and craters coalesce.

Hurley HJ: Diseases of the eccrine sweat glands. In Moschella SL, Hurley HJ (eds): Dermatology, 3rd ed, pp 1514–1537. Philadelphia, WB Saunders, 1992.

Jenkin WM, Craft CW: Management of idiopathic plantar hyperhidrosis. J Am Podiatr Assoc 73:475–480, 1983.

Kero M, Niemi KM: Epidermolysis bullosa. Int J Dermatol 25:75–82, 1986.

Lemont H, Simon W: Granuloma annulare: Case reports of superficial and deep forms. J Am Podiatr Med Assoc 77:82–85, 1987.

Lemont H, Pearl B: Juvenile plantar dermatosis. J Am Podiatr Med Assoc 82:167–169, 1992.

Levit F: Treatment of hyperhidrosis by tap water iontophoresis. Cutis 26:192–194, 1980.

McGrath JA, Ishida-Yamamoto A, Tidman MJ, Heagerty AHM, Schofield OMV, Eady RAJ: Epidermolysis bullosa simplex (Dowling-O'Meara): A clinicopathological review. Br J Dermatol 126:421–430, 1992.

Menghini CL, Bonifazi E: An Atlas of Pediatric Dermatology. Chicago, Year Book Medical Publishers, 1986.

Owens DW, Freeman RG: Perforating granuloma annulare. Arch Dermatol 103:64–66, 1971.

Pasternack WA, Vara ML: Rapid ossification in a subungual osteochondroma. J Foot Surg 27:334–338, 1988.

Payne CME, Wilkinson JD, McKee PH, Jurecka W, Black MM: Nodular prurigo: A clinicopathological study of 46 patients. Br J Dermatol 113:431–439, 1985.

Steinhart A: Disorders of keratinization. In McCarthy DJ, Montgomery R (eds): Podiatric Dermatology, pp 96–105. Baltimore, Williams & Wilkins, 1986.

Stevens AM, Johnson FC: A new eruptive fever associated with stomatitis and ophthalmia. Am J Dis Child 24:526–533, 1922.

Weber RP: Recurrent bullous eruption on the feet in a child. Proc R Soc Med 19:72–76, 1926.

PSYCHOCUTANEOUS DISORDERS

INTRODUCTION

Psychocutaneous skin disorders are thought to be psychosomatic or neurogenic. They are divided into three main groups: (1) the *primary group*, in which the disease is an emotional condition and the skin disorder is only a part of its expression; (2) the *secondary group*, in which the disease is organic but affects the person emotionally; and (3) the *collaborative group*, in which the emotional and organic disorders combine to cause the skin disease.

The important element of emotional factors in the development and duration of many skin disorders is well known. The physician's attitude toward the patient, the method of examination, and the medication prescribed may all have a marked influence on the resolution of the skin disease. The physician must be able to distinguish between psychological factors causing disease and those that aggravate or prolong preexisting disease. It is important to recognize and distinguish between the hostile patient, who may vent his or her anger against the physician, and the contemptuous patient, who may show open disrespect for the physician's decisions, when they present with psychocutaneous disorders.

Recalcitrant dermatoses may be a manifestation of a symbolic transition object, similar to the baby blanket of a young child. Psychologically, patients use their skin eruptions to assure themselves that they are separate persons with their own boundaries.

Three separate, recognized physiological phenomena that appear to be of importance with respect to emotional associations are isolated hyperhidrosis, pruritus, and vascular changes of the skin. Localized hyperhidrosis of the palms, soles, and axillae is usually a response to emotional status. External thermal stimuli do not cause appreciable sweating in these areas. Complica-

tions of this disorder include secondary bacterial, fungal, or reactional hyperkeratotic disorders, such as dyshidrotic eczema.

Pruritus is the direct result of stimulation of the fine nerve endings at the dermoepidermal junction. Itching can be increased or decreased by psychological factors. When patients with severe pruritus are in relaxed states, their scratching ceases. Conversely, itching increases significantly with mental stress. The discussion of disturbing topics can lead to an exacerbation of itching and scratching in patients with eczematous dermatoses. From this observation, one could conclude that pruritus is capable of being intensified or modified by the patient's emotional status.

Vascular changes in the skin secondary to anxiety and other emotional states are poorly understood. It does appear, however, that neural and chemical factors are much more important than hormonal influences in this response. An emotion generated in the cerebral cortex may stimulate a vascular response of vasodilatation in the skin and acute anxiety may produce vasoconstriction, all of which may be relieved by relaxation or biofeedback.

PRIMARY GROUP

In this group, the primary disease is the emotional disorder (psychosis) and the dermatological state is merely an expression of the illness. This is the category in which most of the clinical expressions of psychocutaneous disorders seen on the lower extremities are found. The patients in this group should be considered emotionally disturbed, and they have some desire to damage the skin. In some cases, the damage to the skin may be due to purely a habit response to

TABLE 17–1 Self-Inflicted Dermatosis

Dermatosis	Dermatologic Features	Psychiatric Features	Findings	Treatment
Neurotic excoriations	May be initiated by pruritus; groups of round or linear lesions and scars	Repetitive self-excoriation; perfectionism, compulsive traits, and depression	Patient may admit inflicting lesions; exclude systemic causes of itching	Empathetic, supportive; amitriptyline; benzodiazepines
Factitial dermatitis	Wide range of lesions, burns, ulcers, blisters; bizarre patterns not characteristic of disease	Immature personality; lesions are an appeal for help	Ratio of female to male is 4:1; sudden appearance of lesions; patient cannot describe history	Empathetic, supportive; avoid direct discussion; occlusive dressings or casts
Lichen simplex chronicus	Created by constant rubbing and scratching; thick oval plaques; severe itching; recurs	Triggered by stress	Biopsy may resemble psoriasis or eczema	Corticosteroids and plastic occlusion; intralesional corticosteroids
Prurigo nodularis	Exaggerated form of lichen simplex chronicus; itchy nodules on legs	Severe pruritus interferes with sleep and activities	Biopsy shows thick epidermis and hyperplasia of nerve fibers	Intralesional corticosteroids; excision; tranquilizers
Delusions of parasitosis	Focal erosions and deep scars	Patients are convinced they are infested; a monosymptomatic hypochondriacal psychosis	Most patients are women older than 50	Psychotherapy; patients who deny have poor prognosis

Modified from Habif TP: Clinical Dermatology: A Color Guide to Diagnosis and Therapy, 2nd ed. St. Louis, CV Mosby, 1990.

release tension. Basically, the skin is normal but the patient is not. Included in this group are neurotic excoriations, factitial dermatitis, compulsive movement dermatoses, delusions of disease, and parasitic phobias (Table 17–1).

NEUROTIC EXCORIATIONS. The patient usually digs into the skin with the fingernails in certain preferred areas such as the back (Fig. 17–1), arms (Fig. 17–2), or legs (Fig. 17–3). The lesions are usually small but may be either deep (Fig. 17–4) or very shallow (Fig. 17–5). The lesions are round or linear, and adjacent scars from previous damage may be present. The patients usually do not deny that they have produced the lesions, but they may state that they have some irresistible desire to remove some tiny skin abnormality or blemish. The patient discovers this "blemish" by very careful inspection with the eyes or fingers rather than an actual symptom that it produces. Young girls may report that they need to remove acne or pigmented lesions that are very ugly.

The extent of this disorder may vary from exacerbation of a preexisting dermatitis to severe disfiguring excoriations of the skin. Areas not easily reached, such as the center of the back, are often spared, providing a valuable clue to the origin of this dermatosis. Right-handed persons tend to produce lesions on the left side of the body, and left-handed persons produce lesions on the right side. Patients with this disorder often manifest a repressed form of aggression and a self-destructive behavior pattern. They are frequently perfectionists and have compulsive traits. Depression may also be seen as a disorder in this group of patients. The

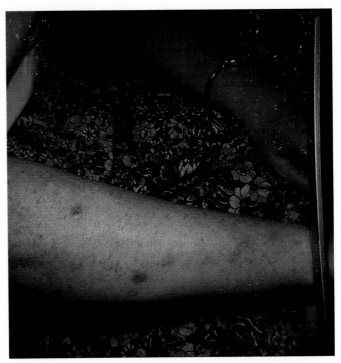

Figure 17–2   Neurotic excoriations. The arms are a common location as shown in this middle-aged woman. (Same patient as in Figure 17–4.)

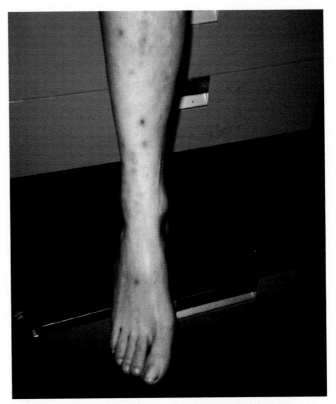

Figure 17–3   Neurotic excoriations. Multiple lesions in a young girl are caused by digging into the skin with her fingernails in an attempt to remove small, relatively inconspicuous blemishes.

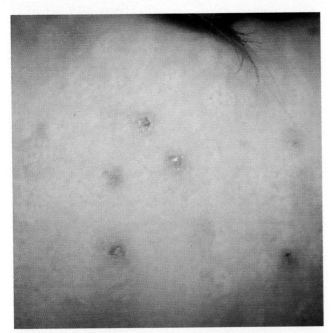

Figure 17–1   Neurotic excoriations. Typical lesions seen on the back in a young girl were acquired while removing "acne blemishes." Note the different stages of healing, ranging from old healed scars to new fresh and bleeding lesions.

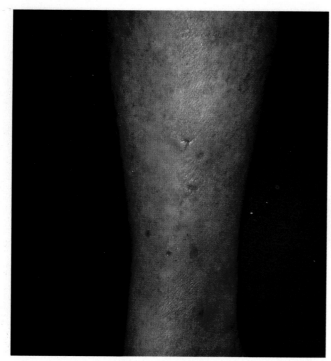

Figure 17–4   Neurotic excoriations. These deep lesions are created by repetitive digging into the skin with the fingernails. Note generalized hair loss from chronic damage to the skin. (Same patient as in Figure 17–2.)

symptom complex does not respond easily to standard treatment, and the patient often continues the compulsive digging for many years. Empathetic and supportive care should be emphasized. Amitriptyline and benzodiazepine may be beneficial in some patients, especially younger girls.

FACTITIAL DERMATITIS. This condition, which is also termed *dermatitis artefacta*, is self-inflicted, but the patient usually maintains a state of denial as to the cause of the problem. The lesions are made to elicit sympathy, escape responsibilities, get out of work duties, or collect disability insurance (Figs. 17–6 through 17–15). The lesions have a clear-cut, bizarre appearance. They are usually seen in circumscribed areas as geometric shapes, and the surrounding skin appears normal. A wide range of lesions may be seen from burns, ulcers, blisters, and scratches. The more common agents of destruction are phenol, silver nitrate, nitric acid, alkali, turpentine, gasoline, lighter fluid, hot metal, lighted cigarette, and injectable substance.

Most of these bizarre lesions resolve very slowly even when small or shallow. Diagnosis may be difficult. If the physician maintains a high suspicion of factitial dermatitis when seeing patients with lesions that do not conform to known disorders, the diagnosis may be made without their knowledge. One helpful diagnostic clue is the disappearance of the lesions under an occlusive dressing, such as a cast, or during constant hospital observation. This is followed by rapid recurrence when no

dressings are present or when the patient is not being observed. This condition is largely confined to women and, interestingly, the nursing profession has a higher incidence than the general population.

In the psychiatric-based group, this disorder is considered an appeal for help. In others, the condition is simply a means of gaining some secondary benefits. This disorder is considered to be a complex and severe condition that requires a psychiatric referral. In most cases, it is not wise to confront patients and accuse them of inflicting the lesions. Confrontation may place the physician in a situation involving a very aggressive and angry patient and may not achieve the goal of directing the patient to psychiatric counseling.

COMPULSIVE MOVEMENTS. Self-injury by prolonged compulsive repetitious movements may produce various types of mutilations, depending on the technique used and the area of injury (Figs. 17–16 through 17–19). These include scaling, crusting, thickening, and hyperpigmentation of the skin involved. In most cases involving the lower extremities, the mechanism of injury is secondary to repetitive rubbing or scratching with the hands or fingernails. On the lower anterior surface of the feet and legs the patient may also use the heel of the opposite foot to produce the same type of lesions.

Lichen simplex chronicus is also in this class and is sometimes referred to as localized neurodermatitis. It is most often seen on the dorsum of the feet (Fig. 17–20), lateral heel area (Fig. 17–21), medial ankle (Fig.

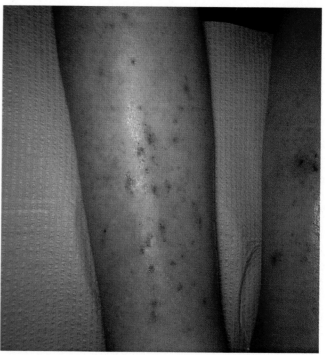

Figure 17–5   Neurotic excoriations. Very fine excoriations are made by rubbing the fingernails across the skin, rather than digging into the skin with the nails.

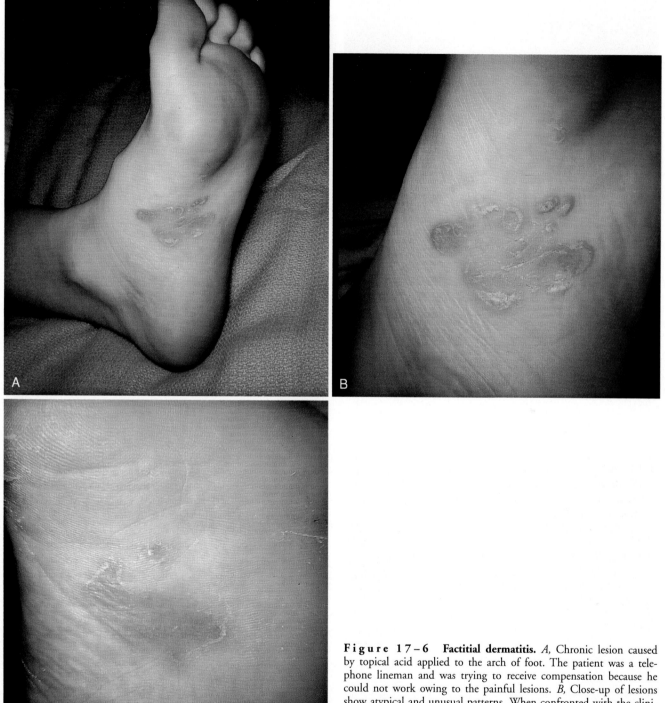

Figure 17–6 Factitial dermatitis. *A,* Chronic lesion caused by topical acid applied to the arch of foot. The patient was a telephone lineman and was trying to receive compensation because he could not work owing to the painful lesions. *B,* Close-up of lesions show atypical and unusual patterns. When confronted with the clinician's suspicions, the patient admitted he had caused these lesions with repeated applications of liquid phenol. *C,* Rapid healing of lesions was seen once the patient stopped applying the acid.

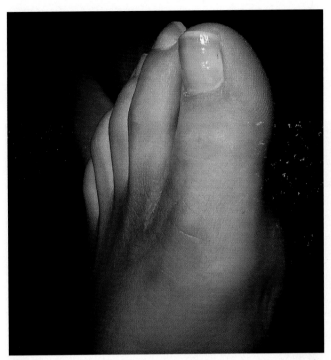

Figure 17–7   Factitial injury. Hyperpigmented lesion on the dorsum of the foot was secondary to injection of a variety of agents by the patient, who was a registered nurse.

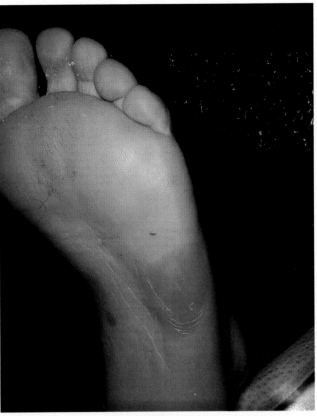

Figure 17–9   Factitial injury. Recurrent blister formed on the styloid region of the foot. It was soon discovered, by a hospital nurse, that the patient was applying lighter fluid to the foot daily.

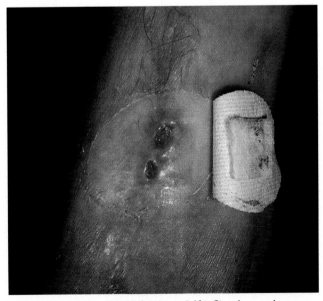

Figure 17–8   Factitial injury. Self-inflicted wounds are seen in the surgical site of a patient on workers' compensation. When the area was covered with an Unna boot dressing it would quickly heal only to recur when the bandages were removed.

17–22), anterolateral ankle (Fig. 17–23), and knee (Fig. 17–24). It is the result of prolonged rubbing or scratching in an isolated area. Prurigo nodularis may be considered a nodular form of lichen simplex chronicus (see Fig. 16–57). These conditions frequently interfere with the patient's abilities to perform certain physical activities and to get a restful night of sleep.

This condition is usually triggered by stress but may result from simple frustration or a subconscious compulsive habit. Understanding the mechanism of action and discussing it openly with the patient is very important. Because much of the compulsive scratching and rubbing occurs at night or without the patient's knowledge, I have found that a corticosteroid-impregnated occlusive tape cover provides both a physical barrier to trauma as well as an effective form of treatment. In resistant cases, the patient may sleep with thin cotton gloves in an attempt to reduce the amount of scratching that occurs subconsciously. Intralesional injections of cortisone and local anesthetic may also be needed in more severe forms of compulsive dermatitis but should be used cautiously to prevent atrophy or other secondary skin changes.

DELUSIONS OF DISEASE. Delusions of disease, especially parasitosis, must be distinguished from a phobia; the latter is a psychoneurotic symptom of lesser import,

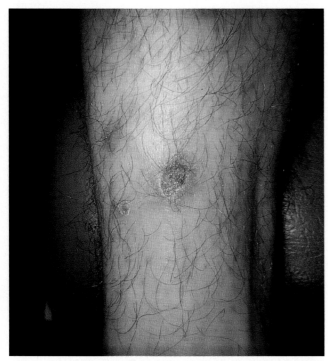

Figure 17–10 **Factitial ulcer.** Chronic, circumscribed ulceration was seen on the skin area of a 52-year-old man. The lesion would clear slightly and then break down repeatedly. The lesion was present for 3 years before discovery of its actual cause. The patient was applying several different caustic materials to the wound each time it began to heal.

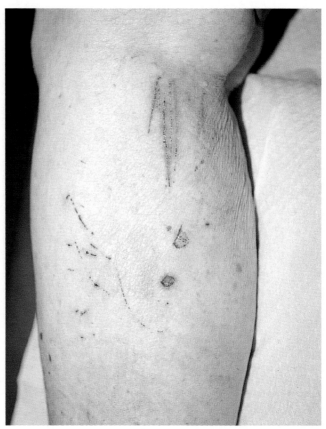

Figure 17–12 **Factitial lesions.** These gouges, scratches, and abrasions were seen in an elderly woman who claimed that the condition was secondary to an internal malignancy. They healed quickly when the patient was confronted by health care workers and the area protected.

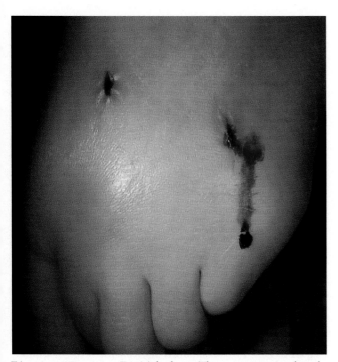

Figure 17–11 **Factitial ulcers.** These spontaneous deep lesions apparently appeared overnight in a hospitalized patient with severe reflex sympathetic dystrophy.

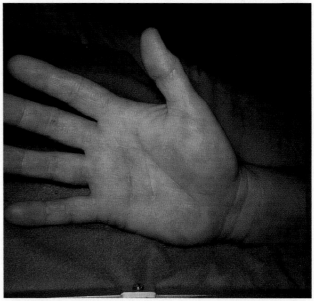

Figure 17–13 **Factitial lesions.** Multiple small burns on the hand were caused by a lighted cigarette. The patient claimed a disability and was unable to work as a janitor due to an "allergy" to wooden handles of brooms and mops.

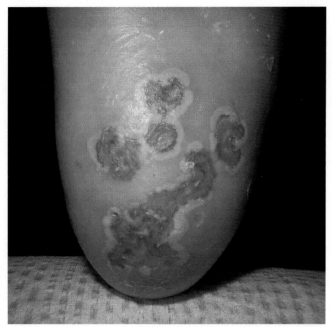

Figure 17–14   Factitial ulcers. An elderly woman with a nonhealing dermatitis on the foot was taken from doctor to doctor by her concerned husband. Bizarre-appearing geometric shapes were seen and later identified as being caused by repeated application of caustic materials. There was a secondary superficial bacterial infection that made the diagnosis even more difficult to determine.

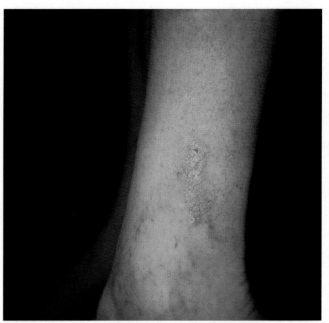

Figure 17–16   Compulsive movements. A single line of hyperpigmented and lichenified tissue may be seen secondary to compulsive scratching with a single finger in the same area.

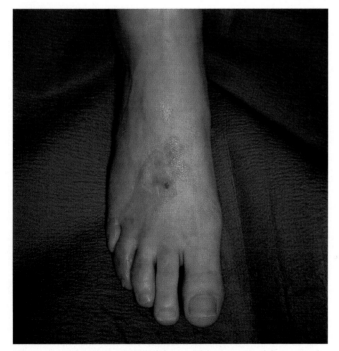

Figure 17–15   Factitial burn. This intentional burn on the foot with hot grease occurred in a young girl with family problems.

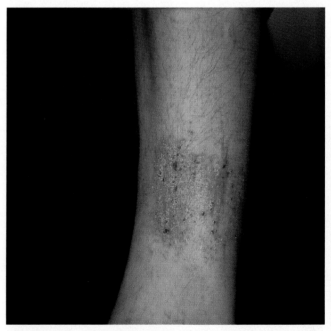

Figure 17–17   Compulsive movements. A localized square patch of scaly, erythematous crusting may be caused by repeated scratching with all four fingers of the same hand at one time.

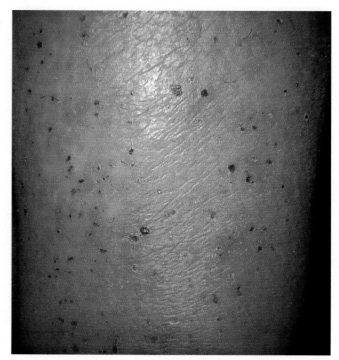

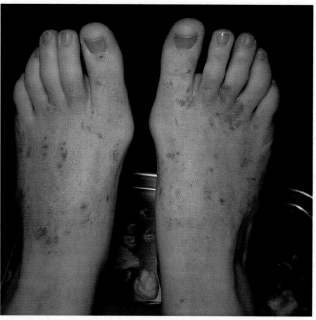

Figure 17–20 Lichen simplex chronicus. Typical lesions seen on the dorsa of both feet are from chronic rubbing and scratching with superficial excoriations.

Figure 17–18 Compulsive movements. Generalized skin changes on the lower leg follow widespread compulsive rubbing and picking at the skin.

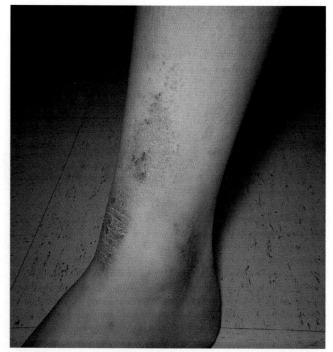

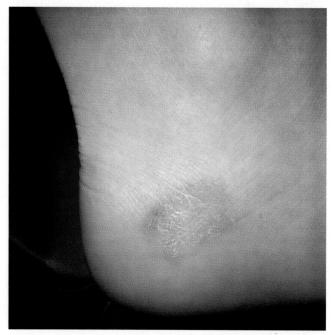

Figure 17–19 Compulsive movements. This lesion is almost always caused by repetitive rubbing of the anterior foot or shin with the heel of the opposite foot.

Figure 17–21 Lichen simplex chronicus. Nummular lichenification is noted on the lateral heel area from chronic rubbing.

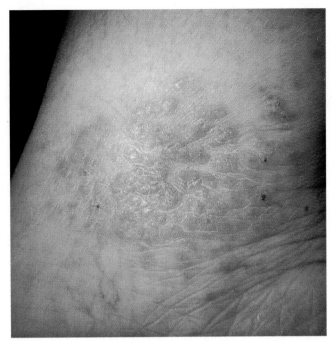

Figure 17–22   Lichen simplex chronicus. Generalized skin changes on the medial ankle follow widespread compulsive rubbing and picking at the skin.

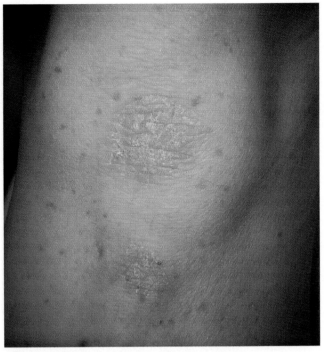

Figure 17–24   Lichen simplex chronicus. Anterior knee lesions are caused by repetitive rubbing in a circular fashion.

whereas the delusion is a psychotic symptom, generally of a serious nature. This condition is frequently classified as a monosymptomatic hypochondriacal psychosis. The characteristic of the delusion of parasitosis is that the patients are totally convinced that they are infested by small parasites and they will dig into the skin to remove the mites (Fig. 17–25).

This is a disorder almost solely of middle-aged or elderly women, but it may occasionally be seen in men.

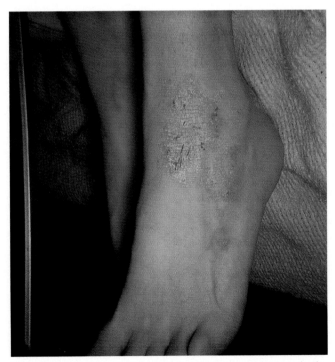

Figure 17–23   Lichen simplex chronicus. Large circular lichenified scaling areas over the anterior and lateral ankle are secondary to chronic rubbing and scratching of the skin.

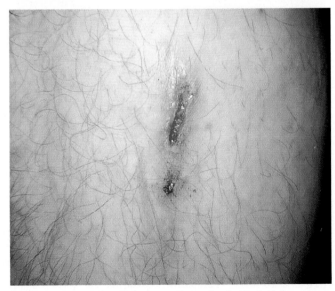

Figure 17–25   Delusions of parasitosis. Typical deep excoriation is produced by the patient digging into the skin to "catch parasites."

The patients are truly deluded in that they tenaciously hold to the belief that they are infested with parasites and they remain convinced even when faced with negative medical examination findings and evaluations showing otherwise. The belief is so fixed that the patient will often bring in proof of an "infestation" in small packets or bathroom cups (Fig. 17–26). The contents of the cup are usually small pieces of epithelial debris that have been scraped or picked from the skin (Fig. 17–27). There may be bits of clothing, carpet, nails, or other materials contained within the debris as well. This group of patients may also have hallucinations, and during the presentation of the collected specimen the patients may insist that they have seen or felt the creatures crawling or burrowing within the skin just before their capture. Some patients will even go so far as to call in the public health department to have the home fumigated. A careful search for parasites by the physician or nurse is always warranted in every case to rule out an actual infestation. Most patients in this category reject all suggestions for psychiatric care and will move on to another clinic or physician, trying to prove that their disease is present.

PARASITIC PHOBIAS. Acarophobia or parasitophobia is a morbid fear of infestation with mites or parasites, but the patients realize that they are free of the condition at the present time. Frequently these patients also have paranoid tendencies. As discussed earlier under the primary group of diseases, there are two main differences in the emotional status of the patients: those who admit that they have traumatized themselves and those who adamantly deny it. The former often have remissions after therapy, whereas the latter usually have very poor prognoses.

SECONDARY GROUP

In this category, the cause is organic but the patient is affected emotionally. There are usually multiple etio-

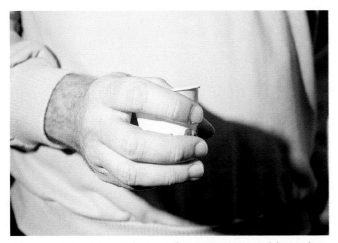

Figure 17–26 **Delusions of parasitosis.** Some delusional patients present with a firmly held cup containing "proof" of their infestations.

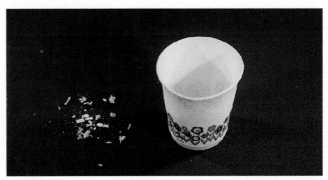

Figure 17–27 **Delusions of parasitosis.** Close inspection of the contents of the cup usually reveals small pieces of skin, fibers, thread, nails, or lint that the patient presents as confirmation of the offending parasites.

logical factors or conditions clearly involving infectious, allergic, genetic, neoplastic, or physical causes. Even though the basic problem is organic and the treatment is symptomatic, the secondary emotional disorders may be very damaging to the patient's psychological status. Acute, painful skin disorders, such as subungual glomus tumors or herpes zoster, may be so disturbing that the patient considers committing suicide. Disfiguring conditions such as von Recklinghausen's disease or mycosis fungoides may also elicit extreme emotional crises.

COLLABORATIVE GROUP

In this category, the emotional and organic disorders combine to cause the skin disease. The emotional relationship to the problem is least understood in this group, and there is a great deal of controversy regarding which conditions should be placed within this classification. Discussion here is limited and is included merely to complete the categories. Included in this classification are verrucae, acne vulgaris, psoriasis, atopic dermatitis, urticaria, dyshidrotic eczema, lichen planus, and herpes simplex.

Psychocutaneous disorders occur in a variety of characteristic and bizarre patterns. Once the physician recognizes the lesions and understands that these psychosomatic problems are necessarily persistent, protracted, and poorly responsive to conservative care, he or she should assist the patient by selective referrals to dermatologists trained to treat psychiatric disorders, psychiatrists, psychologists, members of the clergy, or family service associations.

BIBLIOGRAPHY

Ackner B: Emotions and the peripheral vasomotor system. J Psychosom Res 1:308–310, 1956.

Dockery GL: Psychocutaneous disorders: Some lower extremity presentations. J Am Podiatr Assoc 72:388–395, 1982.

Doran AR, Roy A, Wolkowitz OW: Self-destructive dermatoses. Psychiatr Clin North Am 8:291–298, 1985.

Fruensgaard K, Jørtshoj A, Nielsen H: Neurotic excoriations. Int J Dermatol 17:761–763, 1978.

Gould WM, Gragg TM: Delusions of parasitosis: An approach to the problem. Arch Dermatol 112:1745–1746, 1976.

Gupta MA, Gupta AK, Haberman HF: The self-inflicted dermatoses: A critical review. Gen Hosp Psychiatry 9:45–52, 1987.

Lyell A: Cutaneous artifactual disease. J Am Acad Dermatol 1:391–407, 1979.

Medansky RS, Handler RM: Dermatopsychosomatics: Classification, physiology, and therapeutic approaches. J Am Acad Dermatol 5:125–136, 1981.

Munro A: Delusional parasitosis: A form of monosymptomatic hypochondriacal psychosis. Semin Dermatol 2:197–202, 1983.

Novak M: Psychocutaneous medicine: How to recognize and handle the hostile dermatologic patient and the contemptuous dermatologic patient. Cutis 25:66–69, 1980.

Novak M: Psychocutaneous medicine: Recalcitrant dermatoses seen as a transition object through the psychiatric periscope. Cutis 27:662–668, 1981.

Simmons DA, Daamen MJ, Harrison JW, Weishaar ME: Hospital management of a patient with factitial dermatitis. Gen Hosp Psychiatry 9:147–150, 1987.

INDEX

ISBN 0-7216-5034-1